W9-ARF-017

Household Safety Sourcebook
Hypertension Sourcebook
Immune System Disorders Sourcebook
Infant & Toddler Health Sourcebook
Infectious Diseases Sourcebook
Injury & Trauma Sourcebook
Kidney & Urinary Tract Diseases &
   Disorders Sourcebook
Learning Disabilities Sourcebook,
   2nd Edition
Leukemia Sourcebook
Liver Disorders Sourcebook
Lung Disorders Sourcebook
Medical Tests Sourcebook, 2nd Edition
Men's Health Concerns Sourcebook,
   2nd Edition
Mental Health Disorders Sourcebook,
   3rd Edition
Mental Retardation Sourcebook
Movement Disorders Sourcebook
Muscular Dystrophy Sourcebook
Obesity Sourcebook
Osteoporosis Sourcebook
Pain Sourcebook, 2nd Edition
Pediatric Cancer Sourcebook
Physical & Mental Issues in Aging
   Sourcebook
Podiatry Sourcebook
Pregnancy & Birth Sourcebook,
   2nd Edition
Prostate Cancer
Public Health Sourcebook
Reconstructive & Cosmetic Surgery
   Sourcebook
Rehabilitation Sourcebook
Respiratory Diseases & Disorders
   Sourcebook
Sexually Transmitted Diseases
   Sourcebook, 2nd Edition
Skin Disorders Sourcebook
Sleep Disorders Sourcebook,
   2nd Edition

Smoking Concerns Sourcebook
Sports Injuries Sourcebook, 2nd Edition
Stress-Related Disorders Sourcebook
Stroke Sourcebook
Substance Abuse Sourcebook
Surgery Sourcebook
Thyroid Sourcebook
Transplantation Sourcebook
Traveler's Health Sourcebook
Vegetarian Sourcebook
Women's Health Concerns Sourcebook,
   2nd Edition
Workplace Health & Safety Sourcebook
Worldwide Health Sourcebook

Teen Health Series

Alcohol Information for Teens
Asthma Information for Teens
Cancer Information for Teens
Diet Information for Teens
Drug Information for Teens
Eating Disorders Information
   for Teens
Fitness Information for Teens
Mental Health Information
   for Teens
Sexual Health Information
   for Teens
Skin Health Information for
   Teens
Sports Injuries Information
   for Teens
Suicide Information for Teens

Hepatitis
SOURCEBOOK

Health Reference Series

First Edition

Hepatitis
SOURCEBOOK

*Basic Consumer Health Information about
Hepatitis A, Hepatitis B, Hepatitis C, and Other
Forms of Hepatitis, Including Autoimmune
Hepatitis, Alcoholic Hepatitis, Nonalcoholic
Steatohepatitis, and Toxic Hepatitis, with Facts
about Risk Factors, Screening Methods, Diagnostic
Tests, and Treatment Options*

*Along with Information on Liver Health, Tips for
People Living with Chronic Hepatitis, Reports on
Current Research Initiatives, a Glossary of Terms
Related to Hepatitis, and a Directory of Sources for
Further Help and Information*

Edited by
Sandra J. Judd

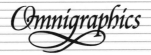

615 Griswold Street • Detroit, MI 48226

Bibliographic Note

Because this page cannot legibly accommodate all the copyright notices, the Bibliographic Note portion of the Preface constitutes an extension of the copyright notice.

Edited by Sandra J. Judd

Health Reference Series

Karen Bellenir, *Managing Editor*
David A. Cooke, M.D., *Medical Consultant*
Elizabeth Barbour, *Research and Permissions Coordinator*
Cherry Stockdale, *Permissions Assistant*
Dawn Matthews, *Verification Assistant*
Laura Pleva Nielsen, *Index Editor*
EdIndex, Services for Publishers, *Indexers*

* * *

Omnigraphics, Inc.

Matthew P. Barbour, *Senior Vice President*
Kay Gill, *Vice President—Directories*
Kevin Hayes, *Operations Manager*
Leif Gruenberg, *Development Manager*
David P. Bianco, *Marketing Director*

* * *

Peter E. Ruffner, *Publisher*

Frederick G. Ruffner, Jr., *Chairman*

Copyright © 2006 Omnigraphics, Inc.

ISBN 0-7808-0749-9

Library of Congress Cataloging-in-Publication Data

Hepatitis sourcebook : basic consumer health information about hepatitis A, hepatitis B, hepatitis C, and other forms of hepatitis, including autoimmune hepatitis, alcoholic hepatitis, nonalcoholic steatohepatitis, and toxic hepatitis, with facts about risk factors, screening methods, diagnostic tests, and treatment options; along with information on liver health, tips for people living with chronic hepatitis, reports on current research initiatives, a glossary of terms related to hepatitis, and a directory of sources for further help and information / edited by Sandra J. Judd.-- 1st ed.
     p. cm.
   Summary: "Provides basic consumer health information about causes, screening, diagnosis and treatments for Hepatitis A, B, and C, and related liver diseases. Includes index, glossary of related terms, and other resources"--Provided by publisher.
   Includes bibliographical references and index.
   ISBN 0-7808-0749-9 (hardcover : alk. paper)
   1. Hepatitis--Popular works. I. Judd, Sandra J.
   RC848.H42H47 2005
   616.3'623--dc22
                                                              2005021573

Table of Contents

Visit www.healthreferenceseries.com to view *A Contents Guide to the Health Reference Series*, a listing of more than 10,000 topics and the volumes in which they are covered.

Part II: Hepatitis Overview

Part III: Hepatitis A Virus (HAV)

Part VI: Other Types of Hepatitis

Part VII: Additional Help and Information

Preface

About This Book

Hepatitis is a disorder in which viruses or other mechanisms produce inflammation in liver cells. It can vary in severity from a minor illness with complete recovery to a life-threatening or lifelong disease. Hepatitis has many different causes. It is most commonly caused by specific viruses which are transmitted through exposure to contaminated food or water or through contact with infected blood products. Hepatitis can also result from an autoimmune condition or from other medical concerns, including drug use, alcoholism, and exposure to chemicals or environmental toxins.

Each year an estimated 61,000 hepatitis A infections occur in the United States, and up to 73,000 Americans are infected with hepatitis B. Additionally, an estimated 30,000 Americans are newly infected with the hepatitis C virus annually; 80 percent will remain chronically infected. The American Liver Foundation currently estimates that more than 4 million Americans have been infected with hepatitis C, and 70% of them don't know it. Hepatitis C causes 10,000 annual deaths in the United States, and the Centers for Disease Control and Prevention estimates that the number will triple in the next twenty years. Yet there is hope for those suffering from hepatitis. Vaccines are available to prevent some forms of the disease, and new research brings us ever closer to a cure.

Hepatitis Sourcebook provides basic consumer health information about hepatitis A, hepatitis B, hepatitis C, and other types of hepatitis, including autoimmune hepatitis, alcoholic hepatitis, nonalcoholic steatohepatitis, and toxin-induced hepatitis. It describes risk factors, prevention, transmission, screening and diagnostic methods, treatment options, and current research initiatives. Tips for coping with chronic hepatitis, a glossary, and resources for additional help and information are also included.

How to Use This Book

This book is divided into parts and chapters. Parts focus on broad areas of interest. Chapters are devoted to single topics within a part.

Part I: Introduction to the Liver begins with a look at the anatomy and physiology of the liver. Basic care of the liver and the symptoms of liver disease are described, along with the effects of alcohol and acetaminophen and the stresses on the liver that accompany pregnancy. The part concludes with a description of the types of tests used in diagnosing liver disease and a discussion of liver biopsy.

Part II: Hepatitis Overview provides a basic overview of the different types of hepatitis and the populations most at-risk for the disease. Methods of hepatitis prevention and available vaccinations are discussed, and the link between hepatitis and cancer of the liver is explained.

Part III: Hepatitis A Virus (HAV) focuses specifically on HAV, including methods of virus transmission, testing, methods of prevention, and HAV vaccination.

Part IV: Hepatitis B Virus (HBV) and Hepatitis D Virus (HDV) provides an overview of HBV, and it includes facts about HDV, which occurs only among people infected with HBV. It discusses transmission, symptoms, prevention, diagnostic testing, pregnancy and pediatric concerns, treatment methods, and recent research. Suggestions are also included for people living with chronic HBV infection.

Part V: Hepatitis C Virus (HCV) focuses on HCV, providing basic facts about virus transmission, screening, diagnosis, and testing. It explains the different HCV genotypes and their implications. The discussion of HCV treatment includes a description of the types of treatment available, the different drugs used in treatment, the use of complementary and alternative medicine, treatment challenges for people in alcohol and drug recovery, side effects of treatment, and new research and clinical trials. The part concludes with a discussion of chronic HCV infection, including disease management, cirrhosis and other complications of chronic infection, and co-infection with the human immunodeficiency virus (HIV).

Part VI: Other Types of Hepatitis covers the less well-known varieties of hepatitis, including hepatitis E, hepatitis G, neonatal hepatitis, autoimmune hepatitis, alcoholic hepatitis, nonalcoholic steatohepatitis, and toxic hepatitis.

Part VII: Additional Help and Information provides a glossary of hepatitis-related terms and a directory of organizations that can provide further information and help in specific areas.

Bibliographic Note

This volume contains documents and excerpts from publications issued by the following U.S. government agencies: Agency for Healthcare Research and Quality (AHRQ); Centers for Disease Control and Prevention (CDC); National Center for Complementary and Alternative Medicine (NCCAM); National Institute of Allergy and Infectious Diseases (NIAID); National Institute of Diabetes and Digestive and Kidney Diseases (NIDDK); and Veterans Affairs National Hepatitis C Program.

In addition, this volume contains copyrighted documents from the following organizations: A.D.A.M., Inc.; American Association for Clinical Chemistry; American Liver Foundation; American Social Health Association; Asian Liver Center at Stanford University; Baylor College of Medicine Office of Public Affairs; Canadian Liver Foundation; eMedicine; Gale Group; Hepatitis B Foundation; Hepatitis C Council of New South Wales; Hepatitis C Support Project; Hepatitis Foundation International; Immunization Action Coalition; Massachusetts Department of Public Health-Bureau of Communicable Disease Control; Medical College of Wisconsin HealthLink; Nemours Foundation; St. Luke's Episcopal Health System; Thomson Micromedex; University of Nottingham School of Nursing and Academic Division of Midwifery; and WebMD Corporation.

Full citation information is provided on the first page of each chapter. Every effort has been made to secure all necessary rights to reprint the copyrighted material. If any omissions have been made, please contact Omnigraphics to make corrections for future editions.

Acknowledgements

Thanks go to the many organizations, agencies, and individuals who have contributed materials for this *Sourcebook* and to medical consultant Dr. David Cooke, verification assistant Dawn Matthews, and document engineer Bruce Bellenir. Special thanks go to managing editor Karen Bellenir and permissions coordinator Liz Barbour for their help and support.

About the Health Reference Series

The *Health Reference Series* is designed to provide basic medical information for patients, families, caregivers, and the general public. Each volume takes a particular topic and provides comprehensive coverage. This is especially important for people who may be dealing with a newly diagnosed disease or a chronic disorder in themselves or in a family member. People looking for preventive guidance, information about disease warning signs, medical statistics, and risk factors for health problems will also find answers to their questions in the *Health Reference Series*. The *Series*, however, is not intended to serve as a tool for diagnosing illness, in prescribing treatments, or as a substitute for the physician/patient relationship. All people concerned about medical symptoms or the possibility of disease are encouraged to seek professional care from an appropriate health care provider.

Locating Information within the Health Reference Series

The *Health Reference Series* contains a wealth of information about a wide variety of medical topics. Ensuring easy access to all the fact sheets, research reports, in-depth discussions, and other material contained within the individual books of the series remains one of our highest priorities. As the *Series* continues to grow in size and scope, however, locating the precise information needed by a reader may become more challenging.

A *Contents Guide to the Health Reference Series* was developed to direct readers to the specific volumes that address their concerns. It presents an extensive list of diseases, treatments, and other topics of general interest compiled from the Tables of Contents and major index headings. To access A *Contents Guide to the Health Reference Series*, visit www.healthreferenceseries.com.

Medical Consultant

Medical consultation services are provided to the *Health Reference Series* editors by David A. Cooke, M.D. Dr. Cooke is a graduate of

Brandeis University, and he received his M.D. degree from the University of Michigan. He completed residency training at the University of Wisconsin Hospital and Clinics. He is board-certified in Internal Medicine. Dr. Cooke currently works as part of the University of Michigan Health System and practices in Ann Arbor, MI. In his free time, he enjoys writing, science fiction, and spending time with his family.

Our Advisory Board

We would like to thank the following board members for providing guidance to the development of this series:

Dr. Lynda Baker,
Associate Professor of Library and Information Science,
Wayne State University, Detroit, MI

Nancy Bulgarelli,
William Beaumont Hospital Library, Royal Oak, MI

Karen Imarisio,
Bloomfield Township Public Library, Bloomfield Township, MI

Karen Morgan,
Mardigian Library, University of Michigan-Dearborn,
Dearborn, MI

Rosemary Orlando,
St. Clair Shores Public Library, St. Clair Shores, MI

Health Reference Series *Update Policy*

The inaugural book in the *Health Reference Series* was the first edition of *Cancer Sourcebook* published in 1989. Since then, the *Series* has been enthusiastically received by librarians and in the medical community. In order to maintain the standard of providing high-quality health information for the layperson the editorial staff at Omnigraphics felt it was necessary to implement a policy of updating volumes when warranted.

Medical researchers have been making tremendous strides, and it is the purpose of the *Health Reference Series* to stay current with the most recent advances. Each decision to update a volume is made on an individual basis. Some of the considerations include how much new information is available and the feedback we receive from people who use the books. If there is a topic you would like to see added to the update list, or an area of medical concern you feel has not been adequately addressed, please write to:

Editor
Health Reference Series
Omnigraphics, Inc.
615 Griswold Street
Detroit, MI 48226
E-mail: editorial@omnigraphics.com

Part One

Introduction to the Liver

Chapter 1

Anatomy and Physiology of the Liver

The Anatomy of the Liver

External Structure

The liver is the largest gland in the body, weighing about 1.4 kg in an adult. It is situated under the diaphragm in the upper abdominal cavity and is held in place by several ligaments. It is a reddish-brown color and comprises of four anatomical lobes. When viewed from the front, the dominant left and right lobes can be seen, which are separated by the falciform ligament.

Situated in a depression on the posterior surface of the liver is the gall bladder, a pear-shaped sac which stores bile synthesized by the liver. The liver performs many vital metabolic functions. It has the ability to store and metabolize useful substances such as nutrients, but it breaks down or detoxifies harmful substances to render them inert and less harmful.

Blood Supply

The liver receives a blood supply from two sources. The first is the hepatic artery, which delivers oxygenated blood from the general circulation.

The second is the hepatic portal vein, delivering deoxygenated blood from the small intestine containing nutrients.

The blood flows through the liver tissue to the hepatic cells where many metabolic functions take place. The blood drains out of the liver via the hepatic vein.

The liver tissue is not vascularized with a capillary network as with most other organs, but consists of blood-filled sinusoids surrounding the hepatic cells.

Internal Structure

The liver lobes are made up of microscopic units called lobules which are roughly hexagonal in shape.

These lobules comprise of rows of liver cells (hepatocytes) which radiate out from a central point. The hepatic cells are in close contact with blood-filled sinusoids and also lie adjacent to canaliculi into which bile is secreted.

Situated around the perimeter of the lobule are branches of the hepatic artery, hepatic portal vein, and bile duct. These cluster together at the "corners" of the lobule, forming what is called the portal triad. At the midpoint of the lobule is the central vein. Blood flows out of the sinusoids into the central vein and is transported out of the liver.

Lobule Activity

The hepatic portal vein and hepatic artery deliver oxygen and nutrients into to the blood sinusoids. This close relationship between the hepatocytes and surrounding blood enables many metabolic processes to take place.

Blood flows out of the sinusoids into the central vein, removing detoxified substances and metabolic end products. The central vein ultimately reunites with the hepatic vein transporting these substances out of the liver.

Bile that is produced by the hepatocytes drains into tiny canals called bile canaliculi (singular *canaliculus*). These drain into bile ducts located around the lobule perimeter.

Hepatocytes

Hepatocytes are the predominant cell type in the liver. An estimated 80 percent of the liver mass is made of these cells. The hepatocytes are round in shape, containing a nucleus and an abundance of cellular organelles associated with metabolic and secretory functions.

Organelles include endoplasmic reticulum (smooth and rough) and Golgi apparatus for secretory functions. Also there are high numbers of mitochondria to provide energy to support the many metabolic functions on the liver.

Some of the hepatocytes lie adjacent to endothelial cells which form the walls of the sinusoids. These two cell types are separated by small space called the space of Disse.

Gall Bladder

Attached to the right lobe of the liver by connective tissue is the gall bladder. Shaped like a pear, it is 7–10 cm long.

Bile produced by the hepatic cells drains out of the lobules via the bile ducts. These unite to form the right and left hepatic ducts, which join cystic duct transporting bile to and from the gall bladder.

The gall bladder concentrates and then stores the bile until it is required to assist in the digestion of fats.

When needed for digestion, bile travels through cystic duct into the common bile duct. This unites with the pancreatic duct to empty bile into the duodenum. Bile flow is under the control of the hormone cholecystokinin, and enters the duodenum through the sphincter of Oddi.

The Physiology of the Liver

Liver Function

The liver receives 30 percent of the resting cardiac output and acts as a giant chemical processing plant in the body. These chemical reactions, called metabolism, are central in the regulation of body homeostasis.

The liver cells, called hepatocytes, contain thousands of enzymes essential to perform vital metabolic functions. They are supermodels in the world of cellular metabolism.

The liver metabolizes both beneficial and harmful substances. It stores nutrients and other useful substances, as well as detoxifying or breaking down harmful compounds. These can then be excreted from the body in bile via the liver; in urine via the kidney, or by other means.

Nutrient Metabolism

The liver is involved in the metabolism of nutrients. It receives digestive products in the form of glucose, amino acids and fatty acids, and glycerol.

The metabolism of carbohydrate, fat, and protein takes place in the liver, although specific functions are carried out by fat depots and skeletal muscle. Metabolic end products are often stored in the liver and utilized at a later stage if required.

How the hepatocytes deal with the nutrients depends on whether each nutrient is in abundance or whether levels are low in the body and they are therefore in demand. The hepatocytes alter their metabolic pathways accordingly.

Carbohydrate

Glucose is a vital energy source for cells, and levels in the blood stream must remain constant. The liver helps maintain blood glucose levels in response to the pancreatic hormones insulin and glucagon.

After a meal, glucose enters the liver and levels of blood glucose rise. This excess glucose is dealt with by glycogenesis in which the liver converts glucose into glycogen for storage. The glucose that is not stored is used to produce energy by a process called glycolysis. This occurs in every cell in the body.

In between meals or during starvation, blood glucose levels fall. The hepatocytes detect this change and restore glucose levels by either glycogenolysis, which converts glycogen back to glucose, or gluconeogenesis, in which nonsugars such as amino acids are converted to glucose.

Fat

The liver is involved in fat metabolism and synthesizes lipoproteins, cholesterol, and phospholipids essential for many body functions. Lipids also provide a valuable alternative energy source to glucose and so the metabolic fate of fats and lipids will depend on the levels of intake in the diet and energy expenditure.

If fat is in excess, the liver prepares for storage. Lipogenesis is the metabolic process in which fats, composed of fatty acids and glycerol, are converted for storage in subcutaneous tissue and other storage depots.

If energy and glucose levels are low, stored fat is converted back into glycerol and fatty acids by a process called lipolysis. This occurs in adipose cells, but the fatty acids and glycerol are transported to the liver for use as an alternative energy supply.

Protein

Amino acids are transported to the liver during digestion and most of the body's protein is synthesized here.

If protein is in excess, amino acids can be converted into fat and stored in fat depots, or if required, made into glucose for energy by gluconeogenesis, which has already been mentioned.

However, before amino acids can be utilized in these ways, the first step is to remove the nitrogen-containing amino group NH_2. This very important metabolic process is called deamination.

In the hepatocytes, NH_2 (the amino group) quickly changes into ammonia NH_3, which is highly toxic to the body. The liver acts fast to convert ammonia into urea that then can be excreted in the urine and eliminated from the body.

Detoxification

The liver is vital for the detoxification and destruction of endogenous and exogenous substances that are harmful to the body.

The liver's own phagocytes, which reside within the lobules, known as Kupffer cells, digest and destroy cellular debris and any invading bacteria.

Other exogenous substances such as drugs and alcohol are detoxified by the liver. Endogenous substances (or those produced by the body) are also dealt with by the liver. Amino acids are deaminated, some hormones are inactivated, and bilirubin, a product of the breakdown of old red blood cells, is also detoxified and rendered harmless by liver metabolism.

Storage

The liver plays an important role as a storage facility. The hepatocytes take up many types of vitamins and minerals from the blood and store them. These include vitamins A, B_{12}, D, E, K, and minerals like iron and copper.

Glycogen, which is formed from excess glucose, is also stored by the liver, although muscle tissue can also store glycogen too.

Bile

The liver synthesizes bile, which is important for fat digestion and is also a route of excretion from the body. Bile consists of water, bile salts, cholesterol, phospholipids, electrolytes, and bile pigments, which give it its typical yellowy-green color.

Bile is stored and concentrated in the gall bladder. The presence of fats in the gut during meals stimulates the gall bladder to empty. Bile enters the duodenum, emulsifying fats into smaller globules, which can then be broken down further by lipase enzymes.

Metabolic wastes and drug products may form part of the bile, which can then be excreted from the body through the digestive tract in the feces. Bilirubin, the toxic end product of hemoglobin breakdown, is excreted from the body in this way.

Chapter 2

Liver Health

Chapter Contents

Section 2.1

Caring for Your Liver

"Caring for Your Liver" is reprinted with permission from Hepatitis Foundation International (HFI). © 2003 Hepatitis Foundation International. All rights reserved. Additional information about HFI is included at the end of this section.

Basic Liver Care

Your liver depends on you to take care of it . . . so it can take care of you. It serves as your body's engine, pantry, refinery, food processor, garbage disposal, and "guardian angel." The trouble is, your liver is a silent partner; when something's wrong it does not complain until the damage is far advanced. So it needs your help every day to keep it healthy and hepatitis-free. To do that, you need to eat a healthy diet, exercise, get lots of fresh air, and avoid things that can cause liver damage.

What Does My Liver Do?

Sadly, people generally have little knowledge of the complexities and importance of the thousands of vital functions their livers perform nonstop.

The liver is about the size of a football—the largest organ in your body. It plays a vital role in regulating life processes. Before you were born, it served as the main organ of blood formation. Now, its primary functions are to refine and detoxify everything you eat, breathe, and absorb through your skin. It is your body's internal chemical power plant, converting nutrients in the food you eat into muscles, energy, hormones, clotting factors, and immune factors.

It stores certain vitamins, minerals (including iron), and sugars; regulates fat stores; and controls the production and excretion of cholesterol. The bile, produced by liver cells, helps you to digest your food and absorb important nutrients. It neutralizes and destroys poisonous substances and metabolizes alcohol. It helps you resist infection and removes bacteria from the blood stream, helping you to stay healthy. Arguably, your liver isn't just your silent partner—it's your best friend.

Three Things to Avoid for Liver Health

Avoid Excessive Alcohol

Most people know that the liver acts as a filter and can be badly damaged by drinking too much alcohol. Liver specialists suggest that more than two drinks a day for men—and more than one drink a day for women—may even be too much for some people.

One of the most remarkable accomplishments of this miraculous organ is its ability to regenerate. (Three-quarters of the liver can be removed and it will grow back in the same shape and form within a few weeks!) However, overworking your liver by heavy alcohol consumption can cause liver cells (the "employees" in the power plant) to become permanently damaged or scarred. This is called cirrhosis.

Avoid Drugs and Medicines Taken with Alcohol

Medicines—especially the seemingly harmless acetaminophen (the active ingredient in Tylenol and other over-the-counter medications)—should never be taken with alcoholic beverages. Many prescribed and over-the-counter drugs and medicines (including herbal medications) are made up of chemicals that could be potentially hazardous to your precious liver cells, especially taken with alcohol.

If you are ill with a virus or metabolic disorder, liver damage may result from the medications you take. In such cases, you should ask your physician about possible liver cell damage.

Avoid Environmental Pollutants

Fumes from paint thinners, bug sprays, and other aerosol sprays are picked up by the tiny blood vessels in your lungs and carried to your liver, where they are detoxified and discharged in your bile. The amount and concentration of those chemicals should be controlled to prevent liver damage. Make certain you have good ventilation, use a mask, cover your skin, and wash off any chemicals you get on your skin with soap and water as soon as possible.

Diet and Your Liver

Overview

Poor nutrition is rarely a cause of liver disease, but good nutrition in the form of a balanced diet may help liver cells damaged by hepatitis viruses to regenerate, forming new liver cells. Nutrition can be an essential part of treatment. Many chronic liver diseases are associated with malnutrition.

Watch the Protein

To quickly determine your daily protein in grams, divide your weight in pounds by 2. Too much daily protein may cause hepatic encephalopathy (mental confusion). This occurs when the amount of dietary protein is greater than the liver's ability to use the protein. This causes a buildup of toxins that can interfere with brain function. Protein is restricted in patients with clinical evidence of encephalopathy. However, controversy exists regarding the type of protein a diet should contain. Vegetable and dairy protein may be tolerated better than meat protein. Medications, such as lactulose and neomycin, may be used to help control hepatitis-related encephalopathy. Due to the body's need for proteins, protein restriction should be undertaken only with a doctor's advice.

Watch the Calories

Excess calories in the form of carbohydrates can add to liver dysfunction and can cause fat deposits in the liver. No more than 30 percent of a person's total calories should come from fat because of the danger to the cardiovascular system. To figure out your daily calorie needs, you'll need a minimum of 15 calories a day for each pound you weigh.

Watch the Salt

Good nutrition also helps to maintain the normal fluid and electrolyte balances in the body. Patients with fluid retention and swelling of the abdomen (ascites) or the legs (peripheral edema) may need diets low in salt to avoid sodium retention that contributes to fluid retention. Avoiding foods such as canned soups and vegetables, cold cuts, dairy products, and condiments such as mayonnaise and ketchup can reduce sodium intake. Read food labels carefully, as many prepared foods contain large amounts of salt. The best-tasting salt substitute is lemon juice.

Watch Vitamins A and D

Excessive amounts of some vitamins may be an additional source of stress to the liver that must act as a filter for the body. Mega-vitamin supplements, particularly if they contain vitamins A and D, may be harmful. Excess vitamin A is very toxic to the liver.

Beware of Alcohol

You'll need to stop drinking completely to give your liver a break—a chance to heal, a chance to rebuild, a chance for new liver cells to grow. This means avoiding beer, wine, cocktails, champagne, and liquor in any other form. If you continue to drink, your liver will pay the price, and if your doctor is checking your liver function tests, it may be hard to determine if a change in a test means there has been damage to your liver due to the disease itself or because of the alcohol.

Beware of Alcohol and Acetaminophen

Acetaminophen is an ingredient in some over-the-counter pain relievers, and is contained in many over-the-counter drugs used for colds or coughs. Taken with alcohol, these products can cause a condition called sudden and severe hepatitis, which could cause fatal liver failure. Clearly, you should never combine these two substances. If you have any doubt about what medicines to take simultaneously, ask your doctor.

Beware of "Nutritional Therapies"

Herbal treatments and alternative liver medicines need to undergo rigorous scientific study before they can be recommended. "Natural" or diet treatments and herbal remedies can be quite dangerous. Plants of the Senecio, Crotalaria, and Heliotropium families, plus chaparral, germander, comfrey, mistletoe, skullcap, margosa oil, mate tea, Gordolobo yerba tea, pennyroyal, and Jin Bu Huan are all toxic to the liver.

About Hepatitis Foundation International

Hepatitis Foundation International (HFI) provides educational materials and training to the public, patients, health educators, and medical professionals about the prevention, diagnosis, and treatment of viral hepatitis, and also provides support to hepatitis patients and researchers. HFI has a variety of materials available through its Liver Wellness/Hepatitis Education program, including the following:

- Videos for lending libraries
- Brochures on liver wellness and hepatitis
- Posters on hepatitis prevention
- Workplace programs

- Teacher and parent information
- Coloring books for children

For more information contact:

Hepatitis Foundation International
504 Blick Drive
Silver Spring, MD 20904-2901
Phone: 301-622-4200
Toll-Free Hotline: 800-891-0707
Fax: 301-622-4702
Website: http://www.HepFI.org

Section 2.2

Symptoms of Liver Disease

Reprinted from "Facts About Your Liver," © 2002 St. Luke's Episcopal Health System. All rights reserved. Reprinted with permission.

The liver is the largest single organ in the human body. In an adult, it weighs about three pounds and is roughly the size of a football. Located in the upper right-hand part of the abdomen, behind the lower ribs, the liver has more than two hundred functions, including:

- converting food into the chemicals the body needs to grow and remain healthy
- eliminating ingested, and internally produced, toxic substances from the blood
- producing bile, a liquid that is essential for digestion
- storing certain vitamins, minerals, and sugars and producing quick energy when it is needed
- controlling the production and excretion of cholesterol
- monitoring and maintaining the proper levels of chemicals and drugs in the blood

- producing immune factors than help the body fight off infection

There are many types of liver disease, and because of the liver's many functions, many can be life-threatening unless treated. Symptoms of liver disease include:

- jaundice (yellowing of the skin and/or eyes)
- dark urine
- gray, yellow, or light-colored stools
- nausea, vomiting, and/or loss of appetite
- vomiting of blood, or bloody or black stools
- abdominal swelling, tenderness, or pain
- prolonged generalized itching
- unusual weight change (an increase or decrease of 5 percent or more within two months)
- sleep disturbances, mental confusion, or coma
- fatigue
- loss of sexual drive or performance

To prevent liver disease, avoid drinking more than two alcoholic drinks per day. Avoid drinking alcohol while taking over-the-counter or prescription drugs. Avoid exposure to industrial chemicals whenever possible, and don't take medications unless they are really necessary. Finally, maintain a good, well-balanced diet.

Chapter 3

Alcohol and the Liver

True or False?

- Many victims of liver disease are not alcoholics.
- Even moderate social drinkers may risk liver damage.
- People who never drink alcoholic beverages may still get serious liver problems.

Answer: All statements are true. How many did you get right?

If you were surprised by the answers, don't be discouraged. You are not alone. Most people are confused about the relationship between alcohol and the liver. The American Liver Foundation has found that there is much misunderstanding on this subject. Because myths can be harmful, here are straight answers to some of the most common questions about alcohol and the liver.

Does alcohol cause liver disease?

Yes, but it is only one of the many causes, and the risk depends on how much you drink and over how long a period. There are more than one hundred liver diseases. Known causes include viruses, hereditary defects, and reactions to drugs and chemicals. Scientists are still investigating the causes for the most serious liver diseases.

How much alcohol can I safely drink?

Because some people are much more sensitive to alcohol than others, there is no single right answer that will fit everyone. Generally, doctors recommend that if you drink, don't drink more than two drinks per day.

Are there dangers from alcohol besides the amount that is consumed?

Yes. Even moderate amounts of alcohol can have toxic effects when taken with over-the-counter drugs containing acetaminophen. If you are taking over-the-counter drugs, be especially careful about drinking and don't use an alcoholic beverage to take your medication. Ask your doctor about precautions for prescription drugs.

Can "social drinkers" get alcoholic hepatitis?

Yes. Alcoholic hepatitis is frequently discovered in alcoholics, but it also occurs in people who are not alcoholics. People vary greatly in the way their liver reacts to alcohol.

What kinds of liver diseases are caused by too much alcohol?

Alcoholic hepatitis is an inflammation of the liver that lasts one to two weeks. Symptoms include loss of appetite, nausea, vomiting, abdominal pain and tenderness, fever, jaundice, and sometimes, mental confusion. It is believed to lead to alcoholic cirrhosis over a period of years. Cirrhosis involves permanent damage to the liver cells. "Fatty liver" is the earliest stage of alcoholic liver disease. If the patient stops drinking at this point, the liver can heal itself.

How can alcoholic hepatitis be diagnosed?

Alcoholic hepatitis is not easy to diagnose. Sometimes symptoms are worse for a time after drinking has stopped than they were during the drinking episode. While the disease usually comes on after a period of fairly heavy drinking, it may also be seen in people who are moderate drinkers. Blood tests may help in diagnosis. Proof is established best by liver biopsy. This involves taking a tiny specimen of liver tissue with a needle and examining it under a microscope. The biopsy is usually done under local anesthesia.

Are men or women more likely to get alcoholic hepatitis?

Women appear to be more likely to suffer liver damage from alcohol. Even when a man and a woman have the same weight and drink the same amount, the woman generally has a higher concentration of alcohol in the blood because she has relatively more body fat and less water than the man, and her body handles alcohol differently.

Do all alcoholics get alcoholic hepatitis and eventually cirrhosis?

No. Some alcoholics may suffer seriously from the many physical and psychological symptoms of alcoholism but escape serious liver damage. Alcoholic cirrhosis is found among alcoholics about 10–25 percent of the time.

Is alcoholic hepatitis different from "fatty liver"?

Yes. Anyone who drinks alcohol heavily, even for a few days, will develop a condition in which liver cells are swollen with fat globules and water. This condition is called "fatty liver." It may also result from diabetes, obesity, certain drugs, or severe protein malnutrition. Fatty liver caused by alcohol is reversible when drinking of alcohol is stopped.

Does alcoholic hepatitis always lead to cirrhosis?

No. It usually takes many years for alcoholic hepatitis to produce enough liver damage to result in cirrhosis. If alcoholic hepatitis is detected and treated early, cirrhosis can be prevented.

Is alcoholic hepatitis dangerous?

Yes. It may be fatal, especially if the patient has had previous liver damage. Those who have had nutritional deficiencies because of heavy drinking may have other ailments. These medical complications may affect almost every system in the body. It is important to recognize and treat alcoholic cirrhosis early, so that these life-threatening consequences are prevented.

How can alcoholic hepatitis be prevented?

The best treatment is to stop drinking. Treatment may also include prescribed medication, good nutrition, and rest. The patient may be instructed to avoid various drugs and chemicals. Since the liver has considerable ability to heal and regenerate, the prognosis for a patient with alcoholic hepatitis is very hopeful—if he or she totally abstains from drinking alcohol.

Is cirrhosis different from alcoholic hepatitis?

Yes. Hepatitis is an inflammation of the liver. In cirrhosis, normal liver cells are damaged and replaced by scar tissue. This scarring keeps the liver from performing many of its vital functions.

What causes cirrhosis?

There are many causes for cirrhosis. Long-term alcohol abuse is one. Chronic hepatitis is another major cause. In children, the most frequent causes are biliary atresia, a disease that damages the bile ducts, and neonatal hepatitis. Children with these diseases often receive liver transplants.

Many adult patients who require liver transplants suffer from primary biliary cirrhosis. We do not yet know what causes this illness, but it is not in any way related to alcohol consumption.

Cirrhosis can also be caused by hereditary defects in iron or copper metabolism or prolonged exposure to toxins.

Should alcoholics receive a liver transplant?

Some medical centers will not transplant alcoholics because they believe a substantial percentage will return to drinking. Other centers require abstinence from drinking at least six months before and after surgery, plus enrollment in a counseling program.

Chapter 4

Acetaminophen Use and Liver Injury

Chapter Contents

Section 4.1

Effects of Acetaminophen on the Liver

The American Liver Foundation believes that warning labels on acetaminophen-containing products should make specific mention of the risk of liver damage. Consumers should be made aware that there are a number of scientific reports that urge that those who regularly consume three or more alcoholic beverages daily should take no more than 2 grams per day of acetaminophen without consulting their physician.

Background

Acetaminophen is generally considered to be safe and effective but, like most drugs, is not entirely without risk. This is particularly true because, unlike most drugs, acetaminophen exhibits a dose-related toxicity and toxic levels may be reached in any individual who takes more than a certain amount. It is recognized that large doses of acetaminophen taken with suicidal intent can lead to liver failure and death. However, recent reports have emphasized the occurrence of unintentional or accidental hepatotoxicity, with liver failure and death in more than 20 percent, typically occurring in moderate to heavy alcohol users.[1,2] In most of these reports the dosage of acetaminophen reported by the patient exceeded the 4 grams per 24 hours limit recommended by the manufacturer, although some patients did report taking doses within this limit. A practical and safe dosage limit for acetaminophen, particularly for alcohol users, has not been established, but is likely to be lower than previously thought.

The Food and Drug Administration (FDA) has held hearings to review the risks of over-the-counter analgesic products. With respect to acetaminophen, reports were submitted of cases of hepatotoxicity in liver failure associated with regular alcohol use and high doses of acetaminophen. Other potential risks were identified with other pain relievers, but not directly related to liver failure. Concern was also raised about gastrointestinal bleeding due to nonsteroidal anti-inflammatory agents if these were used as substitutes for acetaminophen.

In response to these concerns, McNeil Consumer Products, the manufacturer of Tylenol, one of the most widely used acetaminophen products, has voluntarily added a warning notice to its packages as follows:

"Alcohol warning: For this and all other pain relievers, including aspirin, ibuprofen, ketoprofen and naproxen sodium. If you generally consume three or more alcohol-containing drinks per day you should consult your physician for advice on when and how you should take pain relievers."

This label is now widely used on many, but not all, acetaminophen-containing products. The FDA recently published a proposed rule that would require all OTC pain relievers to carry an alcohol warning.

The American Liver Foundation believes that warning labels on acetaminophen-containing products should make specific mention of the risk of liver damage. Consumers should be made aware that there are a number of scientific reports that urge that those who regularly consume three or more alcoholic beverages daily should take no more than 2 grams per day of acetaminophen without consulting their physician.

Risks of Acetaminophen and Alcohol Use

The manufacturer has set the maximum dosage of acetaminophen at 4 grams per day. While acetaminophen is generally a safe and effective drug when taken at recommended doses, several medical authorities recommend that the maximum therapeutic dose be lowered for individuals who drink excessive amounts of alcohol.

Neil Kaplowitz, M.D., in his 1996 medical textbook, says: "Therefore, chronic alcoholics may develop serious liver injury with therapeutic doses of acetaminophen greater than 2 grams per day."[3] Hyman J. Zimmerman, M.D., and Willis C. Maddrey, M.D., in a review article on this subject concluded: "it is our view that individuals that take more than 60 grams a day of alcohol should take no more than 2 grams per day of acetaminophen."[2] This amount of alcohol would be the equivalent of approximately 6 ounces of hard liquor, 4 bottles of beer, 19 ounces of wine, or 12 ounces of fortified wine each day. Note that the FDA currently recommends that patients regularly consuming alcohol consult their physician.

Individuals who have been diagnosed with hepatitis and other liver diseases do not appear to be at greater risks for using recommended doses of acetaminophen.

Recommendations for Enhanced Public Awareness

The American Liver Foundation (ALF) urges manufacturers of acetaminophen to develop, in consultation with FDA, consumer-friendly language that warns of the possibility that regular use of alcohol may increase the risk of liver damage from acetaminophen. Warnings should be reasonably visible in readable type on the package, on the container, and in advertising.

Because it is reported that there are over three hundred products containing acetaminophen, ALF will secure a comprehensive list of such products and make it available through ALF's national hotline (1-800-GO LIVER).

ALF urges the implementation of an education campaign with special attention being given to language barriers and socioeconomic or educational levels, addressing:

- *General public:* a broad-based education campaign stressing proper use of acetaminophen and the hazards of excessive dosing associated with regular alcohol use should be implemented.

- *Health care professionals (e.g., physicians, pharmacists, nurses):* to improve and reinforce their understanding about acetaminophen preparations, the proper use of this drug, the hazards of excessive dosing, and groups at greater risk of liver injury.

The Need for Additional Data

Federal agencies (e.g., CDC, NIH, FDA) should initiate additional research to try to define the risk factors, molecular and cellular mechanisms of, and improved prevention and treatments of, acetaminophen toxicity.

ALF will discuss with CDC and FDA national surveillance projects and registries for acetaminophen toxicity. ALF agrees with the need for more scientific data to permit determination of when a case of hepatotoxicity is really acetaminophen related.

The role of fasting and other underlying conditions on the susceptibility to acetaminophen liver toxicity in those who regularly consume alcohol needs to be explored.

References

1. Schmidt FV, Rochling FA, Casey DL, Lee WM, Acetaminophen toxicity in an urban county hospital. *N. Engl J Med* 1997; 337: 1112–17.

2. Zimmerman HJ, Maddrey W. Acetaminophen hepatotoxicity with regular intake of alcohol: Analysis of instances of therapeutic misadventure. *Hepatology* 1995; 22: 767–73.

3. Kaplowitz N., Drug metabolism and hepatotoxicity, In Kaplowitz N, ed. *Liver and biliary diseases* (Williams and Wilkins, 1996), 112–20.

ALF does not make recommendations concerning treatment for individuals, and suggests that a physician be consulted before pursuing any course or change of treatment.

The American Liver Foundation acknowledges the following physicians for the assistance they provided in preparing this position statement:

- Bruce R. Bacon, M.D., Saint Louis University School of Medicine

- Adrian M. Di Bisceglie, M.D., Saint Louis University School of Medicine

- Neil Kaplowitz, M.D., University of Southern California

- Craig J McClain, M.D., University of Kentucky

- William M Lee, M.D., University of Texas Southwestern Medical School

- Ronald J Sokol, AIM, University of Colorado School of Medicine

- John M. Vierling, M.D., Cedars-Sinai Medical Center

- Paul B. Watkins, M.D., University of Michigan Medical Center

- Hyman Zimmerman, M.D., George Washington University School of Medicine

Section 4.2

Understanding Acetaminophen-Caused Liver Toxicity

"'CAR' Drives Understanding of Acetaminophen Poisoning," October 11, 2002, is reprinted with permission from the Baylor College of Medicine Office of Public Affairs. © 2002 Baylor College of Medicine.

Baylor College of Medicine researchers have identified a protein known as CAR (constitutive androstane receptor) that regulates liver toxicity caused by the common pain-reliever acetaminophen. Their findings are published in the October 11, 2002, issue of the journal *Science*, and will point the way to new treatments for poisoning with similar compounds.

Acetaminophen is found in Tylenol and many other medications. Advisors to the Food and Drug Administration urged the agency in September 2002 to require a stronger warning label on such products.

"Our work explains an important, but unexpected, component of acetaminophen toxicity and adds a new mechanism to the process. It also suggests a new approach to treating hepatotoxicity," said David D. Moore, Ph.D., professor of molecular and cell biology at Baylor College of Medicine.

When a person takes acetaminophen, the liver produces small amounts of a potentially harmful compound called NAPQI (N-acetyl-p-benzoquinone imine). Normally, the liver uses another chemical called glutathione to quickly neutralize NAPQI.

"The problem occurs when you run out of glutathione," said Moore.

An overdose of acetaminophen can cause depletion of glutathione and land a person in the hospital. "Acetaminophen toxicity is the number one cause of hospital admission for liver failure in the United States," he said.

CAR is a receptor that regulates the response of the liver to drugs and other foreign compounds. When it is activated, the liver increases its ability to modify such compounds and eliminate them from the body. This is normally a protective response. In some cases, however, it can also result in harmful effects, for example, by increasing the production of toxic byproducts like NAPQI.

Using a mouse bred to lack CAR, Moore and his co-workers showed that the receptor was critical to the medication's toxicity.

"We found out that high doses of acetaminophen activate CAR, and that CAR then activates target genes that increase toxicity," said Moore. "This generates a vicious cycle in which acetaminophen actually worsens its own toxicity. Because of the absence of this cycle, mice without CAR are partially resistant to high doses of acetaminophen."

When mice that have CAR were given a drug called androstenol, which reverses the receptor's activity, they were even more resistant to toxic effects of acetaminophen. Androstenol could even protect the liver if it was given an hour after a high dose of acetaminophen. However, mice that lacked CAR showed no protective effect.

The current treatment for acetaminophen overdose relies on a compound that replenishes the glutathione in the liver. This treatment is effective if it is given in time.

Blocking CAR "would provide a completely different approach to acetaminophen toxicity and possibly to the toxicity of other agents for which no drug treatment is currently available," said Moore.

Unfortunately, there is no drug yet that efficiently blocks the human form of CAR. Studies to identify such an inhibitor are under way.

Others involved in the Baylor studies were graduate student Jun Zhang and postdoctoral associates Wendong Huang, Steven S. Chua, and Ping Wei.

Chapter 5

Pregnancy and the Liver

How does pregnancy affect the liver? Are there changes in liver function?

Pregnancy has little effect on a normal liver. There are no significant changes in liver function; however, certain markers of liver function may alter slightly during normal pregnancy. For example, blood levels of the protein albumin will decrease during pregnancy because of dilution of the expectant mother's blood. In addition, the blood test for alkaline phosphatase, usually taken as an indicator of liver disease, will increase during normal pregnancy because of a production of this marker by a normal placenta. This small change does not indicate liver disease.

At what stage of fetal development does a liver start functioning? What are the stages of development for the child's liver?

The liver first appears in a developing fetus as early as the third week of pregnancy, although liver function probably does not begin until the sixth to tenth week of pregnancy. Liver function continues to develop over the remainder of pregnancy, but the liver's ability to handle such compounds as bilirubin and bile acids is still not fully mature even at the time of birth. Adult-level liver function probably develops by six to twelve months of age. During childhood, liver function is essentially that of the normal adult, except that the liver is appropriately smaller in the young child compared to an adult.

Should pregnant women be tested for hepatitis B and C?

It is now recommended that all pregnant women be tested during the last two to three months of pregnancy for the presence of the hepatitis B virus. Babies born to women carrying the hepatitis B virus are at considerable risk of contracting hepatitis B immediately after delivery. Preventive measures given to babies include vaccination against the hepatitis B virus right after birth and administration of a special gamma globulin preparation for immediate protection. These measures prevent 90–95 percent of transmission and provide the baby with long-term protection.

Babies born to women carrying the hepatitis C virus are very unlikely to contract hepatitis C, although transmission can occur. There is no specific preventive treatment available. Therefore, currently, there are no recommendations to test women for hepatitis C.

Can women who are infected with viral hepatitis become pregnant?

Yes, especially if their liver has not been seriously damaged.

Should babies be vaccinated for hepatitis B?

If the mother does not carry the hepatitis B virus but other family members do, then babies and young children should probably be vaccinated as early as possible. It is now recommended that all children ultimately receive vaccination against hepatitis B as well, since it is a preventable infection that may occur at any time.

Can mothers who are infected with hepatitis B or C breastfeed their babies?

Mothers who are infected with hepatitis B may breastfeed their babies, especially if the babies have received appropriate vaccination. It is not known whether the hepatitis C virus can be transmitted in breast milk. This, however, seems to be a low risk.

Can a nursing mother take interferon, the drug for hepatitis B or C, or will it harm the baby?

A nursing mother may take interferon for hepatitis B or C. It is not known, however, whether the interferon will have any effects on the nursing baby. Because interferon treatment of chronic hepatitis B or C is elective, it would probably be wise to give a mother interferon before she becomes pregnant or after she has finished nursing.

Can a woman with autoimmune hepatitis become pregnant and give birth to a healthy baby?

Yes. However, if the autoimmune hepatitis is active, women are much less fertile and are likely to have many complications during pregnancy. Thus, it is recommended that women with autoimmune hepatitis first receive appropriate treatment to obtain control of their disease before they become pregnant. They are frequently treated with prednisone, an anti-inflammatory drug that depresses the immune system, which is considered to be safe during pregnancy. Women with uncontrolled serious autoimmune hepatitis and those who have already developed cirrhosis from autoimmune hepatitis may experience complications of liver disease during pregnancy, and their babies are at a higher risk of premature delivery and fetal death. Those babies who are born, however, are normal.

Women with autoimmune hepatitis who require continued use of prednisone to maintain remissions may well be able to become pregnant and carry a fetus to term. However, they should continue use of prednisone during pregnancy as the disease may flare up.

Why do some pregnant women experience itching and jaundice?

During pregnancy some women experience the onset of itching (pruritus) and jaundice, usually related to an impaired bile flow. It arises because of the changes in the liver's ability to handle chemicals called bile acids and bilirubin, and to make bile, probably from the effects of large doses of the hormone estrogen (which normally increases during pregnancy). Certain women have an inherited susceptibility to these effects of estrogen. Women who have had impaired bile flow in pregnancy may develop a similar disorder if they take oral contraceptives. For the mother the disorder is mild, although the itching can be very bothersome. In some severe cases the fetus may become distressed and there is a risk of premature delivery and a low but increased risk of early fetal death or stillbirths. In general, the disease is moderate to mild, and neither the mother nor the baby suffers any lasting consequences.

What is Wilson disease and how does it affect pregnant women?

Wilson disease is an inherited defect that results in the body storing too much copper, which then becomes toxic to the liver, brain, and other organs. Women with untreated Wilson disease have difficulty becoming pregnant, and experience more miscarriages and spontaneous abortions. In addition, in untreated and symptomatic Wilson disease both the mother and fetus are considered at high risk during pregnancy. Women with Wilson disease that has been well controlled, and in whom body copper levels have been reduced to near normal, regain fertility and may have normal, uneventful pregnancies and healthy babies.

Are there any other liver diseases that can affect pregnant women and their babies?

In addition to the diseases mentioned, women with less common diseases, such as primary biliary cirrhosis, primary sclerosing cholangitis, and alcoholic liver disease, among others, may consider pregnancy. In general, women in which liver disease has produced severe liver damage, particularly cirrhosis or serious liver dysfunction, are less fertile. These women and their babies are at higher risk of complications during pregnancy. In addition, three rare liver disorders may have serious consequences for pregnant women and their babies. They are intrahepatic cholestasis of pregnancy (impaired bile flow), toxemia-related disease with the HELLP syndrome, and acute fatty liver of pregnancy.

What is toxemia (preeclampsia) and how does it affect the liver?

Toxemia (or preeclampsia) is a fairly common disorder that occurs late in pregnancy and includes high blood pressure, kidney dysfunction, and the development of leg swelling or edema. In approximately 10 percent of women with preeclampsia, the liver is also affected, with development of blood clots and bleeding into the liver. In mild cases, liver function remains normal, although liver blood tests may be abnormal. In severe cases, large parts of the liver may be destroyed, leading to symptoms similar to severe viral hepatitis. In extremely severe cases, there may be major bleeding into parts of the liver or abdomen, a life-threatening situation.

What is the HELLP syndrome?

The HELLP syndrome is part of the liver disease that affects women with preeclampsia. It derives its name from the abbreviations for hemolysis (breakdown of red blood cells), elevated liver tests, and low platelets in the blood. This occurs in approximately 10 percent of all women with preeclampsia, and may be mild (diagnosed through abnormal blood tests) or may develop into severe liver damage. The disease stops immediately after delivery, and the liver generally heals itself within days to weeks. While the disease is ongoing, the mother is at risk of complications of liver damage and bleeding, and the baby is at risk of premature delivery or stillbirth.

Do oral contraceptives have an adverse effect on the liver?

Oral contraceptives have little adverse effect on the liver in most women. They may, however, cause increased growth of an uncommon liver tumor called a liver cell adenoma. Adenomas are benign liver tumors and do not spread outside the liver. Very large adenomas, however, may rupture and bleed. Thus, oral contraceptives probably should not be used by women who have significant adenomas. Oral contraceptives also may causes itching, jaundice, and cholestasis (decreased bile flow) in women with a genetic susceptibility to the effects of estrogens. Although estrogens are normal female sex hormones, at high levels they may interfere with bile formation in some women. If a woman taking an oral contraceptive develops this estrogen-induced cholestasis, the contraceptives should be discontinued. No lasting effect on the liver is anticipated.

Can a woman who has had a liver transplant become pregnant?

Women who have had a successful liver transplant with good liver function can become pregnant. Fertility returns within a few months after the transplant, and such women have successfully carried normal pregnancies to term. Only a few women who have had a transplant have gone on to become pregnant, however, so it is not known whether the ability to become pregnant and to carry a normal baby to term is completely normal. In addition, although the drugs used for immunosuppression after liver transplantation are thought to be relatively safe for the developing baby, absolute safety cannot be guaranteed.

Can someone with cirrhosis become pregnant?

Yes, although it is much more difficult because of the markedly decreased fertility. If they do become pregnant, they may be able to give birth to a healthy baby. The mother, however, may experience complications of liver failure during pregnancy, and the baby is at higher risk of premature delivery, spontaneous abortion, miscarriage, and stillbirth. Those children who are born, however, are generally healthy.

Is it safe for a pregnant woman to drink moderate amounts of alcohol?

No, because it can damage the unborn child. Moderate alcohol consumption (one to two drinks) probably does not affect the liver of an otherwise normal pregnant woman, but even moderate doses may cause damage to the fetus. In addition, for any woman with liver disease, it makes sense to avoid taking in substances such as alcohol that are known to cause liver toxicity in may people.

Chapter 6

Understanding Liver Function Tests

Chapter Contents

Section 6.1

Liver Function Tests: An Overview

Reprinted from "Liver Function Tests," Nemours Foundation, reviewed and updated September 2002. This information was provided by KidsHealth, one of the largest resources online for medically reviewed health information written for parents, kids, and teens. For more articles like this one, visit www.KidsHealth.org, or www.TeensHealth.org. © 2002 The Nemours Center for Children's Health Media, a division of The Nemours Foundation.

Liver function tests (LFTs) measure liver injury, rather than liver function. They are a group of blood tests that measure substances in the blood that reflect whether the liver has been injured and the extent of the injuries. Sometimes these tests are also called a liver panel. The tests usually include the following: alanine transaminase (ALT), aspartate transaminase (AST), alkaline phosphatase (ALP), albumin, total protein, and total and direct bilirubin.

The liver is a complex organ, located in the upper right corner of the abdomen, which has many vital roles. The liver stores fuel for the body that has been produced from sugars, and it is involved in the processing of fats and proteins. Bile produced by the liver is involved in the digestion and absorption of fat in the intestines. The liver also makes proteins that are essential for blood clotting, and it helps remove poisons and toxins from the body.

When a blood sample is collected from a child to measure LFTs, the skin is cleaned with alcohol first, then a needle is inserted into a vein and blood is drawn into specific tubes. These blood samples are then sent to a laboratory and processed by machines. The tests are done simultaneously, which takes about twenty minutes. Emergency test results are reported within an hour. For routine tests processed at the site of collection, results are usually available within three to six hours. If samples are shipped to a central processing facility, they are usually available the next day.

The Liver Function Tests

Alanine Transaminase (ALT)

Alanine transaminase is an enzyme that is important in the processing of proteins. This enzyme is found in large amounts in the liver, and small amounts of this enzyme are also found in the heart, muscle, and kidney. When the liver is injured or inflamed, the levels of ALT in blood usually rise; therefore, this test is done to check for signs of liver disease. The ALT is elevated, for example, in some viral infections of childhood that may affect the liver, such as mononucleosis.

Aspartate Transaminase (AST)

Aspartate transaminase is an enzyme that plays a role in many aspects of body metabolism. This enzyme is found in many body tissues including the heart, muscle, kidney, brain, and lung. It is also present in the liver. If there is cell injury or death in any of these tissues, AST is released into the bloodstream; therefore, elevated AST levels can be seen in a variety of conditions, including liver disease. For example, the AST may be elevated in viral hepatitis, mononucleosis, or following a heart attack.

Alkaline Phosphatase (ALP)

Alkaline phosphatase is an enzyme found in the liver and bone. Blood levels of the enzyme are elevated in some types of liver disease. Children—especially teens—normally have higher blood levels of ALP than adults. This is related to rapid growth of their bones. Compared to the transaminases, alkaline phosphatase tends to be higher in diseases associated with injury to the bile-secreting part of the liver's activity.

Albumin and Total Protein

Albumin and total protein levels in the blood reflect the protein-building function of the liver. Found throughout the body, proteins perform many functions: hold cells together, carry information from place to place, control chemical reactions, fight infections, transport oxygen, and much more. Albumin is a protein made by the liver, found in large amounts in the blood. In fact, it's similar to the protein in egg whites. In some types of liver disease, the ability of the organ to make proteins is affected. In these cases the blood levels of total protein and albumin are low. Low total protein and albumin levels are also seen in kids who are malnourished.

Because most proteins, including albumin, have fairly long half-lives, the liver's incapacity to produce proteins must last weeks to months to be reflected in lowered blood levels of total protein or albumin.

Total and Direct Bilirubin

Total and direct bilirubin levels in blood are also measured as part of the liver function tests. Bilirubin is the chemical substance that gives bile, a fluid produced by the liver, its yellow-green color. Jaundice, the yellow discoloration of the skin seen in some types of liver disease, occurs because high levels of bilirubin accumulating in the blood lead to some of the substance becoming deposited in the skin. Bilirubin is produced from hemoglobin, which is released when red blood cells break down. The liver takes bilirubin and attaches conjugated sugar molecules to it so it can leave the body through the urine. This type of bilirubin is called conjugated direct (because it can be measured directly in a water solution) bilirubin. In liver disease, bilirubin levels in blood can become high. Measurements of total and direct bilirubin can be helpful in diagnosing specific liver problems.

Section 6.2

Alanine Transaminase (ALT)

Reprinted from "ALT," © 2005 A.D.A.M., Inc. Reprinted with permission.

Alternative Names

SGPT; Serum glutamate pyruvate transaminase; Alanine transaminase

Definition

A test that measures the amount of ALT in serum.

How the Test Is Performed

Adult or child: Blood is drawn from a vein (venipuncture), usually from the inside of the elbow or the back of the hand. The puncture site is cleaned with antiseptic, and a tourniquet (an elastic band) or blood pressure cuff is placed around the upper arm to apply pressure and restrict blood flow through the vein. This causes veins below the tourniquet to distend (fill with blood). A needle is inserted into the vein, and the blood is collected in an airtight vial or a syringe. During the procedure, the tourniquet is removed to restore circulation. Once the blood has been collected, the needle is removed, and the puncture site is covered to stop any bleeding.

Infant or young child: The area is cleansed with antiseptic and punctured with a sharp needle or a lancet. The blood may be collected in a pipette (small glass tube), on a slide, onto a test strip, or into a small container. Cotton or a bandage may be applied to the puncture site if there is any continued bleeding.

How to Prepare for the Test

Infants and children: The physical and psychological preparation you can provide for this or any test or procedure depends on your child's age, interests, previous experiences, and level of trust.

How the Test Will Feel

When the needle is inserted to draw blood, some people feel moderate pain, while others feel only a prick or stinging sensation. Afterward, there may be some throbbing.

Why the Test Is Performed

This test is used to determine if a patient has liver damage. ALT is an enzyme involved in the metabolism of the amino acid alanine. ALT is in a number of tissues but is in highest concentrations in the liver. Injury to the liver results in release of the enzyme into the blood.

Normal Values

Normal range can vary according to a number of factors, including age and gender. Consult your physician or lab for interpretation.

What Abnormal Results Mean

Greater-than-normal levels may indicate:

- hepatitis (viral, autoimmune)
- use of hepatotoxic drugs
- hepatic (liver) ischemia (blood deficiency)

- cirrhosis
- hepatic tumor

What the Risks Are

- excessive bleeding
- fainting or feeling light-headed
- hematoma (blood accumulating under the skin)
- infection (a slight risk any time the skin is broken)
- multiple punctures to locate veins

Special Considerations

Veins and arteries vary in size from one patient to another and from one side of the body to the other. Obtaining a blood sample from some people may be more difficult than from others.

Section 6.3

Aspartate Aminotransferase (AST)

Reprinted from "AST," © 2005 A.D.A.M., Inc. Reprinted with permission.

Alternative Names

Aspartate aminotransferase; Serum glutamic-oxaloacetic transaminase; SGOT

Definition

A test that measures the amount of the enzyme AST in serum.

How the Test Is Performed

Adult or child: Blood is drawn from a vein (venipuncture), usually from the inside of the elbow or the back of the hand. The puncture site is cleaned with antiseptic, and a tourniquet (an elastic band) or blood pressure cuff is placed around the upper arm to apply pressure and restrict blood flow through the vein. This causes veins below the tourniquet to distend (fill with blood). A needle is inserted into the vein, and the blood is collected in an airtight vial or a syringe. During the procedure, the tourniquet is removed to restore circulation. Once the blood has been collected, the needle is removed, and the puncture site is covered to stop any bleeding.

Infant or young child: The area is cleansed with antiseptic and punctured with a sharp needle or a lancet. The blood may be collected in a pipette (small glass tube), on a slide, onto a test strip, or into a small container. Cotton or a bandage may be applied to the puncture site if there is any continued bleeding.

How to Prepare for the Test

Spurious increases in AST may occur in pregnancy and after exercise.

Infants and children: The physical and psychological preparation you can provide for this or any test or procedure depends on your child's age, interests, previous experiences, and level of trust.

How the Test Will Feel

When the needle is inserted to draw blood, some people feel moderate pain, while others feel only a prick or stinging sensation. Afterward, there may be some throbbing.

Why the Test Is Performed

AST is in high concentration in heart muscle, liver cells, skeletal muscle cells, and to a lesser degree, in other tissues. Although elevated serum AST is not specific for liver disease, it is used primarily to diagnose and monitor the course of liver disease (in combination with other enzymes such as ALT, ALP, and bilirubin). It has also been used to monitor patients with heart attacks, but it is much less specific than CPK isoenzyme and LDH isoenzyme for this purpose.

Normal Values

The normal range is 10 to 34 international units per liter (IU/L).

What Abnormal Results Mean

Diseases that affect liver cells cause the release of AST. The AST/ALT ratio (with both elevated) is usually greater than two in patients with alcoholic hepatitis.

An increase in AST levels may indicate:

- acute hemolytic anemia
- acute pancreatitis
- acute renal failure
- hepatic (liver) cirrhosis
- hepatic (liver) necrosis (tissue death)
- hepatitis
- infection mononucleosis
- liver cancer
- multiple trauma
- myocardial infarction (heart attack)
- primary muscle disease
- progressive muscular dystrophy
- recent cardiac catheterization or angioplasty
- recent convulsion
- recent surgery
- severe deep burn
- skeletal muscle trauma

What the Risks Are

- excessive bleeding
- fainting or feeling light-headed
- hematoma (blood accumulating under the skin)
- infection (a slight risk anytime the skin is broken)
- multiple punctures to locate veins

Special Considerations

Veins and arteries vary in size from one patient to another and from one side of the body to the other. Obtaining a blood sample from some people may be more difficult than from others.

Section 6.4

Alkaline Phosphatase (ALP)

Reprinted from "ALP," © 2005 A.D.A.M., Inc.
Reprinted with permission.

Definition

This is a blood test that measures the amount of the enzyme ALP (alkaline phosphatase).

How the Test Is Performed

Blood is drawn from a vein or from a capillary on the heel, finger, toe, or earlobe. The laboratory centrifuges the blood to separate the serum from the cells. The ALP test is done on the serum.

How to Prepare For the Test

Fast for six hours.
Your health care provider may advise you to discontinue drugs that may affect the test, such as:

- antibiotics
- narcotics
- methyldopa
- propranolol
- cortisone
- allopurinol
- tricyclic antidepressants
- chlorpromazine
- oral contraceptives (birth control pills)
- anti-inflammatory analgesics
- androgens
- tranquilizers

- some antiarthritic drugs
- oral antidiabetic drugs.

Why the Test Is Performed

Alkaline phosphatase is an enzyme found in all tissues. Tissues with particularly high concentrations of ALP include the liver, bile ducts, placenta, and bone.

Damaged or diseased tissue releases enzymes into the blood, so serum ALP measurements can be abnormal in many conditions, including bone disease and liver disease. Serum ALP is also increased in some normal circumstances (for example, during normal bone growth) or in response to a variety of drugs.

There are multiple varieties of ALP, called isoenzymes. Different types of isoenzymes, each with different structures, are found in different tissues (for example, liver and bone ALP isoenzymes have different structures) and can be quantified separately in the laboratory. To differentiate the location of damaged or diseased tissue in the body, ALP isoenzyme testing must be done.

Normal Values

The normal range is 44 to 147 IU/L (international units per liter).

Normal values may vary slightly from laboratory to laboratory. They also can vary with age and gender.

What Abnormal Results Mean

Higher-than-normal ALP levels may indicate:

- anemia
- biliary obstruction
- bone disease
- healing fracture
- hepatitis
- hyperparathyroidism
- leukemia
- liver diseases
- osteoblastic bone cancers
- osteomalacia

- Paget disease
- rickets.

Lower-than-normal ALP levels (hypophosphatasemia) may indicate:

- malnutrition
- protein deficiency.

Additional conditions under which the test may be performed:

- alcoholic liver disease (hepatitis/cirrhosis)
- alcoholism
- biliary stricture
- giant cell (temporal, cranial) arteritis
- multiple endocrine neoplasia (MEN) II
- renal cell carcinoma

Special Considerations

The ALP levels vary with age and gender. It is normal for young children experiencing rapid growth and for pregnant women to have high levels of ALP.

Section 6.5

Albumin

Reprinted from "Albumin-Serum," © 2005 A.D.A.M., Inc.
Reprinted with permission.

Definition

This test measures the amount of albumin in serum, the clear fluid portion of blood.

How the Test Is Performed

Blood is drawn from a vein (venipuncture) or capillary. The blood sample is placed in a centrifuge to separate the cells from the serum.

How to Prepare for the Test

The health care provider will advise you, if necessary, to discontinue drugs that may affect the test. Drugs that can increase albumin measurements include anabolic steroids, androgens, growth hormone, and insulin.

Why the Test Is Performed

This test helps in determining if a patient has liver disease or kidney disease, or if not enough protein is being absorbed by the body.

Albumin is the protein of the highest concentration in plasma. Albumin transports many small molecules in the blood (for example, bilirubin, calcium, progesterone, and drugs). It is also of prime importance in maintaining the oncotic pressure of the blood (that is, keeping the fluid from leaking out into the tissues). This is because, unlike small molecules such as sodium and chloride, the concentration of albumin in the blood is much greater than it is in the extracellular fluid.

Because albumin is synthesized by the liver, decreased serum albumin may result from liver disease. It can also result from kidney disease, which allows albumin to escape into the urine. Decreased albumin may also be explained by malnutrition or a low-protein diet.

Normal Values

The normal range is 3.4 to 5.4 g/dL.
Normal values may vary slightly from laboratory to laboratory.

What Abnormal Results Mean

Lower-than-normal levels of albumin may indicate:

- ascites
- burns (extensive)
- glomerulonephritis
- liver disease (for example, hepatitis, cirrhosis, or hepatocellular necrosis "tissue death")
- malabsorption syndromes (for example, Crohn disease, sprue, or Whipple disease)
- malnutrition
- nephrotic syndrome.

Additional conditions under which the test may be performed:

- diabetic nephropathy/sclerosis
- hepatic encephalopathy
- hepatorenal syndrome
- membranous nephropathy
- tropical sprue
- Wilson disease

Special Considerations

If you are receiving large amounts of intravenous fluids, the results of this test may be inaccurate.
Albumin will be decreased during pregnancy.

Section 6.6

Bilirubin

Reprinted from "Bilirubin," © 2005 A.D.A.M., Inc. Reprinted with permission.

Alternative Names

Total bilirubin; Unconjugated bilirubin; Indirect bilirubin; Conjugated bilirubin; Direct bilirubin

Definition

Bilirubin is a breakdown product of hemoglobin. Total and direct bilirubin are usually measured to screen for or to monitor liver or gall bladder dysfunction.

How the Test Is Performed

Blood is drawn from a vein (venipuncture) or capillary. The laboratory centrifuges the blood to separate the serum from the cells, and the bilirubin test is done on the serum.

How to Prepare for the Test

Fast for at least four hours before the test. Your health care provider may instruct you to discontinue drugs that affect the test.

Drugs that can increase bilirubin measurements include allopurinol, anabolic steroids, some antibiotics, antimalarials, azathioprine, chlorpropamide, cholinergics, codeine, diuretics, epinephrine, meperidine, methotrexate, methyldopa, MAO inhibitors, morphine, nicotinic acid, oral contraceptives, phenothiazines, quinidine, rifampin, salicylates, steroids, sulfonamides, and theophylline.

Drugs that can decrease bilirubin measurements include barbiturates, caffeine, penicillin, and high-dose salicylates.

Why the Test Is Performed

This test is useful in determining if a patient has liver disease or a blocked bile duct.

Bilirubin metabolism begins with the breakdown of red blood cells by phagocytic cells. Red blood cells contain hemoglobin, which is broken down to heme and globin. Heme is converted to bilirubin, which is then carried by albumin in the blood to the liver. In the liver, most of the bilirubin is conjugated (chemically attached to) with a glucuronide before it is excreted in the bile. Conjugated bilirubin is called direct bilirubin; unconjugated bilirubin is called indirect bilirubin. Total serum bilirubin equals direct bilirubin plus indirect bilirubin.

Conjugated bilirubin is excreted into the bile by the liver and stored in the gall bladder or transferred directly to the small intestines. Bilirubin is further metabolized by bacteria in the intestines to urobilins, which contribute to the color of the feces. A small percentage of these compounds are reabsorbed and eventually appear in the urine, where they are referred to as urobilinogen.

Normal Values

- direct bilirubin: 0 to 0.3 mg/dl
- total bilirubin: 0.3 to 1.9 mg/dl

Normal values may vary slightly from laboratory to laboratory.

What Abnormal Results Mean

Jaundice is the discoloration of skin and sclera of the eye, which occurs when bilirubin accumulates in the blood at a level greater than approximately 2.5 mg/dl. Jaundice occurs because red blood cells are being broken down too fast for the liver to process, because of disease in the liver, or because of bile duct blockage.

If the bile ducts are obstructed, direct bilirubin will build up, escape from the liver, and end up in the blood. If the levels are high enough, some of it will appear in the urine. Only direct bilirubin appears in the urine. Increased direct bilirubin usually means that the biliary (liver secretion) ducts are obstructed.

Increased indirect or total bilirubin may indicate:

- erythroblastosis fetalis
- Gilbert's disease
- hemolytic anemia
- hemolytic disease of the newborn
- physiological jaundice (normal in newborns)
- sickle cell anemia

- transfusion reaction
- pernicious anemia
- resolution of a large hematoma.

Increased direct bilirubin may indicate:

- bile duct obstruction
- cirrhosis
- Crigler-Najjar syndrome (very rare)
- Dubin-Johnson syndrome (very rare)
- hepatitis.

Additional conditions under which the test may be performed:

- biliary stricture
- cholangiocarcinoma
- cholangitis
- choledocholithiasis
- hemolytic anemia due to G6PD deficiency
- hepatic encephalopathy
- idiopathic aplastic anemia
- idiopathic autoimmune hemolytic anemia
- immune hemolytic anemia
- secondary aplastic anemia
- drug-induced immune hemolytic anemia
- thrombotic thrombocytopenic purpura
- Wilson disease

Special considerations

Interfering factors:

- hemolysis of blood will falsely increase bilirubin levels
- lipids in the blood will falsely decrease bilirubin levels
- bilirubin is light-sensitive; it decomposes in light

Chapter 7

Liver Biopsy: What You Need to Know

Chapter Contents

Section 7.1

Liver Biopsy: An Overview

Reprinted from "Liver Biopsy," National Institute of Diabetes and Digestive and Kidney Diseases (NIDDK), National Institutes of Health, NIH Publication No. 05-4731, November 2004.

In a liver biopsy, the physician examines a small piece of tissue from your liver for signs of damage or disease. A special needle is used to remove the tissue from the liver. The physician decides to do a liver biopsy after tests suggest that the liver does not work properly. For example, a blood test might show that your blood contains higher than normal levels of liver enzymes or too much iron or copper. An x-ray could suggest that the liver is swollen. Looking at liver tissue itself is the best way to determine whether the liver is healthy or what is causing it to be damaged.

Preparation

Before scheduling your biopsy, the physician will take blood samples to make sure your blood clots properly. Be sure to mention any medications you take, especially those that affect blood clotting, like blood thinners. One week before the procedure, you will have to stop taking aspirin, ibuprofen, and anticoagulants.

You must not eat or drink anything for eight hours before the biopsy, and you should plan to arrive at the hospital about an hour before the scheduled time of the procedure. Your physician will tell you whether to take your regular medications during the fasting period and may give you other special instructions.

Procedure

Liver biopsy is considered minor surgery, so it is done at the hospital. For the biopsy, you will lie on a hospital bed on your back with your right hand above your head. After marking the outline of your liver and injecting a local anesthetic to numb the area, the physician will make a small incision in your right side near your rib cage, then insert the biopsy needle and retrieve a sample of liver tissue. In some cases, the physician may use an ultrasound image of the liver to help guide the needle to a specific spot.

You will need to hold very still so that the physician does not nick the lung or gallbladder, which are close to the liver. The physician will ask you to hold your breath for five to ten seconds while he or she puts the needle in your liver. You may feel pressure and a dull pain. The entire procedure takes about twenty minutes.

Two other methods of liver biopsy are also available. For a *laparoscopic biopsy*, the physician inserts a special tube called a laparoscope through an incision in the abdomen. The laparoscope sends images of the liver to a monitor. The physician watches the monitor and uses instruments in the laparoscope to remove tissue samples from one or more parts of the liver. Physicians use this type of biopsy when they need tissue samples from specific parts of the liver.

Transvenous biopsy involves inserting a tube called a catheter into a vein in the neck and guiding it to the liver. The physician puts a biopsy needle into the catheter and then into the liver. Physicians use this procedure when patients have blood-clotting problems or fluid in the abdomen.

Recovery

After the biopsy, the physician will put a bandage over the incision and have you lie on your right side, pressed against a towel, for one to two hours. The nurse will monitor your vital signs and level of pain.

You will need to arrange for someone to take you home from the hospital since you will not be allowed to drive after having the sedative. You must go directly home and remain in bed (except to use the bathroom) for eight to twelve hours, depending on your physician's instructions. Also, avoid exertion for the next week so that the incision and liver can heal. You can expect a little soreness at the incision site and possibly some pain in your right shoulder. This pain is caused by irritation of the diaphragm muscle (the pain usually radiates to the shoulder) and should disappear within a few hours or days. Your physician may recommend that you take Tylenol for pain, but you must not take aspirin or ibuprofen for the first week after surgery. These medicines decrease blood clotting, which is crucial for healing.

Like any surgery, liver biopsy does have some risks, such as puncture of the lung or gallbladder, infection, bleeding, and pain, but these complications are rare.

Section 7.2

Frequently Asked Questions about Liver Biopsy

Liver biopsy is a diagnostic procedure used to obtain a small amount of liver tissue, which can be examined under a microscope to help identify the cause or stage of liver disease.

What are the different ways a liver biopsy can be performed?

The most common way a liver sample is obtained is by inserting a needle into the liver for a fraction of a second. This can be done in the hospital, and the patient may be sent home within three to six hours if there are no complications. The physician determines the best site, depth, and angle of the needle puncture by physical examination or ultrasound. The skin and area under the skin are anesthetized, and a needle is passed quickly into and out of the liver. Approximately half of individuals have no pain afterward, while another half will experience brief localized pain that may spread to the right shoulder.

Another technique used for liver biopsy is guiding the needle into the liver through the abdomen or chest using various imaging techniques. This approach is used when there are localized tumors identified by ultrasound or computed tomography (CT). Either ultrasound or CT scanning is used to pinpoint the site of the tumor and guide the needle to this specific area through the abdomen or chest. After this procedure, the patient is usually allowed to go home the same day.

Less commonly used biopsy techniques are laparoscopy, transvenous or transjugular liver biopsy, and surgical liver biopsy. With laparoscopy, a lighted, narrow tubular instrument is inserted through a small incision in the abdominal wall. The internal organs are moved away from the abdominal wall by gas that is introduced into the abdomen. Instruments may be passed through this lighted instrument or through separate puncture sites to obtain tissue samples from several different areas of the liver. Patients who undergo this procedure may be discharged several hours later.

Transvenous or transjugular liver biopsy may be performed by a radiologist in special circumstances, for example when the patient has a significant problem with blood clotting (coagulopathy) or a large amount of fluid within the abdomen (ascites). For this reason, transjugular liver biopsy is recommended for patients with advanced cirrhosis. With this procedure, a small tube is inserted into the internal jugular vein in the neck and radiologically guided into the hepatic vein, which drains the liver. A small biopsy needle is then inserted through the tube and directly into the liver to obtain a sample of tissue.

Finally, liver biopsy may be done at the time a patient undergoes an open abdominal operation, enabling the surgeon to inspect the liver and take one or more biopsy samples as needed.

When is a liver biopsy used?

Liver biopsy is often used to diagnose the cause of chronic liver disease that results in elevated liver tests or an enlarged liver. It is also used to diagnose liver tumors identified by imaging tests. In many cases, the specific cause of the chronic liver disease is highly suspected on the basis of blood tests, but a liver biopsy is used to confirm the diagnosis as well as determine the amount of damage to the liver. Liver biopsy is also used after liver transplantation to determine the cause of elevated liver tests and determine if rejection is present.

What are the dangers of liver biopsy?

The primary risk of liver biopsy is bleeding from the site of needle entry into the liver, although this occurs in less than 1 percent of patients. Other possible complications include the puncture of other organs, such as the kidney, lung, or colon. Biopsy, by mistake, of the gallbladder rather than the liver may be associated with leakage of bile into the abdominal cavity, causing peritonitis. Fortunately, the risk of death from liver biopsy is extremely low, ranging from 0.1 percent to 0.01 percent.

In order to reduce the risk of bleeding, the coagulation status is assessed in all patients prior to a biopsy. If the prothrombin (coagulating) time is too slow or the platelet count is low, a standard biopsy is not recommended. Vitamin K or fresh frozen plasma may be used to correct clotting abnormalities in such instances. Another alternative in this situation would be a transjugular biopsy.

Are there alternatives to liver biopsy?

The primary alternative to liver biopsy is to make the diagnosis of a liver disease based on the physical examination of the patient, medical history, and blood testing. In some cases, blood testing is quite accurate in giving the doctor the information to diagnose chronic liver disease, while in other circumstances a liver biopsy is needed to assure an accurate diagnosis.

Do liver biopsies ever need to be repeated?

In most circumstances, a liver biopsy is performed only once to confirm a suspected diagnosis of chronic liver disease. Occasionally, liver biopsy is repeated if the clinical condition changes or to assess the results of medical therapy, such as drug treatment of chronic viral hepatitis with interferon or prednisone therapy of autoimmune hepatitis. Patients who have undergone liver transplantation often require numerous liver biopsies in the early weeks to months following the surgery to allow accurate diagnoses of whether the new liver is being rejected or whether other problems have developed.

Part Two

Hepatitis Overview

Chapter 8

What You Need to Know about Hepatitis

Introduction

Hepatitis is a disorder in which viruses or other mechanisms produce inflammation in liver cells, resulting in their injury or destruction. The liver is the largest organ in the body, occupying the entire upper right quadrant of the abdomen. It performs over five hundred vital functions. Among them are the following:

- It processes all of the nutrients the body requires, including proteins, glucose, vitamins, and fats.

- The liver manufactures bile, the greenish fluid stored in the gallbladder that helps digest fats.

- One of the liver's major contributions to life is to render harmless potentially toxic substances, including alcohol, ammonia, nicotine, drugs, and harmful by-products of digestion.

- Old red blood cells are removed from the blood by the liver and spleen, and the iron contained in them is recycled to the bone marrow to make new red blood cells.

The esophagus, stomach, and large and small intestine, aided by the liver, gallbladder, and pancreas, convert the nutritive components of food into energy and break down the non-nutritive components into waste to be excreted.

Damage to the liver can impair these and many other processes. Hepatitis varies in severity from a self-limited condition with total recovery to a life-threatening or lifelong disease. It can occur from many different causes:

- In the most common hepatitis cases, specific viruses incite the immune system to fight off infections (called viral hepatitis). Specific immune factors become overproduced that cause injury.

- Hepatitis can also result from an autoimmune condition, in which abnormal immune factors attack the body's own liver cells.

- Inflammation of the liver can also occur from medical problems, drugs, alcoholism, chemicals, and environmental toxins.

No matter what the cause of hepatitis, it can take either an acute (short term) or chronic form (persistent). In some cases, acute hepatitis develops into a chronic condition, but chronic hepatitis can also occur on its own. Although chronic hepatitis is generally the more serious condition, patients having either condition can experience varying degrees of severity.

Acute Hepatitis

Acute hepatitis can begin suddenly or gradually, but it has a limited course and rarely lasts beyond one or two months. Usually there is only spotty liver cell damage and evidence of immune system activity, but on rare occasions, acute hepatitis can cause severe, even life-threatening, liver damage.

Chronic Hepatitis

The chronic forms of hepatitis persist for prolonged periods. Experts usually categorize chronic hepatitis by indications of severity as one of the following:

- *Chronic persistent hepatitis:* Chronic persistent hepatitis is usually mild and nonprogressive or slowly progressive, causing limited damage to the liver.

- *Chronic active hepatitis:* Chronic active hepatitis involves extensive liver damage and cell injury beyond the portal tract.

Viral Hepatitis

Most cases of hepatitis are caused by viruses that infect liver cells and begin replicating. They are defined by the letters A through G:

- Hepatitis A, B, and C are the most common viral forms of hepatitis. Investigators are still looking for additional viruses that may be implicated in hepatitis unexplained by the current known viruses.

- Other hepatitis viruses include hepatitis E and hepatitis G. Like hepatitis A, hepatitis E is caused by contact with contaminated food or water. It is not serious except in pregnant women, when it can be life threatening. Hepatitis G is always chronic with probably the same modes of transmission as hepatitis C, but to date it does not appear to have serious effects.

Scientists don't know exactly how these viruses actually cause hepatitis (inflammation in the liver). As the virus reproduces in the liver, a number of proteins and enzymes, including many that attach to the surface of the viral protein, are also produced. Some of these may be directly responsible for liver damage. Researchers are investigating elevated levels of specific immune factors, including T-cell subtypes in the liver of hepatitis C and B patients. T-cells are important infection fighters in the immune system that in some cases can release powerful inflammatory agents (e.g., tumor necrosis factor and interferon gamma) that can cause considerable damage, leading to hepatitis B or C.

Autoimmune Chronic Hepatitis

Autoimmune chronic hepatitis accounts for about 20 percent of all chronic hepatitis cases. Like other autoimmune disorders, this condition develops because a genetically defective immune system attacks the body's own cells and organs (in this case the liver) after being triggered by an environmental agent, probably a virus. Suspects include the measles virus, a hepatitis virus, or the Epstein-Barr virus, which causes mononucleosis. It is also possible that a reaction to a drug or other toxin that affects the liver also triggers an autoimmune response in susceptible individuals. In about 30 percent of cases, autoimmune hepatitis is associated with other disorders that involve autoimmune attacks on other parts of the body.

Hepatitis Caused by Alcohol and Drugs

Alcohol. About 10 to 35 percent of heavy drinkers develop alcoholic hepatitis. In the body, alcohol breaks down into various chemicals, some of which are very toxic in the liver. After years of drinking, liver damage can be very severe, leading to cirrhosis in about 10 to 20 percent of cases. Although heavy drinking itself is the major risk factor for alcoholic hepatitis, genetic factors may play a role in increasing a person's risk for alcoholic hepatitis. Women who abuse alcohol are at higher risk for alcoholic hepatitis and cirrhosis than are men who drink heavily. High-fat diets may also increase the risk in heavy drinkers.

Drugs. Because the liver plays such a major role in metabolizing drugs, hundreds of medications can cause reactions that are similar to those of acute viral hepatitis. Symptoms can appear anywhere from two weeks to six months after starting drug treatment. In most cases, they disappear when the drug is withdrawn, but, in rare circumstances, they may progress to serious liver disease. Among the drugs most prominently cited for liver interactions are halothane, isoniazid, methyldopa, phenytoin, valproic acid, and the sulfonamide drugs. Notably, very high doses of acetaminophen (Tylenol) have been known to cause severe liver damage and even death, particularly when used with alcohol.

Nonalcoholic Fatty Liver Disease (NAFLD)

Nonalcoholic fatty liver disease (NAFLD) affects between 10 and 24 percent of the population and covers a number of conditions, notably nonalcoholic steatohepatitis (NASH). NAFLD has features similar to alcohol-induced hepatitis, particularly a fatty liver, but it occurs in individuals who do not consume significant amounts of alcohol. Severe obesity and diabetes are the major risk factors and may pose a risk for more severe conditions. NAFLD may also occur in conjunction with small intestine surgery or other factors.

NAFLD is usually benign and very slowly progressive. In certain patients, however, it can lead to cirrhosis, liver failure, or liver cancer.

Weight reduction and management of any accompanying medical condition are the primary approaches to nonalcoholic fatty liver disease. To date, however, there is no effective treatment for NAFLD. Drugs, such as fibrates, used to lower triglycerides or those that increase insulin levels, such as metformin, may help protect against liver damage. Other drugs showing some promise include ursodiol and betaine. Vitamin E may help reduce liver injury.

Diagnosis

In people suspected of having or carrying viral hepatitis, physicians will measure certain substances in the blood.

- *Bilirubin:* Bilirubin is one of the most important factors indicative of hepatitis. It is a red-yellow pigment that is normally metabolized in the liver and then excreted in the urine. In patients with hepatitis, the liver cannot process bilirubin, and blood levels of this substance rise. (High levels of bilirubin cause the yellowish skin tone known as jaundice.)

- *Liver Enzymes* (*Aminotransferases*): Enzymes known as aminotransferases, including aspartate (AST) and alanine (ALT), are released when the liver is damaged. Measurements of these enzymes, particularly ALT, are the least expensive and least invasive tests for determining severity of the underlying liver disease and monitoring treatment effectiveness. Enzyme levels vary, however, and are not always an accurate indicator of disease activity. (For example, they are not useful in detecting progression to cirrhosis.)

General Tests to Determine Causes of Viral Hepatitis

Radioimmunoassays

To identify the particular virus causing hepatitis, blood tests called radioimmunoassays are performed. Typically, radioimmunoassays identify particular antibodies, which are molecules in the immune system that attack specific antigens. (Antigens are any molecules that the body considers threatening or dangerous and which can be targeted by antibodies.) Some of these tests can pinpoint hepatitis antigens directly. These tests, however, have limitations:

- There may not be sufficient numbers of antibodies to be detectable by blood tests for up to weeks or months after hepatitis develops. Blood tests that are taken too early, then, may miss these signs of infection.

- Antibodies also persist after patients recover, so a positive antibody test can indicate a previous infection but does not necessarily determine if the infection is active.

- The assays for individual hepatitis viruses may differ.

Polymerase Chain Reaction

In some cases of hepatitis C, a polymerase chain reaction (PCR) may be performed. PCR is able to make multiple copies of the virus's genetic material to the point where it is detectable.

Liver Biopsies

A liver biopsy may be performed for acute viral hepatitis caught in a late stage or for severe cases of chronic hepatitis. No laboratory tests for enzyme or viral levels can truly determine the actual damage to the liver. A biopsy helps determine treatment possibilities, the extent of damage, and the long-term outlook.

The biopsy requires abdominal surgery, most often laparoscopy. This procedure requires general anesthesia and involves the following steps:

- The physician makes one or more small incisions (about 0.5–1.0 inch) in the abdomen.

- Carbon dioxide or nitrous oxide is delivered through the incision to inflate the abdomen so that the involved area is visible.

- The surgeon inserts a thin tube, called a laparoscope, which contains a tiny camera. Surgical instruments are also inserted through the incision to remove the liver tissue for biopsy.

- It takes about an hour.

A less invasive procedure, called a minilaparoscopy, uses a smaller scope and may prove to reduce the time of the procedure.

Screening for Liver Cancer

Patients with cirrhosis are usually screened for liver cancer using tests for a substance called alpha-fetoprotein (AFP) and ultrasound. It is not known, however, if such screening has much impact on survival, since it is not very sensitive and has a high rate of false positives (suggesting the presence of cancer when it is not actually present). Screening is not necessary in patients without cirrhosis.

Hepatitis B and D

Hepatitis B and D were formerly called serum hepatitis. Hepatitis B is mainly transmitted through blood transfusions, contaminated needles, and sexual contact. Blood screening has reduced the risk from transfusions. It can also be passed from cuts, scrapes, and other breaks in the skin. Hepatitis D virus can replicate only by attaching to hepatitis B and therefore cannot exist without the B virus being present.

Risk Factors for Hepatitis B

About 1.2 million Americans are chronically infected with HBV and between 20 percent and 30 percent acquired the infection when they were children. Men are at higher risk than women. Fortunately, in the United States the number of new infections has declined dramatically—by 67 percent between 1990 and 2002. In 2002, 8,064 cases were reported compared to over 20,000 in 1990. The greatest decrease has occurred in children. Among young adults and people living in the Northeast, however, the incidence has increased since 1999. This may indicate that sexual activity is an important route for viral transmission and that the protective effect of the vaccine has not yet reached older, high-risk groups. Also, as with hepatitis A, the increase in travelers to underdeveloped nations may be responsible for the steady rate.

HBV is far more common overseas, and about six hundred thousand people die each year from conditions, such as liver cancer or cirrhosis, that are related to chronic hepatitis B. Nearly 70 percent of these infections were acquired during infancy or early childhood.

The following are some people at risk:

• Drug users who share needles.

• Children of infected mothers. Pregnant women with hepatitis B can transmit the virus to their babies. Even if they are not infected at birth, unvaccinated children of infected mothers run a 60 percent risk of developing it before age five. Children are more likely than adults to become chronic carriers, although between 6 percent and 12 percent of children spontaneously recover each year.

• People with multiple sex partners or other high-risk sexual behavior.

• Hospital workers and others exposed to blood products. Contaminated medical instruments, including fingerstick devices used for more than one individual, have been known to transmit the virus.

• Staff members of institutions for mentally impaired people.

- Prisoners.

- Emigrants from areas where the disease rate is high. (International travelers who spend long periods in such areas may also be at risk.)

People at highest risk for becoming chronic carriers of the virus are the following:

- Children infected before they are five, including newborns, most of whom become carriers.

- Infected people with damaged immune systems, such as AIDS patients.

Risk Factors for Hepatitis D

Hepatitis D occurs only in people with hepatitis B. It is not common in the United States, and the incidence of this hepatitis is declining rapidly overseas. Experts anticipate that it will be extremely rare in the near future. Those who recover from hepatitis B are immune to further infection from both hepatitis B and D viruses.

Lifestyle Precautions for Preventing Hepatitis B and C Virus Transmission

The following are some precautions for preventing the transmission of HBV or HCV:

- All objects contaminated by blood from patients with hepatitis B or C must be handled with special care. (Restrictions on food preparation are not necessary for these hepatitis viruses.)

- Patients with viral hepatitis should abstain from sexual activity or take strict precautions if they cannot. Infected patients should use condoms and contraceptives that prevent passage of the virus, possibly even in relationships that last for years. Women partners or infected women should abstain from sexual activity during menstruation. Either partner with infections that cause bleeding in the genital or urinary areas should avoid sexual activity until the infection is no longer active.

- Couples with an infected partner or people sharing a household with an infected person should avoid sharing personal items, such as razors or toothbrushes.

66

There is no evidence that the viruses can be passed through casual contact, or other contact without exposure to blood, including kissing, hugging, sneezing, or coughing or by sharing eating utensils or drinking glasses. People infected with chronic hepatitis B or C should not be excluded from work, school, play, and childcare or any social or work settings on the basis of their infection.

Symptoms of Hepatitis B

Symptoms appear long after the initial infection, usually four to twenty-four weeks later. Many patients may not even experience them or they may be mild and flu-like. About 10 percent to 20 percent of patients have a fever and rash. Nausea is not common. Sometimes there is general aching in the joints. The pain can resemble arthritis, affecting specific joints and accompanied by redness and swelling.

Outlook for Patients with Hepatitis B

The virus does not kill cells directly, but seems to activate cells in the immune system, which cause inflammation and damage in the liver.

Acute Form

Acute hepatitis B is generally mild, but it can be lethal in about 1 percent of patients. Patients who are co-infected with hepatitis D or C are at risk for serious complications. In patients whose immune systems are severely compromised, such as in AIDS, there is risk of a rapidly progressive form of HBV called fibrosing cholestatic hepatitis. Even patients with mild symptoms can remain chronically infected with the virus.

Chronic Form

About 70 percent of patients infected with hepatitis B will eventually eliminate the virus without any treatment. The rest will progress to chronic hepatitis. Hepatitis B can also become chronic without an acute stage. The risk for developing a chronic form of hepatitis D is the same as for hepatitis B alone.

The great majority of people with hepatitis B have a good long-term outlook, especially children infected with the virus. Still, about 5 percent to 10 percent eventually develop cirrhosis, and worldwide, approximately two million people die each year from hepatitis B, globally

67

making it the ninth leading cause of death. Co-infection with hepatitis D or C increases the risk for cirrhosis. HBV also poses a risk for liver cancer. In Asia about 15 percent of people who have chronic hepatitis B develop liver cancer, but this high rate is not seen in other parts of the world. Diet may play a role in a higher or lower risk for liver cancer.

Specific Tests for Identifying Hepatitis B

A diagnosis of hepatitis B relies on measuring the liver enzymes aspartate (AST) and alanine (ALT), which are released when the liver is damaged, assays to identify the viral DNA, and a liver biopsy.

Physicians then must determine if the condition is chronic but inactive or whether it is more aggressive. This is suggested by identifying a specific antigen called HBsAg, which is a protein that is found in the blood in early stages of hepatitis B and suggests the presence of viral replication. Most people develop antibodies to this antigen during convalescence. Their condition is referred to as HBeAG negative or anti-HBe and suggests that infection is on the wane. About 5 percent to 10 percent of people do not clear the infection but become carriers of the antigen (called HBsAG-positive). Evidence of its persistence for more than six months suggests that the condition is chronic.

Tests have been developed that can identify specific genetic types of hepatitis B virus (designated A to G). It is not clear how significant they are in treating patients with HBV.

It is important to remember, however, that viral levels are not an accurate measure of actual liver damage. Only a biopsy can determine this.

To diagnose hepatitis D using an antibody test, hepatitis B must already have been identified.

Preventing Hepatitis B and Its Transmission

General precautions for preventing hepatitis B when traveling are the same as those for hepatitis A. In infected people, measures for preventing transmission are similar to those for hepatitis C.

Vaccinations for Prevention of Hepatitis B

Several inactivated virus vaccines, including Recombivax HB, GenHevac B, Hepagene, and Engerix-B, can prevent hepatitis B (HBV) and are safe even for infants and children. A triple-antigen hepatitis B vaccine (Hepacare) is proving to be effective for people who do not respond to the standard vaccines. Vaccination programs are also proving to reduce the risk for liver cancer. A combination vaccine (Twinrix) that contains Engerix-B and Havrix, a hepatitis A vaccine, is now approved for people with risk factors for both hepatitis A and B.

Until recently, the vaccine contained a mercury-based preservative called thimerosal. In response to concerns, professional organizations recommended suspending vaccinations in infants with noninfected mothers. In September 1999, a thimerosal-free vaccine became available and medical centers are now urged to continue vaccinations. Unfortunately, even after the thimerosal-free vaccine became available, a number of hospitals still haven't restored vaccination of all infants. This is a safe vaccine and it is reducing the need for hospitalization in children. Parents should be sure their children are immunized.

Candidates for HBV Vaccinations.

Experts now recommend that all infants and children not previously vaccinated be immunized by the time they reach the seventh grade.

Typical schedules for hepatitis B vaccinations in childhood are as follows:

- All infants should receive the hepatitis B vaccine soon after birth and before hospital discharge. (The first dose may also be given by age two months if the mother has no evidence of infection.) The second dose should be given at one to four months (at least four to six weeks after first dose); and the third between six and eighteen months (at least sixteen weeks after first dose and eight weeks after second dose). A fourth dose may also be given as part of a combination vaccine. This is a safe vaccine, even in newborns, and parents should be sure their infants are immunized.

- Infants of mothers infected with HBV should be treated with immune globulin plus the hepatitis vaccine within twelve hours of birth. The second dose should be given at one to two months and the third at six months. Infants should be tested for antibody status at nine to fifteen months to see if they are chronic virus carriers or need to be re-vaccinated.

- When it is not known if a mother is infected or not, the infant should receive the vaccine within twelve hours of birth. The mother's blood should then be tested right away. If she is infected, the infant should receive immune globulin as soon as possible (no later than a week).

- Children who are between eleven and twelve and who have not been immunized should receive two or three doses of the vaccine (depending on the brand) given over a few months.

Hepatitis B vaccine protection lasts at least eight to ten years. Booster shots after that may be recommended depending on continuing risk, such as sexual exposure. In fact, a 2002 study suggested that there is risk for infection in teenagers who were vaccinated in infancy, although protection against chronic hepatitis B may be maintained. The following adults are at very high risk and should be vaccinated:

- Healthcare and public safety workers who may be exposed to blood products. Such individuals have a risk for hepatitis B virus that ranges from 15 percent to 30 percent.

- People in the same household as HBV-infected individuals. (Unvaccinated people who have had intimate exposure to people with HBV may be protected with immune globulin, which is sometimes administered with the vaccine.)

- Travelers to developing countries.

- Patients who require transfusions and have not been infected with HBV. (Those with blood clotting disorders should have the vaccination administered under the skin, not injected in the muscle.)

- Sexually active homosexual or heterosexual individuals with multiple partners or who engage in high-risk sexual behavior.

- People with any sexually transmitted diseases.

Other people at risk who would benefit from vaccinations are the following:

- Patients and workers in mental institutions and morticians.

- Patients on hemodialysis. (People on hemodialysis may need larger doses or boosters; they also may need to be re-vaccinated if blood tests indicate they are losing immunity.)

- People who use injected drugs.

- Pregnant women at risk for the virus should be vaccinated; there is no evidence that the vaccine is dangerous to the fetus.

- People receiving treatments or who have conditions that suppress the immune system may need the vaccination, although its benefits for this group are unclear except for those at high risk, such as people with HIV or spleen abnormalities.

The regimen in adults is typically three doses given over six months. One study reported that older adults would benefit from a fourth dose without incurring serious side effects. People with alcoholism may need high doses.

A small percentage of people do not develop immunity even after a vaccine has been given repeatedly. A more potent vaccine is proving to be effective in these people; it loses its effect after five years in about a third of those who receive it.

Soreness at the injection site is the most common side effect. There have been some reports of nerve inflammation after vaccinations for hepatitis B, and there has been some concern about three small studies associating the vaccine with an insignificant increase in multiple sclerosis. Studies in 2001, however, have found no evidence to support these concerns. Nonetheless, some groups oppose the vaccination in children who are not in high-risk groups. It should be strongly stressed that worldwide sixty-five million people with chronic hepatitis are expected to die from liver disease, and vaccinations are saving lives. For example, in Taiwan, where infection rates are high and infants are at risk for hepatitis B from infected mothers, vaccination programs have significantly reduced the risk for liver cancer.

Treatments for Chronic Hepatitis B

Interferon alpha and nucleoside analogues are the important treatments at this time for hepatitis B. At this time, interferon alpha-2b is the standard agent but experts expect the nucleoside analogue lamivudine to replace it as the primary agent. Lamivudine is not only effective, it is less expensive than the interferon. Most likely, the best approach in the future will be combinations of these and other agents to achieve the greatest possible viral reduction and to minimize the chances of drug resistance.

Interferon Alpha for Hepatitis B

Interferon alpha-2b (Intron) is the standard drug for hepatitis B. It has eliminated the virus and sustained significant remission in 25 percent to 40 percent of patients with chronic hepatitis B. The drug is usually taken by injection every day for sixteen weeks. (It does not appear to be effective for hepatitis D.) Unfortunately, even in hepatitis B, the virus recurs in almost all cases, although this recurring mutation may be weaker than the original strain.

Administering the drug for longer periods may produce sustained remission in more patients while still being safe. Interferon is also effective in eligible children, although long-term effects are unclear. A 2001 study suggested that it may temporarily disrupt growth, but it should be noted that hepatitis itself, even without interferon treatment, can compromise growth.

Lamivudine and Other Nucleoside Analogues

Nucleoside analogues are drugs that can block viral replication, and they are important in hepatitis B. The primary agent used in hepatitis is lamivudine (Zeffix). It can be taken orally, has few severe side effects, and is less expensive than interferon. Experts expect it to become the first-line treatment for hepatitis B. Famciclovir is an alternative. Newer nucleoside analogues, adefovir (Hepsera) and entecavir, may prove to be even more effective than the older agents.

Lamivudine has reduced viral count in over half of hepatitis B patients who have taken it as sole therapy for about a year. It also appears to significantly reduce the risk for liver damage and cirrhosis, and appears to be effective and safe in patients with decompensated cirrhosis. The drug even suppresses hepatitis B viral replication in HIV-positive patients and liver transplant recipients. It appears to be effective for children as well as adults. It is not yet clear if it protects against liver cancer, particularly in patients who have harbored the virus since childhood.

A major problem with lamivudine is the development of mutated viral strains that become resistant to the drug, particularly in areas where the virus is common. The specific genetic hepatitis B strain may be an important marker for predicting resistance. Combinations with interferons may be able to help control viral breakthroughs from mutated viruses and help sustain its effectiveness. Other nucleosides, such as adefovir and entecavir, are proving to be effective in patients who become resistant to lamivudine.

Lamivudine causes muscle aches and chills but does not appear to have some of the distressing side effects of interferon, such as depression, hair loss, weight loss, or a drop in white blood cells (leukopenia). Of some concern, however, is eventual resistance to the drug in many patients.

Investigative Therapies

A number of drugs are being studied that boost the body's own immune system to fight the virus.

- *Thymosin Alpha 1 (Zadaxin)*, also called thymalfasin, is a synthetic version of a peptide derived from the thymus gland (which is responsible for maturation of immune factors call T-cells). It is injected and has few side effects. It appears to be safe for hepatitis B patients when used alone or in combination. Combinations with interferon and nucleoside analogues are showing promise.

- *Vaccines as Treatments:* Some hepatitis B vaccines, including Hepagene, are being investigated for treating and preventing hepatitis B.

Some important research is targeting agents that inhibit RNA—the genetic molecules that serve as messengers for regulating cellular processes. In animal studies on hepatitis B, scientists were able to turn off viral replication by targeting HBV RNAs.

Liver Transplantation

If the disease progresses to the point where it becomes life-threatening, liver transplantation may be an option. It is not foolproof, however. Viral recurrence is high in hepatitis B patients, although it can be significantly reduced using monthly infusions of hepatitis B immune globulin (HBIg), particularly when used with lamivudine. These injections may need to be administered life long. Eventually, about 40 percent of patients develop resistance to lamivudine. In such events, alternative agents, such as adefovir, are proving to be effective.

Hepatitis C

Each year about thirty thousand new cases of hepatitis C occur. It is the most common blood-borne infection in the country. Until blood screening began in 1990, the primary mode of known transmission was through transfusions. It is also transmitted through contaminated needles and possibly through sexual transmission. The cause of transmission is unknown in 40 percent of cases.

About 4 million Americans have had an initial HCV infection and an estimated 2.7 million are currently chronically infected. Hepatitis C also affects 170 million people worldwide. Most people with chronic

HCV, however, are unaware that they have it, and experts believe that over the next twenty years there will be a fourfold increase in diagnosed cases in the United States. It is currently not possible to predict which patients will develop the chronic form of hepatitis C.

Ethnic Groups

In general, HCV occurs most commonly in non-Caucasian men between the ages of thirty and forty-nine years. Over 6 percent of African Americans are infected with HCV, which is about two to three times the risk for Caucasians.

Other High-Risk Groups

Some other specific groups are at higher than normal risk:

- *Intravenous drug users.* Intravenous drug use has been the greatest risk factor for HCV since the early 1980s. It accounts for 60 percent of new cases and 20 percent to 50 percent of chronic infections. Individuals who engage in this activity have a risk for infection that is between 50 percent and 80 percent. Intravenous drug use, particularly in people who also drink alcohol heavily, poses a higher risk for severe complications. Intranasal cocaine use also increases the danger. Needle exchange and educational programs have reduced the risk for HIV transmission and should have similar benefits for preventing HCV.

- *People who had transfusions before 1992.* Although transfused blood has been tested for both hepatitis B and C since the early 1990s, individuals given transfusions before then, even decades before, may still be at risk. Such individuals are urged to be tested. Hepatitis C can exist for decades without symptoms, and nearly three hundred thousand people who had transfusions before 1992, including many who were children at the time, may have been infected. Of some reassurance was a 1999 study of people who had transfusions when they were children. After an average of twenty years, only 8 percent tested positive for hepatitis C and only three people showed signs of any liver abnormalities. These results suggest that the virus may be less aggressive in children than in adults, but further observations are needed to learn if the infection remains mild beyond age thirty.

- *Homeless people and prison inmates.* Among the homeless and people in prison the HCV prevalence may be as high as 40 percent.

- *Infants of infected mothers.* The risk for transmission to an infant during pregnancy is about 2 percent but increases to 4 percent to 7 percent during delivery. The highest rates of infection (20 percent) are in mothers who are also HIV positive. It is not clear if Cesarean section delivery in infected mothers offers protection. Avoiding fetal scalp monitoring and prolonged labor may reduce the risk. (Breastfeeding does not increase the risk.)

- *Organ transplant recipients.*

- *Sexual transmission.* Although HCV can be transmitted sexually, the risk is much less than with hepatitis B or other sexually transmitted diseases. For example, the risk for transmitting the HCV within a monogamous relationship is only about 2 percent to 3 percent. The risk is 4 percent to 6 percent for partners of people who have high-risk sex (e.g., those with multiple partners or sex workers). Of note, the risk for women becoming infected through sexual transmission may be three times that of men.

- *Hospital workers.* It should be strongly noted that health care providers in general are at very low risk. The risk of infection from a needle stick is now believed to be about 2 percent. (It is not yet clear if this poses any significant risk to patients.)

- *Children who survive cancer.*

- *Body piercing or tattoos.* Possibly people who have had body piercing or tattoos with contaminated equipment.

Symptoms of Hepatitis C

Most patients with hepatitis C do not experience symptoms. If they appear at all, symptoms develop about a month or two after a person is infected. Symptoms of progressive chronic viral hepatitis may be very subtle. In some patients, itchy skin is the first symptom. Overall, fatigue is the most common symptom. Many patients do not experience any symptoms at all. In fact, chronic hepatitis C can be present for ten to thirty years and in some cases cirrhosis or liver failure can develop before patients experience any clear symptom.

Some evidence suggests, however, that patients with chronic hepatitis C often experience an impaired quality of life, mostly from fatigue. Fatigue can impair daily function, vitality, and mood in ways that are similar to other chronic diseases. The severity of the fatigue is not necessarily related to the degree of liver injury. Some patients develop pain in small joints in the body (such as the hand) that may

75

be nearly indistinguishable from symptoms of rheumatoid arthritis, fibromyalgia, or carpal tunnel syndrome. Other nonspecific symptoms include abdominal discomfort, loss of appetite, depression, and difficulty in concentration.

Outlook for Patients with Hepatitis C

Acute Form

Acute hepatitis C is rarely recognized, since there are no symptoms in up to 80 percent of these patients. An estimated 15 percent to 30 percent of acute cases clear up without becoming chronic. Early treatment with interferons can significantly reduce the risk for progression to chronic hepatitis.

Chronic Form

About 60 percent to 85 percent of infected people develop chronic hepatitis. This poses a risk for cirrhosis, liver cancer, or both.

- Overall, between 10 percent and 15 percent of patients with chronic hepatitis C develop cirrhosis. The risk varies widely, however.

- Of these patients, 4 percent eventually develop liver cancer. (Liver cancer rarely develops without cirrhosis first being present.)

It should be noted, however, that even in patients with cirrhosis, survival rates in one study were nearly 80 percent at ten years. Still, over five thousand deaths are currently attributed annually to hepatitis C and the rate continues to climb. Furthermore, 140,000 people were hospitalized in 1998 for HCV, leading many experts to believe that hepatitis C is indirectly responsible for many more deaths than reported.

Patients with chronic hepatitis C may be also at higher risk for non-liver disorders including the following:

- Cryoglobulinemia (a disorder in which protein clumps form in the blood). This can cause skin rash and ulcers, kidney problems, arthritis, and sensations (such as tingling or pain) in the hands and feet. People with such symptoms may have particular difficulties with interferon, which can have similar side effects.

- Porphyria cutanea tarda (a disorder that causes skin color and texture changes and sensitivity to light.)

- Certain autoimmune disorders, particularly hypothyroidism and rheumatoid arthritis.

- Some experts believe that hepatitis C may infect the central nervous system in certain patients, possibly accounting for the fatigue, depression, or both experienced by patients who have even relatively mild cases.

- Certain non-Hodgkin lymphomas.

High-Risk Chronic Hepatitis C Patients

The risk for cirrhosis varies widely among different patient groups. The following factors influence risk for disease progression to cirrhosis.

- Overall the risk for progression is highest in men—particularly African Americans—who were older at the time of infection. The risk is much lower in women and children (2 percent to 4 percent).

- Moderate to heavy alcohol users. (Alcohol may actually promote viral replication. Even one or two alcoholic drinks a day increase the risk for liver injury in HCV patients.)

- Co-infection with hepatitis B. Co-infection with B significantly affects the outcome of these patients and may be more common than previously believed. This co-condition may cause superinfections with very serious consequences, reduce these patients' responses to interferon therapy, and increase their risk of liver cancer. Patients with hepatitis C should be immunized against hepatitis B.

- Co-infection with HIV.

- A history of transfusions. (In one report, the risk in middle-aged patients with a history of transfusions was 20 percent to 30 percent.)

- Having type 2 diabetes.

- Having large iron stores in the liver.

- High exposure to toxic chemicals or environmental contaminants.

Because there are millions of Americans now infected with chronic hepatitis C, experts have been justifiably concerned that there will be a significant number of cases of liver failure and liver cancer in the coming years. Computer analyses have suggested that mortality rates from HCV-related cirrhosis or liver cancer will double or triple over the next twenty years. Fortunately, improved therapies may significantly reduce these discouraging estimates.

Specific Tests for Identifying Hepatitis C and Determining Its Severity

Tests for Liver Enzymes

Blood tests showing elevated liver enzymes, particularly alanine aminotransferase (ALT), plus symptoms of hepatitis (e.g., jaundice, fatigue) are often the first signs of acute hepatitis. In chronic hepatitis, however, liver enzymes may be normal or fluctuate. They also can be elevated even after the virus has cleared.

Tests to Identify the Virus

The standard first test for diagnosing hepatitis C is known as enzyme-linked immunosorbent assay (ELISA or EIA). The antibody for hepatitis C is used to identify the virus but it may not show up for six weeks to a year after the onset of the disease, so its absence is not necessarily an indication of a healthy liver. A test called an immunoblot assay (called RIBA) may also be used to confirm the presence of the virus. An accurate home test (Hepatitis C Check) is now available. It supplies a lancet for obtaining a drop of blood, which is sent to the laboratory for EIA and possibly RIBA analysis. Results take about a week.

Tests to Identify Genetic Types and Viral Load

Additional tests called HCV RNA assays may be used to confirm the diagnosis. They use a polymerase chain reaction (PCR) to detect the RNA (the genetic material) of the virus. Such tests may be performed if there is some doubt about a diagnosis but the physician still firmly believes the virus is present.

HCV RNA assays also determine virus levels (called viral load). Such levels do not reflect the severity of the condition or speed of progression, as they do for other viruses, such as HIV. However, high viral loads suggest a poorer response to treatment with interferons.

Such techniques may also be used to determine the genotype of the virus, which can be helpful in determining a treatment approach. There are six main genetic types of HCV and more than ninety subtypes. They do not appear to affect the rate of progression of the disease itself, but they can differ significantly in their effects on response to treatment. Genotype 1 is the most difficult to treat and is the cause of up to three-quarters of the cases in the United States. The other common genetic types are types 2 (15 percent) and 3 (7 percent), which are more responsive to treatment.

Liver Biopsy

Only a biopsy can determine the extent of injury in the liver. Some experts are now recommending biopsies for all chronic hepatitis C patients, regardless of severity, because of the risk for liver damage even in patients without symptoms. If a biopsy does not show any scarring and liver enzymes are normal, patients can be assured that the outlook is very favorable.

Prevention of Hepatitis C

No vaccines are available, but immune globulin helps protect against developing hepatitis C after transfusions. Periodic doses of immune globulin in sexual partners of infected people also appear to confer protection. In infected people, measures for preventing transmission are similar to those for hepatitis B.

Treatments for Hepatitis C

Interferons Alone and in Combination with Ribavirin for Hepatitis C

The current gold standard for treating chronic hepatitis C is a once-weekly injection of the interferon called pegylated interferon in combination with oral ribavirin (a nucleoside analogue). Patients are typically treated for twenty-four to forty-eight weeks depending on certain factors, such as the genotype. Interferons are also used for patients with acute hepatitis C to prevent the development of the chronic form.

Interferons are natural proteins that activate certain immune functions in the body and have anti-viral properties. Ribavirin is poor at inducing initial responses alone but it can double sustained response rates when combined with an interferon.

A number of natural and synthetic interferons are available:

• Natural interferons were the first used for HCV and include interferon alpha-2a (Intron) and interferon alpha-2b (Roferon).

79

Rebetron is the combination of interferon alpha-2b and ribavirin.

- Pegylated interferons (PegINF) are long-acting formulations of interferon. They include alfa-2b (Peg-Intron) or alfa-2a (Pegasys). Both are now available in combination with ribavirin. (Rebetol is the alfa-2b combination.) The combination is now considered the gold standard for treating HCV. Response rates of up to 51 percent with genotype 1 and over 80 percent with genotypes 2 and 3 have been reported. PegINFs may even help patients with cirrhosis. Whether the combination treatment protects against future liver cancer is still unclear. (A higher total dose, rather than a longer duration of treatment, may be the critical factor for protection.)

- Alfacon-1 (Infergen), also called consensus interferon, is a genetically modified interferon. A combination of alfacon-1 with ribavirin is proving to help some patients who were nonresponsive to ribavirin with interferon.

Side Effects of the Combination Treatment

The side effects of the combination include those of both interferon and ribavirin. Interferon side effects may occur more often in the combination treatment. Ribavirin used in the combination treatment adds the following specific side effects:

- Hemolytic anemia. This complication is reversible and usually stabilizes after a month or two of treatment. However, some patients may become so anemic that they have to withdraw. Since anemia can worsen heart disease, patients with a history of significant heart problems should not be treated with ribavirin. Other nucleoside analogues, including levovirin and viramidine, are under investigation that may have a lower risk for anemia than ribavirin.

- Skin disorders.

- Coughing and shortness of breath.

- Emotional and neurologic symptoms, such as severe sleep disturbances, depression, and anxiety.

- Gastrointestinal symptoms (heartburn and weight loss).

- Temporary thyroid dysfunction (either over- or underactivity). The presence of hypothyroidism (low activity) is, in fact, associated with long-term remission of hepatitis.

Overall, the significant side effects of the combination treatment include flu-like symptoms, blood disorders (e.g., hemolytic anemia and low white blood cell counts), and psychologic and neurologic symptoms (particularly depression). Side effects from the combination result in treatment discontinuation in 10 percent to 14 percent of patients. The most frequent reason cited in the United States is depression. Of note, combination of both drugs poses a very high risk for birth defects in children whose mothers used the drugs while pregnant.

Determining Treatment Success

Physicians gauge treatment success and approaches based on the patient's response to the treatments:

- *Early Response.* These are patients who respond to the drug right away. This means that their viral count drops very rapidly within the first few weeks of treatment and is still undetectable at twelve weeks. (One difficulty in deciding when to stop treatment even in responders is the inability to predict at twelve weeks which of these patients will relapse and which ones will have sustained response.)

- *Sustained Response.* Patients who are free of the virus longer than six months are considered to be sustained responders. The overall sustained response rates with the current standard combination of pegylated interferon and ribavirin is over 50 percent, with certain factors predicting higher or lower response rates.

- *Relapse.* In relapse, the virus comes back and requires retreatment. This occurs most likely because of the development of mutant strains that may be resistant to the drugs used or because the original dose was too low.

- *Nonresponse.* Patients are considered to be nonresponders if the virus is still detectable twelve weeks after interferon alone or twenty-four weeks after combination therapy. Retreating these patients has achieved only a 15 percent response. Those who achieved a response called breakthrough at some point in the initial treatment may be more likely to respond. (During a breakthrough there is a temporary reduction in liver enzymes or disappearance of the virus.) Alfacon-1 (Infergen) may be beneficial for some nonresponding patients. Patients should also ask their physician about any clinical trials that might be appropriate.

People at Risk for Poor Response to Combination Treatment

The following patients have a higher chance for a lower response to combination treatment with interferon and ribavirin:

- People who are at high risk in the first place for aggressive hepatitis C.

- Having a high viral count.

- Having a specific genetic type of the virus affects the response to treatment. Those with genotypes 2 or 3 who are given the current standard treatment (pegylated interferon plus ribavirin) can now achieve a sustained response of over 80 percent. Unfortunately, the response is lower in those with genotype 1. In one 2003 study, the sustained response rates in patients with genotype 1 were 39 percent in Caucasian patients and 26 percent in African Americans (which were the highest response rates reported at that time for this latter group). Young people with type 1 have a much higher response rate than older patients.

- Being African American also poses a risk for poor response. African Americans are less responsive to treatment than Caucasians and Asians. The reasons for this are unclear.

Failure can be due to other, modifiable factors, which should be assessed before stopping treatment, particularly in patients who had interferon alone. They include the following:

- Interferon dose is too low.

- Patient did not comply fully with the treatment.

- Patient was consuming alcohol.

- Treatment time was too short. Some evidence suggests that response can significantly improve for many patients with genotype 1 if treatment time is extended to forty-eight weeks.

Even if viral levels persist, there is some evidence the interferon treatment may still have benefits. For example, patients with normal liver enzyme levels appear to have almost no risk for liver damage, even if viral levels persist after treatment. Also of note, there is some evidence that interferon still reduces liver scarring and may even reduce the risk for liver cancer in some patients, even if the treatment does not eliminate the virus. More research is needed, however, to confirm these early findings.

Investigative Drugs for Hepatitis C

The current drugs used for HCV still do not meet the needs of all patients. They are expensive, have significant side effects, do not work in half the patients who take them, and are unsuitable in many others. Investigation then is ongoing to find better solutions. Some showing promise include the following:

- *IMPDH Inhibitors.* Mycophenolate mofetil and VX-497 are agents that inhibit an enzyme known by its brief name, IMPDH, which may block replication of the hepatitis C virus. If effective, they would most likely be used in combination with interferon and ribavirin.

- *Amantadine (Symmetrel)* is an anti-viral agent being investigated in various combinations. For example, triple therapy with amantadine, pegylated interferon, and ribavirin is showing particular promise. In some cases, the side effects of amantadine can be severe, and include vertigo, insomnia, nervousness, and depression. They are particularly disabling among older patients who receive inappropriately high doses.

- *Thymosin Alpha 1 (Zadaxin),* also called thymalfasin, is a synthetic version of a peptide derived from the thymus gland (which is responsible for maturation of immune factors call T-cells). It is being used for hepatitis B and is under investigation for hepatitis C in combinations with natural interferons and pegylated interferon.

- *Protease Inhibitors.* Novel protease inhibitors (similar to those used for HIV) are under investigation for hepatitis C patients who fail other treatments. These agents are based on molecular therapies that target proteins involved in viral reproduction.

Other agents under investigation include vaccines, genetic therapies known as antisense oligonucleotides or monoclonal antibodies, and drugs that will help prevent or reduce progression of liver scarring or progression to liver cancer. Even if successful, none of these agents would be available for some years.

Of interest are studies using phlebotomy (which is simply drawing blood) to reduce iron levels. In one study, maintenance therapy with this procedure reduced liver inflammation and possibly slowed progression of cirrhosis.

Liver Transplantation for Hepatitis C

If the disease progresses to the point where it becomes life-threatening, liver transplantation may be an option. In fact, nearly 40 percent of liver transplant patients are infected with hepatitis C. In any case, liver transplantation is not a cure for hepatitis C. The virus nearly always returns. One study of patients with hepatitis C reported five-year risks for viral recurrence of 80 percent and for cirrhosis of 10 percent. Retreatment with antiviral agents at this point is being investigated.

Description of Interferons

Interferons are natural proteins that activate certain immune functions in the body and have anti-viral properties. The natural interferons being used for chronic hepatitis B, C, or both are called type I interferons. They are given by injection, need to be taken three times a week, and include the following:

- Interferon alpha 2b (Intron A). Used for both hepatitis B and C.

- Interferon alpha 2a (Roferon-A). Mostly used for hepatitis C.

- Interferon alfa-n1 (Wellferon). Approved but mostly used in Canada for hepatitis C.

Newer synthetic interferons have been developed that are showing some advantages over the natural forms:

- *Pegylated interferon (PegINF).* Pegylated interferons employ a small molecule called polyethylene glycol (PEG), which attaches to a protein and extends the activity of the interferon. This action allows the drug to be taken only once a week. Agents available include pegylated interferon alfa-2b (Peg-Intron) and alfa-2a (Pegasys).

- *Interferon alfacon-1 (Infergen).* This agent is referred to as a consensus interferon (CIFN) because it was genetically developed using the most commonly occurring amino acid sequences from each of the natural type 1 alpha interferons. It is five to ten times more biologically active than natural type 1 interferons. CIFN is usually given three times a week when used as initial treatment.

84

Interferon Candidates

The best candidates for interferon treatments are those at greatest risk for cirrhosis. Factors suggesting a higher risk for cirrhosis include the following:

- Detectable virus levels as determined by an assay test.

- High levels of aminotransferase enzyme for more than six months. (Those with normal liver enzyme levels appear to have almost no risk for liver damage, even if the virus is evident. In the latter case, however, the disease may progress in some patients. Whether to treat these patients is still under debate.)

- Indication of liver scarring on biopsy.

Patients who are not good candidates for interferon and are usually ineligible are the following:

- Women who are pregnant or planning to become pregnant soon.

- Patients with advanced cirrhosis. (It is unclear if the drug improves survival in patients with advanced cirrhosis and, in any case, it may be dangerous for them.)

- Patients with fluid in the abdomen.

- Patients with anemia or risk factors for anemia should not take the combination treatments, although they may be candidates for interferon alone.

The response of children to interferon may be better than those in adults, although large studies are needed to confirm this and to uncover any possible long-term complications of the drugs. At this time, children are given interferons only as part of clinical trials.

A number of patients are currently ineligible for treatment because of the high risk for noncompliance and because of the severe psychiatric effects of the drugs. They include patients with psychiatric and medical problems and substance abusers. Some experts suggest that many of these individuals may be eligible and there should be greater efforts to determine more candidates. For example, many alcohol and drug users have been successfully treated even if they have not consistently abstained or if they were on methadone at the time. It is unclear whether treatment is useful in active drug users, although this should be considered on a case-by-case basis. Even moderate alcohol use can compromise treatment and accelerate disease progression.

Disease Recurrence

In both hepatitis B and C, the disease often persists or returns despite treatment. The virus continually generates many "mutant viruses" that differ just slightly from the parent virus. These mutated viruses may be resistant to interferons and so, over time, the drugs become ineffective.

Side Effects and Complications

Common side effects of any interferon are flu-like symptoms (fever, chills, muscle aches) that usually occur within six hours and gradually decline over a week or two. (Pegylated interferon may pose a higher risk for these symptoms than the natural interferons.)

Chronic or more serious effects include the following:

• Emotional and mental changes. Depression can be very severe and cases of suicidal thoughts have been reported. Other mental and emotional symptoms include anxiety, amnesia, confusion, irritability, impaired concentration, decreased alertness, memory problems, and mental slowing.

• Changes in sensation.

• Weight loss.

• Skin rashes.

• Hair loss.

• Gastrointestinal problems, including nausea, vomiting, and diarrhea, and, in severe cases intestinal bleeding and ulcers.

• Fatigue and general weakness.

• Back pain.

• Complications in the lungs, including exacerbation of asthma. In severe cases, interferon can cause shortness of breath, inflammation in the lungs, and pneumonia.

• Possible negative effects on cholesterol and lipid levels.

• Heart rhythm disturbances, which, in rare cases, can be serious.

• Mild anemia.

• Interferon often causes a drop in platelet and white blood cell counts, increasing susceptibility to bacterial infections. Growth factors are being investigated to reduce this effect.

- May trigger an autoimmune response, possibly causing anemia, diabetes, lupus-like symptoms, hypothyroidism, or even autoimmune hepatitis.

- Complications in the eye, including bleeding that, in some cases, may lead to loss of vision if not detected promptly.

- Rare reports of acute pancreatitis.

- In children, interferon therapy temporarily disrupts growth.

Patients have a difficult time with prolonged therapy. Over 20 percent drop out if treatment lasts longer than two years. Depression is the most common reason for withdrawal.

A number of different methods for delivering interferons are under investigation to help reduce some of the problems with injections. They include oral compounds and the use of pumps, controlled release implants, encapsulation in tiny fatty or synthetic spheres, and other methods.

Hepatitis A

About one-third of the U.S. population has antibodies to hepatitis A, indicating previous infection by the virus. The hepatitis A virus infects up to 200,000 Americans every year and causes symptoms in about 134,000 of them. Almost 30 percent are children under age fifteen.

Hepatitis A (formerly called infectious hepatitis) is excreted in feces and transmitted by contaminated food and water. Eating shellfish taken from sewage-contaminated water is a common means of contracting hepatitis A. Infected people can transmit it to others if they do not take strict sanitary precautions. Hepatitis A is infectious for two to four weeks before symptoms develop and for a few days afterward.

Among the people at risk for passing the infection along or being infected are the following:

- *International travelers.* Hepatitis A is the hepatitis strain people are most likely to encounter in the course of international travel. In fact, in spite of the availability of a vaccine, the increase in travel to underdeveloped countries has kept the incidence of hepatitis A steady in Western nations. The incidence may even be increasing.

- *Day care employees and children.* It is estimated that between 11 percent and 16 percent of hepatitis A cases occur among day care employees and children who attend day care. The risk for children attending day care is very low, however, if hygienic precautions are used, particularly when changing babies and handling diapers.

- *Sexually active homosexual men.*

- *Intravenous drug users.*

- *Health care, food industry, and sewage workers.*

A fly may act as a mechanical vector of diseases such as Hepatitis A, which means the fly carries the infective organism on its feet or mouth parts and contaminates food or water which a person then consumes. A biological vector actually develops an infective organism in its body and passes it along to its host, usually through its saliva. A fly can be a biological vector, as in the transmission of leishmaniasis by the sand fly.

Symptoms of Acute Hepatitis

Symptoms of acute viral hepatitis may begin suddenly or develop gradually. They may be so mild that patients mistake the disease for the flu. They include the following:

- Nearly all patients experience some fatigue and often have mild fever.

- Gastrointestinal problems are very common, including nausea, vomiting, a general feeling of discomfort in the abdomen, or a sharper pain that may occur in the upper right area of the abdomen. This pain tends to increase during jerking movements, such as climbing stairs or riding on a bumpy road.

- GI problems can lead to loss of appetite, weight loss, and dehydration.

- After about two weeks, dark urine and jaundice (a yellowish color in the skin and whites of the eyes) develops in some, but not all, patients. (Children tend not to develop jaundice.)

- About half of all hepatitis patients have light-colored stools, muscle pain, drowsiness, irritability, and itching, usually mild.

- Diarrhea and joint aches occur in about a quarter of patients.

- The liver may be tender and enlarged and most people have mild anemia.

- In about 10 percent of patients, the spleen is enlarged.

Preventing Hepatitis A Infections When Traveling to High-Risk Countries

Travelers should take the following precautions:

- Be vaccinated against hepatitis A and possibly B if traveling for long periods of time to countries where epidemics occur.

- Use only carbonated bottled water for brushing teeth and drinking. (It should be noted that ice cubes can carry infection.) Boiling water is the best method for eliminating infectious agents. There is some debate about how long to boil, but bringing the water to a good boil for at least a minute generally renders it safe to drink.

- Heated food should be hot to the touch and eaten promptly.

- Don't buy food from street vendors.

- Beware of sliced fruit that may have been washed in contaminated water. Travelers themselves should peel all fresh fruits and vegetables.

- Avoid dairy products.

- Avoid raw or undercooked meat and fish.

Vaccinations for Hepatitis A

Two vaccines (Havrix, Vaqta) are now available and both are very safe and effective for preventing hepatitis A (HAV). They can be given along with immune globulin and other vaccines. A 2001 study also strongly suggested they may be used interchangeably (i.e., if one is given as the first vaccination, the other may be safely used as the booster). A combination vaccine (Twinrix) that contains both Havrix and Engerix-B (a hepatitis B vaccine) is now approved for people with risk factors for both hepatitis A and B.

Candidates for HAV Vaccinations

Vaccinations for hepatitis A are recommended for the following individuals:

- People in specific populations where outbreaks occur. Indeed, a 2001 study showed that widespread vaccination of children in one county in California led to dramatic decreases in the number of outbreaks among all adults in the community at large.

89

Daycare centers are highly associated with such outbreaks, although risks in such centers vary widely depending on the community, so universal immunization in daycare centers is not recommended.

- Sexually active homosexual men.

- Patients with any form of chronic hepatitis. (It should be noted that the HAV vaccination should be given to patients before they reach advanced stages of liver disease, when there is a lower rate of response.)

- Health care workers exposed to the virus.

- Travelers to developing countries. (Travelers should also receive immune globulin if they are visiting high-risk areas within four weeks of the vaccination.)

- Experts now recommend routine vaccinations for children and adolescents in high-risk states. These states are Arizona, Alaska, California, Idaho, Nevada, New Mexico, Oklahoma, Oregon, South Dakota, Utah, Washington, Missouri, Texas, Colorado, Arkansas, Montana, and Wyoming.

- People who have had intimate exposure to patients with hepatitis A may be protected with immune globulin or possibly with the vaccine itself.

- People with chronic liver disease, including those with hepatitis C, should also be vaccinated, particularly if they have not been exposed to hepatitis A, since the infection can cause liver failure in these patients.

Side Effects

Although there are few side effects, allergic responses from the vaccination can occur. Hair loss has been reported in a very few people after a second administration. There may be pain at the injection site. (Havrix causes more pain at the injection site than Vaqta.)

Symptoms of Hepatitis A

Symptoms are usually mild, especially in children, and generally appear between two and six weeks after exposure to the virus. Adult patients are more likely to have fever, jaundice, and itching that can last one to several months.

General Outlook for People Infected with Hepatitis A

This is the least serious of the common hepatitis viruses. It does not directly kill liver cells and there is no risk for a chronic form. Fulminant hepatitis is the only major concern, but even if it develops, it is almost always less dangerous than with other viral types. Only one in a thousand patients are at risk for death from this complication. If hepatitis A infection occurs in patients with hepatitis C, however, superinfections can occur, even without cirrhosis, leading to a life-threatening form of fulminant hepatitis. (Infection of patients with hepatitis B who do not have cirrhosis does not appear to be as dangerous.)

Specific Tests for Hepatitis A

Radioimmunoassays are generally used to identify IgM antibodies, first produced to fight hepatitis A. They appear early in the course of the disease and usually can be identified as soon as symptoms appear. IgM antibodies disappear during recovery, but those known as IgG antibodies persist, and their presence can be used to indicate a previous infection.

Treatments and Measures to Prevent Transmission of Hepatitis A

The primary goals for managing acute viral hepatitis are to provide adequate nutrition, to prevent additional damage to the liver, and to prevent transmission to others.

Precautions for Preventing Transmission of Hepatitis A

Because hepatitis A (and also hepatitis E) are usually passed through contaminated food, people with these viruses should not prepare food for others; unfortunately, these viruses are most contagious before symptoms appear.

- Using hot water when cleaning utensils or clothing is essential. Heating a contaminated article for a minute kills the virus. Simple household bleach is effective for disinfecting hard surfaces. Sterilizing is not necessary. Still, even with strong precautions, utensils used by the patient for eating and cooking should be kept separate from those used by others.

- Abstain from sexual activity or take strict precautions.

- Abstain from alcohol. Moderate drinking (one or two drinks per evening) after recovery is not harmful for most people.

Outlook

In most cases of acute viral hepatitis, recovery is complete and the liver returns to normal within two to eight weeks. In a small number of cases of hepatitis B or C, the condition can be prolonged and recovery may not occur for a year. About 5 percent to 10 percent of these patients will experience a flare-up of symptoms in a milder form before full recovery. A few of these patients may go on to develop chronic hepatitis. People who have been infected with a hepatitis virus continue to produce antibodies to that specific virus. This means that they cannot be reinfected with the same hepatitis virus again. Unfortunately, they are not protected from other types.

Serious consequences of acute viral hepatitis are rare, but can be life threatening if they occur. Pregnant women with acute hepatitis B, C, or E are at higher risk for complications of acute hepatitis.

In very rare cases, within two months of onset of acute hepatitis, a very serious condition known as fulminant hepatitis can develop. In this event, the liver fails with catastrophic consequences. The following events may develop:

- A large, swollen abdomen (known as ascites) and a peculiar hand-flapping tremor (called asterixis).

- These symptoms may be followed by stomach and intestinal bleeding and mental confusion, stupor, or coma caused by brain injury (encephalopathy).

No medications, including corticosteroids, have any effect against the condition itself. Liver transplantation is currently the only lifesaving treatment for fulminant acute hepatitis and has survival rates of up to 60 percent. Without liver transplantation, the chance of survival is only 20 percent.

Other serious and rare consequences of acute viral hepatitis are aplastic anemia (which can be fatal), pancreatitis, hypoglycemia, and polyarteritis, a serious inflammation of blood vessels.

General Prognosis for Chronic Hepatitis

Chronic Persistent Hepatitis

Chronic persistent hepatitis is usually mild and nonprogressive or slowly progressive, causing limited damage to the liver. Cell injury in such cases is usually limited to the region of portal tracts, which contains vessels that carry blood to the liver from the digestive tract. In some cases, however, more extensive liver damage can occur over long periods of time and progress to chronic active hepatitis.

Chronic Active Hepatitis

If damage to the liver is extensive and cell injury occurs beyond the portal tract, chronic active hepatitis can develop. Significant liver damage has usually occurred by this time. Nearly every bodily process is affected by a damaged liver, including digestive, hormonal, and circulatory systems. Symptoms can significantly impair daily life.

- *Cirrhosis.* If liver cells are destroyed between the portal tract and the central veins in the liver, progressive cell damage can build a layer of scar tissue over the liver, resulting in the condition known as cirrhosis. In such cases, the entire liver is threatened with malfunction and failure. If cirrhosis develops, the average survival time is about ten years. The risk for cirrhosis is much higher in patients with hepatitis C than in those with hepatitis B.

- *Liver Cancer.* The risk for liver cancer in patients with cirrhosis is about 14 percent but varies widely depending on the cause of hepatitis. (Liver cancer is rare in patients who do not develop cirrhosis.)

Symptom Management

The primary goals for managing viral hepatitis are to provide adequate nutrition, to prevent additional damage to the liver, and to prevent transmission to others. For mild cases of acute viral hepatitis, no drug therapy or other treatment is either available or necessary. Hospitalization is needed only for people at high risk for complications, such as pregnant women, elderly people, patients with other serious conditions, or those who have severe nausea and vomiting and need to have fluids administered intravenously.

The following tips may be useful:

- In some cases, the physician may prescribe drugs that have minimal impact on the liver to alleviate the symptoms of hepatitis, such as nausea or severe itching.

- All patients should abstain from alcohol and sexual contact during the acute phase.

- Although most patients with hepatitis experience fatigue and require more rest than usual, they can be as physically active as they want without affecting recovery. In fact, patients should be encouraged to be as active as they can.

- Depression is common, particularly in people used to an active life. Patients should be reassured that in the great majority of hepatitis cases, recovery is complete.

- The liver processes many types of medications, so as soon as hepatitis is diagnosed, the patient should stop taking all drugs, including over-the-counter medications, except those a physician specifically prescribes or recommends. Of special note, ibuprofen (Advil, Motrin) apparently increases liver enzymes in hepatitis C patients and therefore should be avoided. Ibuprofen is one of the common painkillers known as nonsteroidal anti-inflammatory drugs (NSAIDs). Other NSAIDs include aspirin and naproxen. The usual alternative to an NSAID is acetaminophen (Tylenol). It should be noted that acetaminophen also can be toxic in the liver, particularly when drinking alcohol.

After the onset of acute hepatitis, periodic visits to the physician for repeat blood tests are necessary, the frequency of which depends on how well the patient feels. If symptoms still occur after three months and laboratory tests still indicate active presence of the virus, the patient should be evaluated every month. If symptoms persist beyond six months, a liver biopsy may be required to determine any liver damage.

Dietary Factors to Protect the Liver

In general, no vitamins or special diets have been proven to be particularly beneficial. The following may be helpful, however:

- Eating many small snacks during the day, with larger ones in the morning, may help prevent weight loss while reducing the severity of nausea. Patients might be able to tolerate high-caloric drinks to supplement their regular diet.

- One small Japanese study suggested that vitamin E might help protect against liver damage in patients with hepatitis C.

- Thiamine binds to iron and helps reduce iron load in the liver. One small study suggested it may be helpful for patients with chronic hepatitis B. Pork is high in the vitamin, but more healthful sources include dried fortified cereals, oatmeal, corn, nuts, cauliflower, sunflower seeds, and vitamin pills.

- Some research suggests that supplements of omega-3 fatty acids (found in fish oil and evening primrose oil) may help protect the diseased liver.

- In one Norwegian study, higher coffee intake was associated with a lower risk for cirrhosis.

Treatment for Chronic Hepatitis

Chronic Hepatitis B and C

Drug treatments for chronic hepatitis B and C are aimed at reducing or preventing liver damage and boosting or modifying the immune system to promote its attack on the viruses. The important agents for treating chronic hepatitis are interferons (particularly interferon alpha) and nucleoside analogues (ribavirin, lamivudine, famciclovir, and adefovir), which act directly against the virus. They are being used as sole therapy and in combinations. These drugs are used differently depending on the specific hepatitis. Other drugs with different mechanisms are also being tested. Smokers with hepatitis C should make every attempt to quit, as research now indicates that smoking is associated with increased severity of the infection.

Autoimmune Hepatitis

Patients with autoimmune hepatitis who have mild symptoms and slight inflammation of the liver do not require any treatment except to alleviate symptoms. They should be monitored, however, for any signs of disease progression. Severe autoimmune hepatitis is a life-threatening condition and requires intensive therapy.

Liver Transplantation

Liver transplantation may be indicated in the following patients:

- Those who have developed life-threatening cirrhosis and who have a life expectancy of more than twelve years.

- Patients with liver cancer that has not spread beyond the liver may also be candidates.

Current five-year survival rates after liver transplantation are between 55 percent and 80 percent, depending on different factors.

Patients also report improved quality of life and mental functioning after liver transplantation. Unfortunately, in about half of all chronic hepatitis patients, the disease recurs after transplantation.

Patients should consider medical centers that have performed more than fifty transplants per year and produced better-than-average results. Unfortunately, in 2003 with 18,000 Americans waiting for a liver donor, only 4,244 liver transplantations were performed. And, given the large number of people with hepatitis C, this situation will almost certainly worsen over the following years.

Warnings on Alternative and So-Called Natural Remedies

Many patients with serious or chronic diseases are now investigating alternative medications. Among the natural substances being investigated for hepatitis are ginseng, glycyrrhizin (a compound in licorice), catechin (found in green tea), and silymarin (found in milk thistle). A 2001 review analyzed studies on ten herbal remedies for hepatitis C. None showed significant benefits except silymarin, which improves liver enzyme levels. Other studies are also reporting benefits on the liver from silymarin.

Alternative or natural remedies are not regulated and their quality is not publicly controlled. In addition, any substance that can affect the body's chemistry can, like any drug, produce side effects that may be harmful. Even if studies report positive benefits from herbal remedies, the compounds used in such studies are, in most cases, not what are being marketed to the public.

There have been a number of reported cases of serious and even lethal side effects from herbal products. In addition, some so-called natural remedies were found to contain standard prescription medication. The following warnings are of particular importance for people with hepatitis:

* Kava (an herb used for anxiety and tension) can be toxic to the liver and cause severe hepatitis and even liver failure if taken excessively.

* Black licorice (not the red candy) can increase blood pressure and may be harmful in people with hypertension.

Autoimmune Hepatitis (AIH)

Autoimmune chronic hepatitis typically occurs in women between the ages of twenty and forty who have other autoimmune diseases, including systemic lupus erythematosus, rheumatoid arthritis, Sjögren syndrome, inflammatory bowel disease, glomerulonephritis, and hemolytic anemia. Some research indicates that the postmenopausal period may be another peak in incidence of AIH among women. About 30 percent of patients are men, however, and in both genders there is often no relationship to another autoimmune disease. In general, no major risk factors have been discovered for this condition.

Symptoms of Autoimmune Hepatitis

About 85 percent of people with chronic active autoimmune hepatitis do not have severe symptoms at all. When symptoms occur, they range from minimal to severe, and include fatigue, jaundice, fever, and weight loss. The liver and spleen are often enlarged. In addition, patients with this condition may experience skin disorders, including palmar erythema (red palms) and spider angioma (a blood-red spot, the size of a pinhead, from which tiny blood vessels radiate like spider legs). Itching is not common, however. The abdomen or legs may be swollen due to the accumulation of fluid.

Tests for Autoimmune Chronic Hepatitis

If a patient experiences symptoms of chronic active hepatitis for six months or more and a virus cannot be identified, then autoimmune hepatitis is usually suspected. There are other autoimmune liver diseases, however, that can confuse a diagnosis. To help confirm this condition, test results may show high levels of immune factors called serum globulins or certain antibodies to liver proteins. In some cases, a successful trial of steroid drugs may be the only way to diagnose autoimmune hepatitis.

Outlook for Autoimmune Hepatitis

Autoimmune hepatitis is usually benign and causes little trouble, although there is a very small risk that it can evolve into the active form. One study reported a ten-year survival rate of 95 percent, which was similar to that for the same age group in the general population. However, if the condition evolves into the chronic active form, five-year survival rate may be only 50 percent if the disease is not treated. (The survival rate can be higher in people with milder symptoms and less liver damage.)

Although very uncommon, severe autoimmune hepatitis can be life-threatening and require intensive therapy, including possibly liver transplantation. The risk for liver failure and bleeding in the stomach and esophagus is highest in the early years after disease onset. This risk diminishes over time but is replaced by an increase in liver cancer rates and bleeding in the stomach and intestines. The risk for liver cancer is not as high, however, as with chronic viral hepatitis.

Treatments for Autoimmune Hepatitis

Patients with autoimmune hepatitis who have mild symptoms and slight inflammation of the liver do not require any treatment except to alleviate symptoms. They should be monitored, however, for any signs of disease progression. Because of effective treatment options and in spite of a high rate of relapse, long-term survival rates in patients with autoimmune hepatitis are excellent. Drugs that block factors in the immune system and help reduce inflammation and symptoms of autoimmune hepatitis are most often used.

Corticosteroids

Corticosteroids, prednisone and prednisolone, are the standard agents used for autoimmune hepatitis. They produce remission of symptoms in about 80 percent of patients with autoimmune hepatitis. For most patients, steroids also reduce symptoms within three months, improve liver function within six months, and restore liver health within two years. Between 10 percent and 20 percent of patients continue to deteriorate despite steroid treatment, although higher doses may help some of these people. (Steroids are generally not useful for chronic hepatitis B or C, and, in fact, suppressing the immune system in these patients can encourage the viruses to replicate more quickly.)

Treatment usually needs to continue for about two years before the disease is in complete remission. Usually, steroids are stopped when disease symptoms have disappeared, when blood tests show that aminotransferase levels are less than two times normal, and when liver biopsies reveal no active cell damage. Steroid medications must be withdrawn very slowly. Patients who are very elderly or who have advanced (decompensated) cirrhosis are not good candidates for this treatment.

Unfortunately, remission rarely lasts more than three years. About half of patients relapse within six months, and only about 20 percent of patients achieve remission (are disease-free) for more than five years. Re-administering prednisone therapy after relapse achieves another remission in 80 percent of patients.

Side effects can be very distressing and sometimes serious; they include weight gain, skin problems, moon-shaped face, high blood pressure, diabetes, cataracts, mental disturbances, infections, and osteoporosis.

Investigative Agents

In severe cases, drugs that block the immune system may be used:

- Azathioprine (Imuran) is often prescribed along with steroids to help reduce severe side effects caused by using steroids alone. Azathioprine also suppresses the immune system and helps prevent relapse, but the drug will not induce remission by itself. In one promising study, patients who continued to use azathioprine after prednisolone was withdrawn had no relapses for at least a year. Unfortunately, long-term use of azathioprine may increase the risk for cancer, although studies indicate that this risk is very low.

- Cyclosporine A (Neoral) is another immunosuppressant and may prove to be a safe and effective alternative to corticosteroids.

Some important research is targeting agents that inhibit RNA—the genetic molecules that serve as messengers for regulating cellular processes. In a 2003 animal study, an agent that targeted RNA specifically affecting cell receptors involved in liver injury protected against autoimmune hepatitis in mice.

Liver Transplantation and Autoimmune Hepatitis

If all therapies fail and the disease becomes life threatening, liver transplantation may be performed. Liver transplantation is problematic, however. In one study, half of patients who received a transplant required re-transplantation within a year. Autoimmune hepatitis recurred in 25 percent of patients studied. (According to one 2000 study, transplantation in these patients may improve accompanying autoimmune disorders in half of patients who experienced it.) Children who develop autoimmune hepatitis after liver transplantation may respond to corticosteroid and azathioprine therapy.

Chapter 9

Hepatitis Statistics and Populations at Risk

Chapter Contents

Section 9.1

Hepatitis and Liver Disease in the United States

"Statistical Overview" is reprinted from "Hepatitis and Liver Disease in the United States," Copyright © 2004 The American Liver Foundation. All rights reserved. Reprinted with permission. For additional information, visit http://www.liverfoundation.org. "Disease Burden from Hepatitis A, B, and C in the United States" is from the Centers for Disease Control and Prevention (CDC), October 2004.

Statistical Overview

- 25,000,000 Americans—one in every 10—are or have been afflicted with liver and biliary diseases.

- 25,000 Americans die each year from chronic liver disease and cirrhosis; 300,000 people are hospitalized each year due to cirrhosis.

- Alcoholic liver disease and chronic hepatitis C are the leading causes of cirrhosis.

- An estimated 25,000 people are infected with the hepatitis C virus each year.

- There are an estimated 3.9 million people who are or have been infected with hepatitis C, 2.7 million of whom are chronically infected; approximately 70 percent of people infected do not know they have the virus.

- 8,000 to 10,000 people die of hepatitis C each year. The Centers for Disease Control and Prevention (CDC) estimate that the number of annual deaths from hepatitis C will triple in the next ten to twenty years.

- Hepatitis B is responsible for 5,000 deaths annually, including 3,000 to 4,000 from cirrhosis and approximately 1,000 to 1,500 from primary liver cancer.

102

* One out of every 250 people is a carrier of hepatitis B and can pass it on to others, often unknowingly.

* Up to 80,000 people are infected with the hepatitis B virus each year.

* Up to 90 percent of pregnant women who are carriers of the hepatitis b virus could transmit the virus to their children. Vaccinations of the newborns would prevent them from becoming carriers.

* Due to the screening of pregnant women for HBV and vaccinations of newborns with the hepatitis B vaccine, there has been a decline in the number of infected newborns.

* Hepatitis B is one hundred times more infectious than HIV, the virus that causes AIDS. There are 500 million hepatitis B viral particles in one teaspoon of blood compared to 5–10 HIV particles.

* The estimated medical and work loss cost per year of hepatitis B is $700 million; the estimated medical and work loss cost per year of hepatitis C is $600 million.

* One out of every 20 people will be infected with hepatitis B in his or her lifetime.

* Approximately 5,000 liver transplants were performed in 2000. Because of the shortage of organs, it is estimated that nearly 1,700 prospective recipients died in 2001 while waiting for a liver for transplantation. There are currently over 18,000 people waiting for a liver transplant.

* You are at a high risk of hepatitis C infection if you: were notified that you received blood from a donor who later tested positive for hepatitis C; have ever injected illegal drugs, even if you experimented a few times many years ago; received a blood transfusion or solid organ transplant before July 1992; received a blood product for clotting problems produced before 1987; have ever been on long-term kidney dialysis; have received a tattoo or body piercing (although considered to be of a lesser degree of risk, contamination of needles is possible).

* You are at a high risk of hepatitis B infection if you: have sex with someone infected with HBV; have sex with more than one partner; are a man, and have sex with a man; live in the same house with someone who has lifelong HBV infection; have a job

that involves contact with human blood; shoot drugs; are a patient or work in a home for the developmentally disabled; have hemophilia; travel to areas where hepatitis B is common.

- Non-Hispanic African Americans have the highest infection rate for hepatitis C; Asian and Pacific Islanders have the highest rate for hepatitis B infection.

Notes on Sources and Methodology for Tables and Figures

Number of Acute Clinical Cases Reported: For hepatitis A and hepatitis B, the number of cases reported to the National Notifiable Disease Surveillance System (NNDSS). Cases of hepatitis C/NANB are also reported to NNDSS (1,150 cases in 2003) but are unreliable for monitoring trends in hepatitis C because these reports include cases based only on a positive lab test for anti-HCV, most of which represent chronic HCV infection. (CDC, Summary of Notifiable Diseases, United States, 2002, *MMWR* 2003; 51[53].)

Estimated Number of Acute Clinical Cases and New Infections: Incidence estimates are derived from catalytic modeling of seroprevalence data from the Third National Health and Nutrition Examination Survey (NHANES III) applied to cases reported to the Nationally Notifiable Disease Surveillance System (NNDSS) (for hepatitis A and hepatitis B) or to the Sentinal Counties Study of Viral Hepatitis (for hepatitis C).

Number of Persons with Chronic Infection: HBV: Margolis HS, Coleman PJ, Brown RE, et al. Prevention of hepatitis B virus transmission by immunization: An economic analysis of current recommendations. *JAMA* 1995; 274(15): 1201–8. HCV: Alter MJ, et al. Prevalence of hepatitis C infection in the United States, 1988 through 1994. *NEJM* 1999; 341:556–62.

Estimated Annual Number of Chronic Liver Disease Deaths: HBV: Margolis HS, Coleman PJ, Brown RE, et al. Prevention of hepatitis B virus transmission by immunization: An economic analysis of current recommendations. *JAMA* 1995; 274(15): 1201–8. HCV: Centers for Disease Control and Prevention. Recommendations for the prevention and control of hepatitis C virus infection and HCV-related chronic disease. *MMWR* 1998; 47(RR-19): 1–39.

Percent Ever Infected: Seroprevalence estimates for HAV, HBV, and HCV come from the Third National Health and Nutrition Examination Survey. HAV: CDC. Prevention of Hepatitis A through active or passive immunization. *MMWR* 1996; 45: RR-15. HBV: McQuillan GM, et al. Prevalence of hepatitis B virus infection in the United States: The National Health and Nutrition and Examination Surveys, 1976 through 1994. *AJPH* 1999; 89(1): 14–18. HCV: Alter MJ et al. Prevalence of hepatitis C virus infection in the United States, 1988 through 1994. *NEJM* 1999; 341:556–62.

Table 9.1. Disease Burden from Hepatitis A, B, and C in the United States

Hepatitis A

	2003	2002	2001	2000
Number of Acute Clinical Cases Reported	7,653	8,795	10,616	13,397
Estimated Number of Acute Clinical Cases	33,000	38,000	45,000	57,000
Estimated Number of New Infections: Current	61,000	73,000	93,000	143,000

Estimated Number of New Infections:	Historical	mean	min	max
	1990–1999	301,000	181,000	373,000
	1980–1989	254,000	221,000	380,000

Number of Persons with Chronic Infection	No chronic infection
Estimated Annual Number of Chronic Liver Disease Deaths	No chronic infection
Percent Ever Infected	33.0%

Hepatitis B

	2003	2002	2001	2000
Number of Acute Clinical Cases Reported	7,526	8,064	7,844	8,036
Estimated Number of Acute Clinical Cases	21,000	23,000	22,000	22,000
Estimated Number of New Infections: Current	73,000	79,000	78,000	81,000

Estimated Number of New Infections:	Historical	mean	min	max
	1990–1999	140,000	79,000	232,000
	1980–1989	259,000	208,000	287,000

Number of Persons with Chronic Infection	1.25 million persons
Estimated Annual Number of Chronic Liver Disease Deaths	5,000
Percent Ever Infected	4.9%

Hepatitis C

	2003	2002	2001	2000
Number of Acute Clinical Cases Reported	No data	No data	No data	No data
Estimated Number of Acute Clinical Cases	4,900	4,800	3,900	6,300
Estimated Number of New Infections: Current	30,000	29,000	24,000	38,000

Estimated Number of New Infections:	Historical	mean	min	max
	1990–1999	67,000	36,000	179,000
	1982–1989	232,000	180,000	291,000

Number of Persons with Chronic Infection	2.7 million persons
Estimated Annual Number of Chronic Liver Disease Deaths	8,000–10,000
Percent Ever Infected	1.8%

Table 9.2. Disease Burden from Hepatitis A in the United States

Year	Reported Acute Cases	Estimated Acute Cases	Estimated Infections
1980	29,087	124,000	234,000
1981	25,802	110,000	223,000
1982	23,404	100,000	228,000
1983	21,534	92,000	221,000
1984	22,038	94,000	232,000
1985	23,211	99,000	228,000
1986	23,429	100,000	239,000
1987	25,280	108,000	255,000
1988	28,506	122,000	305,000
1989	35,822	153,000	380,000
1990	31,522	135,000	373,000
1991	24,219	104,000	288,000
1992	23,112	99,000	274,000
1993	24,238	104,000	284,000
1994	26,796	115,000	333,000
1995	31,582	135,000	356,000
1996	31,032	133,000	335,000
1997	30,021	128,000	341,000
1998	23,229	99,000	243,000
1999	17,047	73,000	181,000
2000	13,397	57,000	143,000
2001	10,616	45,000	93,000
2002	8,795	38,000	73,000
2003	7,653	33,000	61,000

Table 9.3. Disease Burden from Hepatitis B in the United States

Year	Reported Acute Cases	Estimated Acute Cases	Estimated Infections
1980	19,014	53,000	208,000
1981	21,151	59,000	229,000
1982	22,176	62,000	239,000
1983	24,319	68,000	267,000
1984	26,116	73,000	281,000
1985	26,612	74,000	287,000
1986	26,106	73,000	283,000
1987	25,915	72,000	287,000
1988	23,175	65,000	253,000
1989	23,421	65,000	255,000
1990	21,277	59,000	232,000
1991	17,911	50,000	193,000
1992	16,126	45,000	175,000
1993	13,361	37,000	144,000
1994	12,517	35,000	133,000
1995	10,805	30,000	113,000
1996	10,637	30,000	112,000
1997	10,416	29,000	110,000
1998	10,258	29,000	109,000
1999	7,694	21,000	79,000
2000	8,036	22,000	81,000
2001	7,844	22,000	78,000
2002	8,064	23,000	79,000
2003	7,526	21,000	73,000

Table 9.4. Disease Burden from Hepatitis C in the United States

Year	Estimated Acute Cases	Estimated Infections
1982	29,500	180,000
1983	30,800	188,000
1984	36,000	219,000
1985	42,700	261,000
1986	43,000	262,000
1987	35,400	216,000
1988	39,400	240,000
1989	47,800	291,000
1990	29,400	179,000
1991	18,400	112,000
1992	12,000	73,000
1993	9,400	57,000
1994	8,900	54,000
1995	5,900	36,000
1996	5,900	36,000
1997	6,300	38,000
1998	6,800	41,000
1999	6,400	39,000
2000	6,300	38,000
2001	3,900	24,000
2002	4,800	29,000
2003	4,900	30,000

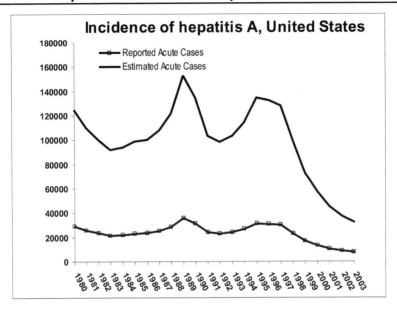

Figure 9.1. Incidence of Hepatitis A, United States

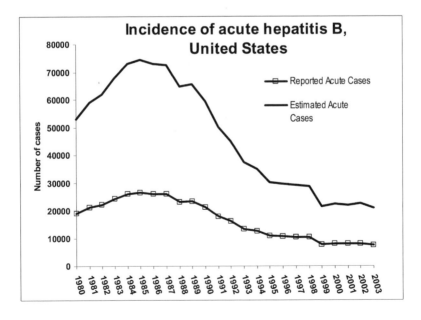

Figure 9.2. Incidence of Acute Hepatitis B, United States

109

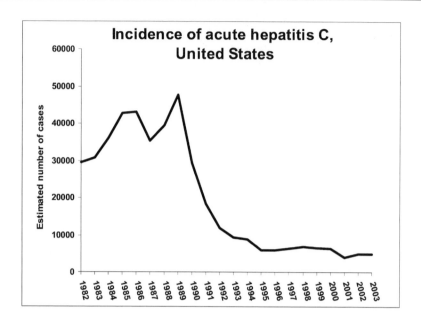

Figure 9.3. *Incidence of Acute Hepatitis C, United States*

Section 9.2

Hepatitis in Children

Reprinted from "Hepatitis," Nemours Foundation, reviewed and updated November 2001. This information was provided by KidsHealth, one of the largest resources online for medically reviewed health information written for parents, kids, and teens. For more articles like this one, visit www.KidsHealth.org, or www.TeensHealth.org. © 2001 The Nemours Center for Children's Health Media, a division of The Nemours Foundation.

Signs and Symptoms

Hepatitis is an inflammatory process involving the liver. Hepatitis, in its early stages, may cause flu-like symptoms. These symptoms may include malaise (a general ill feeling), fever, muscle aches, loss of appetite, nausea, vomiting, diarrhea, and jaundice. Some people may have no symptoms at all and may not even know they're infected.

If hepatitis progresses, its symptoms begin to point to the liver as the source of illness. Chemicals normally secreted by the liver begin to build up in the blood. This causes jaundice (a yellowing of the skin and whites of the eyes), foul breath, and a bitter taste in the mouth. Urine turns dark or "tea-colored," and stools become white, light, or "clay-colored." There also can be abdominal pain, which may be centered below the right ribs (over a tender, swollen liver) or below the left ribs (over a tender spleen).

Description

The word *hepatitis* simply means an inflammation of the liver, without pinpointing a specific cause. Someone with hepatitis may be suffering from one of several disorders, including a viral infection of the liver; liver injury caused by a toxin (poison); liver damage caused by interruption of the organ's normal blood supply; or trauma.

Most commonly, hepatitis is caused by one of three viruses: the hepatitis A virus; the hepatitis B virus; or the hepatitis C virus. In some cases, mononucleosis can also result in hepatitis.

In children, the most common form of hepatitis is hepatitis A, also called "infectious hepatitis." This form is caused by the hepatitis A virus (HAV), which lives in the stools of infected individuals. When someone touches or eats anything that is contaminated with HAV-infected stool, the virus can pass into the body through the mouth. This makes it easy for HAV to spread in overcrowded, unsanitary living conditions. HAV also spreads in contaminated water, milk, and foods, especially in shellfish. Because hepatitis A can be a mild infection, particularly in children, it is possible for some people to be unaware that they have had the illness. In fact, although medical tests show that about 40 percent of urban Americans have had hepatitis A, only about 5 percent recall being sick.

Hepatitis B, also called "serum hepatitis," is caused by the hepatitis B virus (HBV). HBV spreads through infected body fluids, such as blood, saliva, semen, vaginal fluids, tears, breast milk, and urine. Infections may occur through a contaminated blood transfusion (uncommon in the United States), shared contaminated needles or syringes for injecting drugs, or sexual activity with an HBV-infected person. HBV-infected mothers can also pass the virus to their newborn babies.

Hepatitis C is spread by direct contact with an infected person's blood. It can be spread by sharing drug needles or getting a tattoo or body piercing with unsterilized tools, blood transfusions (especially ones that occurred before 1992; since then the U.S. blood supply has been routinely screened for the disease), or from mother to newborn. Hepatitis C is also a common threat in kidney dialysis centers. Less commonly, it is spread through sexual contact. Rarely, people living with an infected person can contract the disease by sharing items that might contain that person's blood, such as razors or toothbrushes.

There are other viruses that can cause hepatitis, including Hepatitis E. These viruses are known as "non-ABC hepatitis" because most of them have not been completely identified.

All of these viral hepatitis conditions can be diagnosed and followed through the use of readily available blood tests.

Incubation

The incubation period for viral hepatitis varies depending on which hepatitis virus causes the disease. For hepatitis A, the incubation period is two to six weeks. For hepatitis B, the incubation period is between one and five months. For hepatitis C, it is estimated that the incubation period is two to twenty-six weeks.

Duration

Children with hepatitis A usually have mild symptoms or are without symptoms. They may be more fatigued than normal, but they are rarely jaundiced. Almost all previously healthy persons who develop hepatitis A will completely recover from their illness in a few weeks or months without long-term complications.

With hepatitis B, 90 to 95 percent of patients recover from their illness completely within six months, without long-term complications. In some cases, however, persons with either hepatitis B or C can go on to develop chronic hepatitis and cirrhosis (chronic degeneration) of the liver. Some persons with hepatitis B or C may also become life-long carriers of these viruses and can spread them to other people.

Contagiousness

Hepatitis A is contagious, and its virus can be spread in contaminated food or water, as well as in unsanitary conditions in child-care facilities or schools. Toilets and sinks used by an infected person should be cleaned with antiseptic cleansers. All persons who live with or care for someone with hepatitis should wash their hands after contact with the infected person. In addition, when traveling to countries where hepatitis A is prevalent, your child should be vaccinated with at least two doses of the hepatitis A vaccine.

Hepatitis B is highly contagious. Its virus can be found in virtually all body fluids, though its main routes of infection are through sexual contact, contaminated blood transfusions, and shared needles for drug injections. Household contact with adults with hepatitis B can put people at risk for contracting hepatitis. Frequent hand washing and good hygiene practices can reduce this risk. Use of the hepatitis B vaccine can greatly decrease the incidence of this infection. Ask your child's doctor about this vaccine.

Hepatitis C is contagious and can be spread through shared drug needles, contaminated blood products, and, less commonly, through sexual contact. Hepatitis C can be spread from mother to fetus during pregnancy, however, the risk of passing hepatitis C to the fetus is about 5 percent. If you are pregnant, contact your doctor if you think you may have been exposed to hepatitis C.

Over the past several years, improved medical technology has almost eliminated the risk of catching hepatitis from contaminated blood products and blood transfusions. But, as tattoos and acupuncture have become more popular, the risk of developing hepatitis from improperly sterilized equipment used in these procedures has increased.

Prevention

In general, to prevent viral hepatitis you should follow good hygiene and avoid crowded, unhealthy living conditions. If you travel to areas of the world where sanitation is poor and water quality is uncertain, extra care is necessary, particularly when drinking and swimming. Never eat shellfish from waters contaminated by sewage. You should also remind children to wash their hands thoroughly after using the toilet and before eating. If someone in the family develops hepatitis, antiseptic cleansers should be used to clean any toilet, sink, potty-chair, or bedpan used by that person.

Since contaminated needles and syringes are a major source of hepatitis infection, you should encourage drug awareness programs in your community and schools. At home, speak to your children frankly and frequently about the dangers of drug use. Also encourage abstinence and safe sex for teens, in order to eliminate their risk of hepatitis infection through sexual contact.

A hepatitis A vaccine is available, and is especially recommended for travelers, sexually active individuals, and people in high-risk occupations, such as health care and child care personnel. If you are planning to travel abroad, consult your doctor in advance so you and your family have enough time to complete the required immunizations. The vaccine is especially useful for staff of child care facilities or schools, family members of infected persons, or sexual partners of someone with hepatitis A.

There is also a hepatitis B vaccine, which should be given to both children and adults as part of routine immunization. Talk to your child's doctor about vaccinations for hepatitis.

When to Call Your Child's Doctor

Call your child's doctor if your child has symptoms of hepatitis, attends a school or child care facility where someone has hepatitis, or has been exposed to a friend or relative with the illness.

If older children volunteer at a first-aid station, hospital, or nursing home, be sure that they are aware of proper safety procedures for preventing contact with blood or body fluids. Such employment may warrant an immunization against HBV. Call your doctor if you believe that your child may have been exposed to a patient with hepatitis.

If you already know that your child has hepatitis, call your child's doctor if you notice any of the following symptoms: confusion or extreme drowsiness, skin rash, or itching. Monitor your child's appetite and digestive functions, and call your child's doctor if appetite decreases, or if nausea, vomiting, diarrhea, or jaundice increase.

Professional Treatment

When symptoms are severe or laboratory tests show liver damage, hospital treatment of hepatitis is sometimes necessary.

Home Treatment

Children with mild hepatitis may be treated at home. Except for using the bathroom, they should rest in bed until fever and jaundice are gone and appetite is normal. Children with a lack of appetite should try smaller, more frequent meals and fluids that are high in calories (like milkshakes). They should eat healthy foods rich in protein and carbohydrates and drink plenty of water.

Section 9.3

Hepatitis Information for African Americans

The Impact of Viral Hepatitis in Our Community

What Is Hepatitis and How Do I Get It?

Viral hepatitis is a liver disease that does not discriminate. It affects millions of people from different backgrounds, cultures, and lifestyles. There are factors, however, that may place African Americans at greater risk than others.

Viral Hepatitis: A National Health Problem

- Estimated new infections of hepatitis A per year in the United States: 20,000–40,000; Estimated infections lasting more than six months: None.

- Estimated new infections of hepatitis B per year in the United States: 80,000; Estimated infections lasting more than six months: 1.25 million (5 percent of all HBV cases).

- Estimated new infections of hepatitis C per year in the U.S.: 25,000; Estimated infections lasting more than six months: 2.7 million (75–85 percent of all HCV cases).

The Hepatitis A Virus (HAV)

HAV infection can cause an acute, flu-like illness with yellowing of the skin (jaundice), nausea and vomiting, fatigue, loss of appetite, abdominal pain, or diarrhea. It lasts from three to six weeks, but can sometimes last for six months. Most patients recover with no serious long-term health problems. Symptoms are more severe in adults than

116

in children, who often have no symptoms. HAV is spread when infected human feces (body waste) is ingested by mouth.

HAV Infection Risk Factors

Fecal (body waste)/Oral contamination:

- Not washing hands after using the bathroom or changing a diaper
- Eating uncooked food prepared by an infected person who did not wash his or her hands after using the bathroom
- Drinking contaminated water
- Having oral/anal sex

The Hepatitis B Virus (HBV)

HBV Infection can cause symptoms similar to HAV. Most adults fight off infection and have no long-term health problems, but in 5 percent of cases it becomes chronic (lasting more than six months) and can then cause cirrhosis (scarring of the liver), liver cancer, and liver failure, resulting in five thousand deaths per year. HBV is spread through contact with infected body fluids or blood.

HBV Infection Risk Factors

Blood and body fluids:

- Having unprotected sex with an infected partner
- Using illegal injection drugs, even once
- Using the razor or toothbrush of an infected person
- Exposure as a health care worker to infected blood or body fluids
- Being born to an infected mother

The Hepatitis C Virus (HCV)

HCV infection becomes chronic in 85 percent of cases, and often has no symptoms until liver damage has occurred after many years of infection. Hepatitis C can cause cirrhosis, liver cancer and liver failure, and is responsible for ten thousand to twelve thousand deaths per year. HCV is spread through blood-to-blood contact.

HCV Infection Risk Factors

Blood-to-blood contact known to transmit infection:

- Using illegal injection drugs, even once
- Having a blood transfusion or organ transplant before July 1992
- Having long-term hemodialysis
- Receiving clotting factor made prior to 1987
- Being injured by a needle or other sharp object that has infected blood on it
- Being born to an infected mother
- Sharing cocaine straws

Blood-to-blood contact that may transmit infection:

- Having unprotected sex with multiple partners or a history of sexually transmitted disease
- Tattooing or body piercing in unsanitary conditions
- Using the razor or toothbrush of an infected person
- Other exposure to infected blood

Increased Hepatitis Risk among African Americans

African Americans may be at increased risk of viral hepatitis for several reasons:

- *Sickle Cell Anemia:* Sickle cell is a genetic blood disorder that affects African Americans almost exclusively—99 percent of all people with sickle cell are African American. Sickle cell requires treatment with blood transfusion. People who received blood transfusions before 1992, when a test to detect HCV became available, are at increased risk for infection with hepatitis C.

- *Health Care Employment:* More than three million African Americans are members of labor unions and work in occupations, such as nursing, health care, and emergency services, that may increase their exposure to HBV and HCV. Health care workers exposed to blood infected with HBV or HCV are at increased risk of infection.

Your health care provider can perform blood tests to determine if you are infected with viral hepatitis. The only way to be sure if you are infected with viral hepatitis is to get tested.

Hepatitis C: An Emerging Epidemic

Over four million Americans have been infected with hepatitis C. Hepatitis C is two to three times more common in African Americans than in whites in the United States, and the complications of hepatitis C—end-stage liver disease, death from cirrhosis, liver cancer—appear to be more common in African Americans.

As many as 70 percent of people infected with the virus do not know that they have it, as they have no (or very vague) symptoms. However, this virus may be causing serious liver damage that will likely not be recognized for several years. Within the next twenty years, hepatitis C is expected to cause more deaths annually than AIDS in the United States.

Although the rate of new infections is now greatly reduced, most of the people with HCV were infected years ago and are unaware of their condition. If they are not tested and evaluated for liver damage and the potential to benefit from treatment, many may develop liver damage and liver failure.

The best way to determine who may be infected is to assess the presence of risk factors for contact with infected blood. Some people may not want to talk about or be able to recall risk factors, such as past drug use.

Getting Tested and Getting Treated

If you think you may have been exposed to viral hepatitis, you should get tested. Blood tests for HAV, HBV, and HCV are available through a physician and, in some cases, through a public health clinic.

Those who test positive for chronic hepatitis B or C may need a liver biopsy (a small piece of liver tissue is taken with a needle) to determine the existence or extent of liver damage. Early diagnosis and management of hepatitis viruses may have long-term health benefits.

Treatment for hepatitis A involves bed rest, good nutrition, and intake of extra fluids. HAV infection does not usually lead to long-term health problems and is rarely fatal.

Treatments are available for chronic hepatitis B and C. Therapy with interferon, lamivudine, or adefovir dipivoxil is available to help people with chronic hepatitis B. Therapy with interferon or pegylated interferon, alone or in combination with ribavirin, can help many people with chronic hepatitis C. Additional treatment options are being developed, and more research is needed to develop hepatitis cures.

Alcohol

If you have viral hepatitis, you should avoid alcohol. Studies show that the use of alcohol substantially increases the risk of serious liver damage in persons with chronic viral hepatitis.

Vaccines Stop the Spread of Some Hepatitis Viruses

Vaccines for hepatitis A and B (there is no vaccine for hepatitis C) can provide long-term protection from these diseases.

The hepatitis A vaccine is recommended for people older than the age of two who:

- Travel to countries with high rates of HAV infection (Mexico, the Caribbean, Central and South America, Africa, the Middle East, Eastern Europe, countries bordering the Mediterranean, and parts of Asia)

- Are children living in communities with high rates of the disease or regular outbreaks

- Have chronic liver diseases, including HBV and HCV infection (HAV can increase liver damage and can be fatal to these patients)

- Engage in oral/anal sex

The HAV vaccine is given in two doses, six to eighteen months apart, and it takes thirty days to take effect. For people already exposed to the virus, immune globulin can reduce the risk of infection if given within fourteen days of exposure.

The hepatitis B vaccine is recommended as a part of the routine schedule of childhood immunizations. Many states require this vaccination for entry into elementary school.

This vaccine was not routinely given to infants until 1991, so children born before then may not be protected. Children up to age eighteen should be immunized. The government's Vaccines for Children Program will pay for immunizations for eligible children up to age eighteen. The Centers for Disease Control and Prevention (CDC) recommends that all pregnant women be tested for hepatitis B so that infections can be prevented in their newborns.

Experts also recommend immunization for:

- Infants born to HBV-infected mothers
- People with chronic liver diseases, including HCV infection
- People who have unprotected sex with more than one sexual partner
- People who are exposed to blood in the workplace, including health care and emergency service workers

Getting Help and Information

Speak with your doctor or contact your local public health department for information about possible free or low-cost testing, vaccination and referral for treatment.

Contact the American Liver Foundation for more information about hepatitis or to find a local chapter or support group.

Section 9.4

Hepatitis in Asian Americans

Reprinted from "Hepatitis B in Asian Americans," © 2003 Asian Liver Center at Stanford University. Reprinted with permission.

Why should Asians and Pacific Islanders (API) be aware of hepatitis B?

Asians have the highest rate of hepatitis B of all ethnic groups. Hepatitis B rates for the API population range up to 15 percent, compared to the 0.3 percent among the general U.S. population. API make up more than half of the 1.3–1.5 million known hepatitis B carriers in the United States. The most common route of infection among API is through perinatal sources. In the United States, API children were found to have low vaccination rates despite national vaccination guidelines and availability. Many children worldwide remain unvaccinated and may become chronic carriers as adults. The

121

World Health Organization (WHO) estimates that there are four hundred million people with chronic hepatitis B, many of whom are not even aware of their condition. Most hepatitis B carriers have no symptoms but they can still transmit the infection and develop liver cancer. Furthermore, the incidence of liver cancer among API ethnic groups is 1.7 to 11.3 times higher than rates among Caucasian Americans.

How is hepatitis B transmitted among Asians and Pacific Islanders?

While hepatitis B can be transmitted by blood transfusions, sharing needles, and unprotected sex, most API individuals become infected as infants or young children. Frequently, transmission of the hepatitis B virus occurs during the birthing process when the virus is passed on from the mother—who is often unaware that she is a carrier—or during early childhood through close personal contact with blood or bodily fluid of infected individuals, such as contact between open wounds or sharing contaminated toothbrushes. However, hepatitis B is not spread by contaminated food or water, as with other types of hepatitis.

Why is hepatitis B often not diagnosed?

The danger of hepatitis B lies in its silent transmission and progression. Many chronic hepatitis B carriers have no symptoms and feel healthy. If the proper tests are not administered, carriers may even appear to exhibit normal blood tests for liver function, granting them a deceptively clean bill of health. Diagnosis of hepatitis B cannot be made unless the doctor orders a specific blood test that tests for the presence of the hepatitis B surface antigen (HBsAg), a marker for chronic infection. Since the detection of hepatitis B is so easily missed, even by doctors, it is up to the patient to specifically request the HBsAg test. Early detection not only benefits the carrier, but will also prevent the infection from being passed silently between individuals of the same and subsequent generations.

How is hepatitis B life-threatening?

One out of four hepatitis B carriers die from liver cancer or cirrhosis (liver damage leads to scarring and eventual death due to liver failure). Some develop cancer as early as thirty years of age. Each year, approximately one million people worldwide, many of whom are

Asians and Pacific Islanders, die from the disease because they are diagnosed at a point too late for possible effective treatment. Because many carriers look and feel healthy even in the early stages of liver cancer, the disease can progress silently without the carrier knowing. Symptoms often appear only during the late stages of the disease. All chronic hepatitis B carriers, whether they feel healthy or sick, are at risk for developing liver cancer or cirrhosis. Hepatitis B is one the largest health threats for Asians. Thus it is important for all API to be checked for hepatitis B and vaccinated if not previously exposed. Also, chronic carriers need to take control of their own health, learn about hepatitis B treatments available, and be regularly screened for liver cancer after a certain age.

Section 9.5

Latinos and Hepatitis

Reprinted from "Latinos and Hepatitis C," by José Azócar, M.D., July 2003, with permission of the Hepatitis C Support Project, http://www.hcvadvocate.org, © 2003. All rights reserved.

Hepatitis C virus (HCV) infection affects an estimated 1.8 percent of Americans (about 3.9–4 million people in the United States). Yet little is known about HCV prevalence and transmission rates in non-Caucasian populations.

To determine whether HCV seroprevalence rates are different in Latinos and Caucasians, my research group conducted a case-control study of Latinos living in a western Massachusetts city. Our research included a prevalence study of HCV antibodies in blood samples from five hundred randomly selected Latino patients receiving medical care at an inner-city health facility in Springfield, Massachusetts. We also conducted a case-control study of HCV transmission risk factors.

HCV Seroprevalence

Blood samples from clinic participants were tested for HCV antibodies using the enzyme immunoassay (EIA). An HCV RNA reverse transcriptase-polymerase chain reaction (RT-PCR) assay was done on positive samples to measure HCV viral load and a restriction fragment length polymorphism (RFLP) test was done to determine genotype; samples that were positive by EIA and negative by PCR were confirmed using a recombinant immunoblot assay (RIBA).

Among the five hundred randomly selected patients in the seroprevalence study, forty tested positive for HCV. Thus, we estimate that the population prevalence rate in this inner-city Latino population is 8 percent—nearly four times greater than the rate previously reported for the population at large. HCV genotype was determined for sixty-four patients. Genotype 1 was most common in this group (75.2%; 62.7% 1a and 12.5% 1b); some patients had genotype 2 (1.5% 2a and 14% 2b), 3a (1.5%), or 4a (7.8%). The proportions of HCV genotypes in our study population were similar to those seen in other ethnic groups in the United States.

Risk Factor Analysis

Known risk factors for hepatitis C include injection and inhaled drug use, needle sharing, tattooing and body piercing, sharing of sharp objects, a history of sexually transmitted diseases, unprotected sexual activity, and sexual activity with multiple partners. Although this list is lengthy, many people with HCV (40% or more by some estimates) lack any of these risk factors, suggesting that the list is likely incomplete.

To investigate this issue, we conducted a parallel case-control study of HCV risk factors that compared 105 HCV-infected Latino patients attending our hepatitis C clinic and 130 uninfected Latino controls receiving routine health maintenance at an adjoining clinic. Participants were interviewed in English or Spanish by trained interviewers using a forty-item risk factor questionnaire divided into nine sections: demographic data, personal history, family history, incarceration history, risk factors for blood exposure, needlestick exposure, drug use history, tobacco and alcohol use, and sexual behavior. Education and counseling were provided after the questionnaire was completed.

All 235 participants in the study were of Puerto Rican ancestry. HCV positive and HCV negative (control) subjects were similar in age (a mean of 39.2 years vs. 42.5 years). Most (80%) lived in Springfield, with the rest residing in neighboring communities such as Chicopee and Holyoke.

Among the 128 men and 107 women in the study, more men (70 individuals, or 54.69%) than women (35 individuals, or 32.71%) were

HCV positive. There were approximately six times more Spanish-speaking than English-speaking individuals, with the HCV prevalence rate somewhat higher among the Spanish speakers. A large proportion (42%) were either divorced, separated, or widowed, while 30 percent were single and 27 percent were married. With respect to education, nearly 60 percent had either high school or some college education and about 40 percent had an eighth-grade education or less. About 70 percent of the group were unemployed, while about 24 percent were either employed or students (7% did not report employment status). Interestingly, those who were divorced/separated/ widowed, had less education, or were unemployed were less likely to have HCV.

We conducted a logistic regression analysis to determine how several risk factors influenced the rates of HCV infection among the Latinos in our population (see Table 9.5).

All forms of drug use were associated with higher HCV seroprevalence in our cohort. As expected, injection drug use was associated with a very high increase in relative risk (OR = 30.40), but nasal inhalation (OR = 26.44) and smoking of drugs (OR = 18.1) were also correlated with higher rates of HCV infection. We also found that using drugs (injected, inhaled, or smoked) during sex was strongly associated with a higher risk of HCV infection (OR = 18.67). Tobacco smoking (OR = 5.19) and alcohol use (OR = 2.20) were less strongly associated with higher HCV seroprevalence.

Almost half of our cohort (114 individuals, or 48%) had a history of incarceration, and more than half (148 individuals, or about 63%) had a history of incarceration within their families. A history of prior incarceration was associated with a large increase in HCV prevalence (OR = 7.79). In particular, those who had received a tattoo in jail had a significantly higher risk of HCV (OR = 8.20). For tattooing in general, the risk was lower (OR = 3.76) than for tattoos done in jail. For body piercing, the risk was lower still (OR = 1.69). We also observed that sharing of sharp objects such as nail clippers, razors, or scissors (OR = 13.75) and prior needlestick accidents (OR = 6.63) both increased the relative risk of HCV.

Along with drug use during sex, having more than one sexual partner during the past year and having a history of sexually transmitted diseases (OR = 4.59) were both associated with an increased risk of HCV.

We looked at the timing of blood transfusions and surgical procedures likely to involve a blood transfusion—before or after the initiation of routine screening of donated blood—and found no significant difference in prevalence rates (OR = 1.89 for transfusion; OR = 0.65 for surgery). However, the number of subjects who had received a transfusion was small (22 individuals) and may not provide an adequate sample size to detect differences.

Interestingly, the presence of a family member with hepatitis C appeared to have a protective effect (OR = 0.29) and was associated with a lower rate of HCV infection.

Table 9.5. Logistic Regression Analyses of Personal and Family History Characteristics of Patients in the Risk Factor Study

Risk Factor	OR	95% CI	P value
Personal exposure			
Intravenous drugs	30.40	13.7–67.3	<0.001[a]
Inhaled drugs	26.44	13.2–53.1	<0.001[a]
History of drug use during sex	18.67	4.25–81.9	<0.001[a]
Smoked drugs	18.13	9.39–35.0	<0.001[a]
Shared objects[b]	13.75	2.90–65.2	0.001[a]
Tattoo done in jail	8.20	3.30–20.4	<0.001[a]
Previous Incarceration	7.79	4.24–14.3	<0.001[a]
Needle accident	6.63	1.42–31.0	0.016[a]
Tobacco smoking	5.19	2.96–9.13	<0.001[a]
History of sexually transmitted diseases	4.59	1.97–10.7	<0.001[a]
Tattoo	3.76	1.98–7.10	<0.001[a]
Alcohol use	2.20	1.28–3.79	0.004[a]
Body piercing	1.69	0.96–2.97	0.068
Blood transfusion	1.89	0.77–4.61	0.163
Surgical procedure[c]	0.65	0.39–1.20	0.109
Family associated exposure			
Family member with HIV	0.63	0.34–1.14	0.125
Family member with hepatitis A	0.66	0.18–2.42	0.529
Family member with hepatitis B	0.48	0.12–1.99	0.313
Family member with hepatitis C	0.29	0.14–0.60	0.001a

Note: OR = Odd ratios, 95% CI = 95% confidence intervals

[a]Significant at P < 0.05.

[b]Sharing objects: refers to sharing of cutting edge objects such as nail clippers, scissors, and razors (among others).

[c]Surgical procedures: included procedures with the potential for the involvement of blood transfusion, such as gunshot wounds and hysterectomy (among others).

Conclusion

As noted previously, Miriam Alter and colleagues found an overall HCV prevalence among the general U.S. population of 1.8 percent based on the Center for Disease Control and Prevention's NHANES III study, which included non-Hispanic whites, non-Hispanic blacks, and Mexican-Americans. In that study, neither sex nor race/ethnicity was independently associated with HCV infection. The strongest factors independently associated with HCV infection were illegal drug use and high-risk sexual behavior; other factors independently associated with HCV included poverty, having twelve or fewer years of education, and a history of divorce or separation.

Our results showed that in an inner-city Latino population the HCV seroprevalence rate—8 percent—was strikingly higher than that previously described for the general population. This difference likely reflects different behavior patterns. Our study cohort was living in a densely populated area, was largely unemployed, had unstable marital status, and had high rates of incarceration within the family. However, our data suggest that low socioeconomic status, low education level, and marital dissolution were not independently associated with HCV infection. These data contrast with the findings of Alter and colleagues described previously.

Studies of Latin American immigrants have shown that they tend to be younger, are more likely to receive tattoos and body piercings, and more often reside in multifamily dwellings. But these characteristics alone would not traditionally put the population at substantially higher risk for HCV infection, were they not accompanied by injection drug use.

We expected to find that injection drug use would put our study population at higher risk for HCV. However, we found that the use of drugs in other forms (inhaled and smoked) also strikingly increased the likelihood of HCV infection, as did high-risk sexual behavior and tattooing.

Tattooing as a risk factor for HCV infection has been controversial. Robert Haley and colleagues reported that individuals who had received a tattoo in a commercial tattoo parlor were nine times more likely to be infected with HCV than people who had not been tattooed, and a study of prisoners in Norway found that tattooing was significantly associated with HCV infection, independent of a history of injection drug use. Our data also showed that people who reported having a tattoo had higher rates of HCV infection. However, while the risk of HCV was greatly increased if the tattoos had been done in jail, the risk was not significantly higher if the tattoos had been done in other settings.

Similar data have been reported with respect to the association between tattooing and HIV in U.S. prisons.

While most prior studies of the epidemiology of HCV transmission have looked at cohorts of blood donors and recipients, our study of a community-based Latino population allowed us to examine the importance of risk factors other than blood transfusion. In the past ten years, intensive screening of donated blood has dramatically decreased transfusion-associated HCV transmission, and our data suggest that blood transfusion and surgical procedures were not significant risk factors for HCV infection in this population.

The high rate of HCV infection in our cohort suggests that there likely will be a large increase in HCV-related chronic liver disease in inner-city Latino populations within the next one or two decades. The presence of many potentially modifiable risk factors in this study suggests that a focus on preventive strategies targeted toward Latinos is extremely important. In our study, subjects who had family members with hepatitis C were less likely to be seropositive themselves, suggesting that awareness of the disease and education about its prevention can have a protective effect. In addition, education should be provided to the Latino population to encourage testing and early treatment of hepatitis C, which could help minimize long-term liver damage. Based on the characteristics of our population, such education should be targeted to individuals of all educational levels and should be provided in both Spanish and English. The prevalence in other Latino populations without a high rate of risk factors for HCV infection, mainly the use of drugs, is more likely to be close to the 1.8 percent found in the general U.S. population.

Selected References

1. Alter MJ. Epidemiology of hepatitis C. *Hepatology*. 1997; 26 (3 Suppl 1): 62S–65S.

2. Alter MJ, Mast EE. The epidemiology of viral hepatitis in the United States. *Gastroenterol Clin North Am*. 1994; 2:437–55.

3. Choo QL, Kuo G, Weiner AJ, Overby LR, Bradley DW, Houghton M. Isolation of a cDNA clone derived from a blood-borne non-A, non-B viral hepatitis genome. *Science*. 1989; 244:359–62.

4. Alter MJ, Margolis HS, Krawczynski K, Judson FN, Mares A, Alexander WI, et al. The natural history of community-acquired hepatitis C in the United States. The Sentinel Counties Chronic

non-A, non-B Hepatitis Study Team. *N Engl J Med*. 1992; 32:1899–1905.

5. Mansell CJ, Locarnini SA. Epidemiology of hepatitis C in the East. *Semin Liver Dis*. 1995; 15:15–32.

6. Abdel-Wahab MF, Zakaria S, Kamel M, Abdel-Khaliq MK, Mabrouk MA. Salama H, et al. High seroprevalence of hepatitis C infection among risk groups in Egypt. *Am J Trop Med Hyg*. 1994; 51:563–67.

7. Chen TZ, Wu JC, Yen FS, Sheng WY, Hwang SJ, Huo TI, et al. Injection with nondisposable needles as an important route for transmission of acute community-acquired hepatitis C virus infection in Taiwan. *J Med Virol*. 1995; 46:247–51.

8. Haley RW, Fischer RP. Commercial tattooing as a potentially important source of hepatitis C infection. Clinical epidemiology of 626 consecutive patients unaware of their hepatitis C serologic status. *Medicine* (Baltimore). 2001; 80:134–51.

9. Holsen DS, Harthug S, Myrmel H. Prevalence of antibodies to hepatitis C virus and association with intravenous drug abuse and tattooing in a national prison in Norway. *Eur J Clin Microbiol Infect Dis*. 1993; 12:673–76.

10. Sun Dx, Zhang FG, Geng YQ, Xi DS. Hepatitis C transmission by cosmetic tattooing in women. *Lancet*. 1996; 347:541.

11. Hayes MO, Harkness GA. Body piercing as a risk factor for viral hepatitis: an integrative research review. *Am J Infect Control*. 2001; 29:271–74.

12. Braithwaite RL, Stephens T, Sterk C, Braithwaite K. Risks associated with tattooing and body piercing. *J Public Health Policy*. 1999; 20:459–70.

13. Conry-Cantilena C, VanRaden M, Gibble J, Melpolder J, Shakil AO, Viladomiu L, et al. Routes of infection, viremia, and liver disease in blood donors found to have hepatitis C virus infection. *N Engl J Med*. 1996; 334:1691–96.

14. Weinstock HS, Bolan G, Reingold AL, Polish LB. Hepatitis C virus infection among patients attending a clinic for sexually transmitted diseases. *JAMA*. 1993; 269:392–94.

15. Prevention CfDCa. Recommendations for prevention and control of hepatitis C virus (HCV) infection and HCV-related chronic disease. *Morb Mortal Wkly Rep.* 1998; 47:1–39.

16. Bureau UC. Justice Statistics. *Bureau of Justice, Statistic Bulletin* 2000; Sept.

17. Bureau UC. Current Population Survey. *Population Characteristics 2000.*

18. Doll DC. Tattooing in prison and HIV infection. *Lancet.* 1988; 1:66–67.

Section 9.6

Hepatitis among Prison Inmates

Reprinted from "Viral Hepatitis and the Criminal Justice System,"
Centers for Disease Control and Prevention (CDC), October 2002.

The unique circumstances of the criminal justice environment create opportunities to reach an underserved population with viral hepatitis prevention and treatment services. However, correctional facilities must grapple with several issues, including uncertainty about who will pay for these services, a lack of screening and treatment guidelines, and a need for staff training.

Viral Hepatitis in the Criminal Justice System

Hepatitis B and C are highly prevalent in correctional facilities. Although the prevalence of hepatitis B virus (HBV) and hepatitis C virus (HCV) infections in correctional facilities is not known with certainty, a number of indications point to their being very common:

- Studies of prison populations in California, Virginia, Connecticut, Maryland, and Texas have found evidence of HCV infection in 29–42 percent of inmates, and national figures for HCV infection among incarcerated populations estimate that 15–30 percent of inmates across the country may be HCV positive.

- A California survey found that half the incoming women and a third of incoming men tested positive for hepatitis B virus infection.

- Injection drug use is the primary transmission route for HCV. High-risk sexual behaviors (such as unprotected sex with multiple partners) and injection drug use are the major transmission routes for HBV. A substantial majority of prison and jail inmates—as much as 80 percent—have serious drug problems, including injection drug use.

Transmission can occur within and beyond the corrections setting. Many inmates already have chronic HBV or HCV infection when they enter prison or jail. Because symptoms are often mild or nonexistent, inmates may not know they are infected and can unwittingly transmit the virus to others through injection drug use, consensual sex, rape, and tattooing with contaminated equipment. Transmission can also occur as a result of sharing personal items, such as razors or toothbrushes. There is also a high risk of transmission to the larger community outside of the facility if an inmate continues to practice high-risk drug use and sexual behaviors after release.

Particular Challenges in Responding to Hepatitis B and Hepatitis C

Awareness of viral hepatitis as an important public health issue is growing, but correctional facilities face a number of unique issues as they try to respond:

- Currently, no specific federal guidelines exist for screening or treating inmates who may be at risk or who are already infected with HBV and HCV, although such guidelines are currently being developed. Such guidelines should provide facilities with assistance in developing and implementing policies for routine screening, immunization, and medical evaluation and management.

- Viral hepatitis prevention measures, including screening, immunization, and treatment, can be expensive. States and communities will need to identify sources for funding these services within correctional facilities, as well as develop policies for continuing care (such as completing immunization or therapy) after the inmate's release.

131

- Variable length of sentences and constant movement of inmates within and between facilities makes ensuring complete immunization, monitoring chronic infections, and establishing and carrying out treatment regimens difficult.

- Antiviral therapy for chronic hepatitis B and chronic hepatitis C is complicated, has limited effectiveness, and is not appropriate for everybody. Facilities that have instituted viral hepatitis treatment programs have found that periodic training and updates for correctional health and pharmacy staff are needed for successful programs. Successful HIV/AIDS treatment programs in correctional facilities also may provide some useful lessons learned.

- Many inmates have other illnesses and conditions, such as HIV, tuberculosis, diabetes, or mental illness. Treatment of an inmate's hepatitis B or hepatitis C may not be the highest priority for the correctional health staff if a beneficial outcome is uncertain.

Despite these challenges, the unique circumstances of the correctional environment create an unparalleled opportunity to reach a population that has been resistant to or unreached by education and interventions and to provide them with beneficial prevention and treatment services:

- Vaccines are available for hepatitis A and hepatitis B, providing a real prevention opportunity.

- Many correctional facilities already have education, prevention, and treatment programs focused on HIV, sexually transmitted diseases, and substance abuse. Viral hepatitis prevention, screening, and treatment messages could build on these existing efforts.

Section 9.7

Hepatitis Information for Injection Drug Users

Hepatitis C is a serious liver disease. If you inject or shoot street drugs, you need to know:

- Hepatitis C is caused by infection with the hepatitis C virus (HCV).

- HCV is blood-borne, meaning that it is spread by blood.

- Sharing needles, syringes, cookers, cotton, water, water glasses, or other containers used for rinsing needles can spread the hepatitis C virus from one person to another.

Shooting drugs is the main risk factor for infection with HCV. Hepatitis C is a life-threatening disease:

- Most people who become infected with HCV develop chronic or long-term hepatitis C.

- Hepatitis C can lead to scarring of the liver, liver cancer, and death.

- Most people who are infected with HCV don't know that they are sick. You can feel fine and still be infected with the hepatitis C virus.

What Can You Do?

Get Tested

Ask your doctor about a hepatitis C test or contact your syringe exchange, harm reduction, or drug treatment program. Your test result is usually available within a few days.

If the test shows that you have hepatitis C, you can:

- Get counseling about what to do next. There are treatment options that can help you.
- Learn how to prevent the spread of HCV to other people.
- Learn how to protect yourself from more harm, by not drinking alcohol and getting vaccinated against hepatitis A and B.

Get Safe

There is no vaccine to prevent hepatitis C, but you can reduce your risk:

- Don't share works (needles, syringes, cookers, cotton, water, water glasses, or other containers used to rinse needles).
- Limit your exposure and the exposure of others to blood. HCV may be found in blood, in syringes, on cookers, on tourniquets (the belt, or whatever you use to tie up before injections), and on other surfaces.
- Soak works in full-strength bleach for ten minutes and then rinse this equipment in water to remove bleach thoroughly. If bleach is not available to you, you can use rubbing alcohol.
- Wear a latex condom during sex.

Get Help

If you want to cut down or stop using drugs, you have many options. Contact a drug treatment or harm reduction program that has trained counselors who can help.

How Is HCV Spread?

HCV is spread by contact with infected blood, which can occur by:

- Sharing works, including needles, syringes, cookers, cotton, water, water glasses, or other containers used to rinse needles.
- Unprotected sex with an infected partner. This does not happen often, but you should still practice safe sex to reduce your risk of HIV (the AIDS virus) and hepatitis B and C.
- Being born to an infected mother.

- Blood transfusions received before July 1992.
- Lack of sanitary conditions.
- Exposure to blood in the workplace through needlestick injuries.

HCV is not spread by:

- Sharing eating utensils or drinking glasses
- Casual contact
- Breast feeding
- Sneezing
- Food or water
- Coughing
- Hugging or kissing

What Are the Symptoms?

Most people with hepatitis C do not have symptoms and they can be infected with HCV and feel fine for many years.

When symptoms do occur with hepatitis C, they feel like the flu and can include:

- Yellowing of the skin (jaundice)
- Tiredness
- Nausea and vomiting
- Diarrhea
- Abdominal pain
- Loss of appetite
- Dark urine, light-colored stool

What Else Do You Need to Know?

There are two other forms of viral hepatitis that you need to know about, that can be prevented by vaccines.

Hepatitis A

- Hepatitis A is very common among people who shoot drugs.

- Hepatitis A is an infectious disease of the liver caused by the hepatitis A virus (HAV). HAV is found in stool and is spread when infected stool gets in the mouth.

- Hepatitis A usually lasts for about three to six weeks, but it makes some people sick for several months.

- Adults who become infected with HAV can become extremely ill, but usually recover with no serious, long-term health problems.

Hepatitis B

- Hepatitis B is very common among people who shoot drugs.

- The hepatitis B virus (HBV) can be spread by having sex with an infected person or by sharing needles or injection equipment with an infected person.

- Most adults fight off infection with HBV, but it becomes chronic (lifelong) in 6 percent of adults.

- Chronic infection with HBV can cause severe liver disease, including scarring of the liver (cirrhosis), liver cancer, and death.

Get Vaccinated

People who shoot drugs should be vaccinated against hepatitis A and hepatitis B. Ask your doctor about getting vaccinated.

Chapter 10

Preventing Hepatitis

This infectious virus is complex—it comes in three primary forms in the United States (A, B, and C) and two less prevalent forms (D and E). Yet there is much you can do to help prevent hepatitis. Safe and effective vaccines exist to prevent Hepatitis A and B. Although hepatitis C does not have a vaccine yet, there are ways to reduce the risk of getting it. Today, about four million people in the United States are afflicted with chronic hepatitis.

Preventing Hepatitis A (HAV)

Vaccinate

Immunization of children (two to eighteen years of age) consists of two or three doses of the vaccine. Adults need a booster dose six to twelve months following the initial dose of vaccine. The vaccine is thought to be effective for at least fifteen to twenty years. Vaccines to prevent HAV infection prior to exposure provide protection against the virus as early as two to four weeks after vaccination.

Other people who should be vaccinated include:

- Users of illegal injected drugs.

- Restaurant workers and food handlers.

- Young people living in dorms or in close contact with others.
- Children living in communities that have high rates of hepatitis.
- Children and workers in daycare centers.
- People engaging in anal/oral sex.
- People with chronic liver disease.
- If you eat raw shellfish frequently, ask your physician about being vaccinated.
- Laboratory workers who handle live hepatitis A virus.

Common Sense Hygiene

Hands should be washed with soap and water following bowel movements and before food preparation.

Traveler Precautions

People who travel to developing countries where sanitary conditions are poor should receive temporary immunity (less than three months) by having immune globulin (IG) administered intramuscularly. For those exposed to HAV, IG should be given as soon as possible and no later than two weeks after initial exposure.

Preventing Hepatitis B (HBV)

Vaccinate

Safe and effective vaccines can prevent HBV. Vaccines provide protection against hepatitis B for fifteen years and possibly much longer. Currently, the Center for Disease Control recommends that all newborns, infants, and eleven- and twelve-year-olds be vaccinated. Two or three injections over a six- to twelve-month period are required to provide full protection.

Newborns exposed to HBV at birth by an infected mother should receive HBIG plus the hepatitis B vaccine within twelve hours of birth and two additional doses of vaccine at one and six to twelve months of age.

All children and adolescents should be vaccinated since most cases of HBV occur in sexually active young adults. Those who engage in high-risk behaviors should be vaccinated as well.

Everyone who handles blood or blood products in their daily work should be vaccinated.

Practice Safe Sex

Use latex condoms. If you have hepatitis, or if you have more than one sex partner within a six-month period, you should consider vaccination. Unvaccinated individuals who have been exposed to HBV-infected persons through unprotected sex or contact with infected blood or body fluids should receive an intramuscular injection of hepatitis B immune globulin (HBIG) within fourteen days of exposure and the hepatitis B vaccine.

Don't Share!

If you are a user of injected drugs, never share drug needles, cocaine straws, or any drug paraphernalia. No one should share anything that could have an infected person's blood on it (e.g., toothbrush, razor, nail clipper, body piercing instruments).

Handle Blood Spills Correctly

If there is a blood spill, even a small one, wipe it up with a 10 percent solution of household bleach (believed to kill the virus).

Preventing Hepatitis C (HCV)

There is no vaccine to prevent HCV. Vaccines for Hepatitis A and B do not provide immunity against hepatitis C (although they should be taken if you get Hepatitis C). In addition, the source of HCV infection remains a mystery in about 10 percent of the cases. That means preventive measures are your first line of defense against HCV.

Preventive actions for HCV are the same as for hepatitis B.

Hepatitis A Vaccination

Is the hepatitis A vaccine safe and effective?

The HAV vaccine, made from inactive hepatitis A virus (synthetic), is highly effective in preventing the hepatitis A infection when given prior to exposure. However, its safety when given during pregnancy has not been determined.

What are the vaccine's restrictions?

Currently, the hepatitis A vaccine is not licensed for children under two years of age in the United States.

Who should be vaccinated against hepatitis A?

Since just about anyone is a candidate to get hepatitis A, it would not be inappropriate for every American older than two to be vaccinated. Those at higher risk for hepatitis A are: users of illegal drugs; individuals who have chronic liver disease or blood clotting disorders (e.g., hemophilia); those who have close physical contact with people who live in areas with poor sanitary conditions; those who travel or work in developing countries (this includes all countries except northern and western Europe, Japan, Australia, New Zealand, and North America except Mexico); men who have sex with other men; and children in populations that have repeated epidemics of hepatitis A (e.g., Alaska natives, American Indians, and certain closed religious communities).

What is the dosage regimen?

Recommended dosages and schedules vary with the patient's age and which specific vaccine is used. Whether you are a child over two or an adult, more than one shot is needed for long-term protection. Check with your doctor or nurse to determine how many shots are needed and when to return for the next dose. The vaccine provides protection for about four weeks after the first injection; a second injection protects you longer, possibly up to twenty years.

Hepatitis B Vaccination

Is the hepatitis B vaccine safe and effective?

Yes. The hepatitis B vaccine has been available since 1982. Use of hepatitis B vaccine and other vaccines is strongly endorsed by the medical, scientific, and public health communities as a safe and effective way to prevent disease and death. Hepatitis B vaccines have been shown to be very safe when given to infants, children, and adults. There is no confirmed evidence that indicates that hepatitis B vaccine can cause chronic illnesses.

Could vaccinations eradicate hepatitis B?

Eradication of hepatitis B is possible through a comprehensive vaccination program. The way to do this is to make sure all newborns and children under nineteen are vaccinated against HBV.

Who should be vaccinated?

All newborns and children up to the age of nineteen, especially adoptees. All individuals living in the same household with a chronically infected individual. Those who are in positions where they are exposed to blood at work or through drug use, or who have multiple sex partners. Individuals with hepatitis C and other chronic liver diseases.

Why is it so important to vaccinate children against hepatitis B?

Parents and guardians are encouraged to have their children vaccinated at an early age to prevent the serious complications that can occur when youngsters under the age of five are infected. HBV, a sexually transmitted disease, is one hundred times more infectious than HIV (the virus that causes AIDS), so teens must be given the HBV vaccine!

What is the Vaccines for Children Program?

The Vaccines for Children Program provides free hepatitis B vaccines to young people under the age of nineteen years who are on Medicaid, who have no insurance, or whose insurance does not cover immunizations.

Can the babies of infected mothers be vaccinated?

Yes. All newborns, especially those whose moms are HBV-infected, should get three vaccination shots for hepatitis B—the first within twelve hours of birth, the second at one to two months, and the third at six months. All women should be screened with the hepatitis B surface antigen test during early pregnancy to determine if they are a carrier (chronically infected) of HBV. It is safe to vaccinate pregnant women. In addition, babies born to infected mothers should receive a shot called H-BIG within twelve hours of delivery. Without the above intervention, 90 percent of babies born to infected mothers will become chronically infected, reducing their life expectancies.

What is the dosage regimen?

HBV vaccines require three injections to obtain long-lasting immunity. Hepatitis B vaccine is given as an intramuscular injection,

141

and can be given to children at the same time as other vaccinations. It can be given in a number of schedules, each of which provides excellent protection. For infants, vaccination can begin at birth. A second dose at one month of age and the third dose at six months of age may be given. The hepatitis B vaccine is also marketed in combination with *Haemophilus influenza* type b (Hib). Check with your physician for proper timing and doses.

About Hepatitis Foundation International

Hepatitis Foundation International (HFI) provides educational materials and training to the public, patients, health educators, and medical professionals about the prevention, diagnosis, and treatment of viral hepatitis, and also provides support to hepatitis patients and researchers. HFI has a variety of materials available through its Liver Wellness/Hepatitis Education program, including the following:

- Videos for lending libraries
- Brochures on liver wellness and hepatitis
- Posters on hepatitis prevention
- Workplace programs
- Teacher and parent information
- Coloring books for children

For more information contact:

Hepatitis Foundation International
504 Blick Drive
Silver Spring, MD 20904-2901
Phone: 301-622-4200
Toll-Free Hotline: 800-891-0707
Fax: 301-622-4702
Website: http://www.HepFI.org

Chapter 11

Vaccinations for Hepatitis

Candidates for Hepatitis A Vaccination

Routine Vaccination

- Children living in areas with high incidence rates of hepatitis A (above the national average). Check with your health department to see if this applies to your area.

High-Risk Populations

- Travelers to developing countries with high rates of hepatitis A, including Mexico
- Men who have sex with men
- Users of illegal drugs
- People who work with hepatitis A virus in research settings
- People who work with infected nonhuman primates
- Recipients of clotting factor concentrates
- People with chronic liver disease (because of risk of fulminant hepatitis A)

Reprinted from "Vaccinations for Hepatitis A and B," National Institute of Diabetes and Digestive and Kidney Diseases, National Institutes of Health, NIH Publication No. 04-425, February 2004.

Table 11.1. Doses and Schedules: Hepatitis A

Havrix[a]

Age: Children age 2 to 18 years

Number of Doses	2
Schedule	0 and 6 to 12 months
Dose	720 ELISA units (0.5 mL)

Age: Adults 18 years and older

Number of Doses	2
Schedule	0 and 6 to 12 months
Dose	1440 ELISA units (1.0 mL)

Vaqta[b]

Age: Children age 2 to 17 years

Number of Doses	2
Schedule	0 and 6 to 18 months
Dose	25 units (0.5 mL)

Age: Adults 17 years and older

Number of Doses	2
Schedule	0 and 6 months
Dose	50 units (1.0 mL)

[a]Inactivated vaccine. Manufactured by SmithKline Beecham Biologicals.

[b]Inactivated vaccine. Manufactured by Merck & Company, Inc.

Postexposure Prophylaxis

Immune globulin (IG) can provide temporary immunity to hepatitis A when given within two weeks of exposure to the hepatitis A virus. The dose is 0.02 mL/kg injected into the gluteal muscle in adults or the anterolateral thigh muscle in children under two years. Concurrent hepatitis A vaccination may also be appropriate in people two years and older. IG protects against the hepatitis A virus for three to five months, depending on dosage.

Candidates for Hepatitis B Vaccination

Routine Vaccination

- All infants, children, and adolescents

High-Risk Populations

- People with multiple sex partners and those who have been recently diagnosed with a sexually transmitted disease

Table 11.2. Doses and Schedules: Hepatitis B

Age: Infants with HBsAg-negative mother
Number of Doses — 3
Schedule — 0 to 2, 1 to 4, and 6 to 18 months
Dose Recombivax HB[a] — 5.0 µg (0.5 mL)
Dose Energix-B[b] — 10 µg (0.5 mL)

Age: Infants with HBsAg-positive mother
Number of Doses — 3
Schedule — Hepatitis B immune globulin and vaccination within 12 hours of birth, then vaccine at 1 to 2 and 6 months
Dose Recombivax HB[a] — 5.0 µg (0.5 mL)
Dose Energix-B[b] — 10 µg (0.5 mL)

Age: Children and adolescents age 1 to 19 years
Number of Doses — 3
Schedule — 0, 1 to 2, and 4 to 6 months
Dose Recombivax HB[a] — 5.0 µg (0.5 mL)
Dose Energix-B[b] — 10 µg (0.5 mL)

Age: Adolescents 11 to 15 years
Number of Doses — 2
Schedule — 0 and 4 to 6 months
Dose Recombivax HB[a] — 10 µg (1.0 mL)
Dose Energix-B[b] — N/A

Age: Adults 20 years and older
Number of Doses — 3
Schedule — 0, 1 to 2, and 4 to 6 months
Dose Recombivax HB[a] — 10 µg (1.0 mL)
Dose Energix-B[b] — 20 µg (1.0 mL)

Age: Immunocompromised adults
Number of Doses — 3
Schedule — 0, 1, and 6 months
Dose Recombivax HB[a] — 40 µg (1.0 mL)
Dose Energix-B[b] — N/A

Age: Immunocompromised adults
Number of Doses — 4
Schedule — 0, 1, 2, and 6 months
Dose Recombivax HB[a] — N/A
Dose Energix-B[b] — 40 µg (2.0 mL)

Note: There should be at least one month between the first and second doses, at least two months between the second and third doses, and at least four months between the first and third doses. For infants, the third dose should not be given before six months of age.

[a]Recombinant vaccine. Manufactured by Merck & Company, Inc.

[b]Recombinant vaccine. Manufactured by SmithKline Beecham Biologicals.

- Sex partners and household contacts of HBV carriers
- Men who have sex with men
- Household contacts of adoptees from countries with high rates of hepatitis B
- Injection drug users
- Travelers to countries with high rates of hepatitis B (staying longer than six months)
- People with occupational exposure to blood
- Clients and staff in institutions for the developmentally disabled
- Patients with chronic kidney failure (including those on chronic hemodialysis)
- Patients receiving clotting factor concentrates
- Inmates of long-term correctional facilities

Postexposure Prophylaxis

Prophylactic treatment for exposure to hepatitis B virus involves either hepatitis B immune globulin (HBIG), hepatitis B vaccine, or a combination of both. The HBIG dose equals 0.06 mL/kg. Efficacy ranges from 70 to 95 percent for different types of exposure.

Table 11.3. Prophylactic Treatment for Exposure to Hepatitis B Virus

Exposure	Treatment
Perinatal	One dose of HBIG given with the first hepatitis B vaccine dose.
Percutaneous or permucosal	HBIG and vaccination depending on vaccination and exposure status.
Sexual	HBIG with or without vaccination for exposure to acute hepatitis B; vaccination alone for chronic exposure.
Household contact	HBIG with vaccination for acute hepatitis B in infants under age twelve months; vaccination alone for chronic.

Combination Vaccine

Twinrix is a vaccine for both hepatitis A and hepatitis B. It combines two FDA-approved vaccines—Havrix, for hepatitis A, and Engerix-B, for hepatitis B. It protects individuals eighteen years of age or older against diseases caused by hepatitis A and hepatitis B viruses. The vaccine is recommended for travelers whose occupation or behavior puts them at high risk for exposure to hepatitis B virus, or who are visiting countries with a high or intermediate rate of both hepatitis viruses, as defined by the Centers for Disease Control and Prevention.

Table 11.4. Twinrix Vaccine

Age: Adults 18 years and older

Number of Doses	3
Schedule	0, 1, and 6 to 12 months
Dose	720 ELISA units (Hepatitis A), 20 µg (Hepatitis B) (1.0 mL total)

Note: Twinrix is manufactured by SmithKline Beecham Pharmaceuticals.

References

Centers for Disease Control and Prevention. Prevention of hepatitis A through active or passive immunization: recommendations of the Advisory Committee on Immunization Practices. *Morbidity and Mortality Weekly Report.* 1999; 48(RR-12).

Centers for Disease Control and Prevention. Hepatitis B virus: a comprehensive strategy for eliminating transmission in the United States through universal childhood vaccination: Recommendations of the Advisory Committee on Immunization Practices. *Morbidity and Mortality Weekly Report.* 1991; 40(RR-13).

Food and Drug Administration. 2001. New Combination Vaccine Approved for Protection against Two Hepatitis Viruses. FDA Talk Paper. Available at: www.fda.gov/bbs/topics/ANSWERS/2001/ANS01084 .html. Accessed February 9, 2004.

The U.S. Government does not endorse or favor any specific commercial product or company. Trade, proprietary, or company names appearing in this chapter are used only because they are considered necessary in the context of the information provided. If a product is not mentioned, this does not mean or imply that the product is unsatisfactory.

Chapter 12

Hepatitis Diagnosis

Chapter Contents

149

Section 12.1

Diagnosing Hepatitis: An Overview

"Diagnosis and Treatment of Viral Hepatitis" is reprinted with permission from Hepatitis Foundation International (HFI). © 2005 Hepatitis Foundation International. All rights reserved. This material is updated frequently. To view the most current information, visit http://www.hepfi.org. Additional information about HFI is included at the end of this section.

Hepatitis A (HAV)

A blood test showing the presence of IgM anti-HAV in serum confirms the diagnosis of acute hepatitis A infection. Symptoms of this virus strain include nausea, vomiting, and diarrhea. Once infected and recovered, the antibodies to the virus provide protection from future infections with HAV. Following this, HAV blood tests will always return a positive result.

Treatment of HAV

Fortunately, 99 percent of those infected will recover without treatment.

Prevention of Hepatitis A

Individuals exposed to hepatitis A through household and close personal contact (anal/oral contact) or who plan to travel to developing countries where sanitary conditions are poor can receive temporary immunity (less than three months) by inoculation with immune globulin (IG) administered intramuscularly. For those exposed to HAV, IG should be given as soon as possible and no later than two weeks after initial exposure. Vaccines to prevent HAV infection prior to exposure provide protection against the virus as early as two to four weeks after vaccination. Hands should be washed with soap and water following bowel movements and before food preparation. Immunization of children (two to eighteen years of age) and adults consists of two doses of the vaccine. The second dose is given six to twelve months following the initial dose of vaccine. The vaccine is thought to be effective for at least fifteen to twenty years.

Other individuals who should be vaccinated include: persons engaging in anal/oral sex; users of illegal injectable drugs; children living in communities that have high rates of hepatitis; certain institutional workers; workers in day-care centers; and laboratory workers who handle live hepatitis A virus. Patients with chronic liver disease and those with clotting factor disorders should be vaccinated against hepatitis A as well.

Hepatitis B (HBV)

Acute HBV infection is diagnosed by a simple blood test detecting the presence of hepatitis B surface antigen (Hbsag) and IgM antibody to hepatitis B core antigen (anti-HBc IgM). These antibodies develop in the blood in the early stages of infection at the time symptoms appear. Antibody to HBsAg (anti-HBs) develops after active infection and serves as an indicator of immunity.

- Anti-HBs +: Indicates individual has been vaccinated, has received immune globulin, is immune, or is an infant who has received antibodies from its mother.

- Anti-HBc +: Indicates past or present infection and lasts indefinitely. Also may be detected in someone who has received immune globulin or an infant who has received antibodies from its mother.

- IgM anti-HBc +: Indicates recent infection with HBV, usually within four to six months.

- HBeAg +: Indicates active viral replication and high infectivity.

- HBsAg +: Indicates acute or chronic HBV. Persistence for six months after acute infection indicates progression to chronic HBV.

Treatment for HBV

While there is no treatment for acute hepatitis B, there are three approved treatments for chronic hepatitis B: interferon alfa-2b and lamivudine, and adefovir dipivoxil. Only patients with active HBV replication are candidates. About 35 percent of patients treated with injections of interferon for four to six months will have a long-term response. The response to oral lamivudine, given for at least one year, may be somewhat lower. Lamivudine is very well tolerated but viral resistance to treatment may occur. Adefovir dipivoxil is less likely to induce resistance but, like lamivudine, must usually be given for prolonged periods. Interferon therapy often results in a number of side effects, including flu-like symptoms, fatigue, headache, nausea and vomiting, loss of appetite, depression, and hair thinning. Because interferon may depress the bone marrow, blood tests are needed to monitor white blood cells, platelets. Liver enzymes are monitored during treatment. Patients with chronic hepatitis B should be vaccinated against hepatitis A.

Prevention of Hepatitis B

Safe and effective vaccines provide protection against hepatitis B for at least fifteen to twenty years and possibly much longer. Three injections over a six- to twelve-month period are usually required to provide full protection. All children and young adults should be vaccinated since most cases of HBV occur in sexually active young adults. Those who engage in high-risk behaviors should be vaccinated as well.

Unvaccinated individuals who have been exposed to HBV-infected persons through unprotected sex or contact with infected blood or body fluids should receive an intramuscular injection of hepatitis B immune globulin (HBIG) within fourteen days of exposure and the hepatitis B vaccine. Newborns exposed to HBV at birth by an infected mother should receive HBIG plus the hepatitis B vaccine within twelve hours of birth and two additional doses of vaccine at one and six to twelve months of age. Infected individuals should practice safe sex. Avoiding contact with infected blood or other body fluids directly or on objects such as needles, razors, toothbrushes, etc. may reduce the risk of transmission. Sores and rashes should be covered with bandages and blood on any surface should be cleaned up with household bleach.

Hepatitis C (HCV)

Infection by the hepatitis C virus can be determined by a blood test that detects HCV antibodies in the blood. This test is not a part of a routine physical, and people must ask their doctor for the hepatitis C test. If the initial test is positive, a second test should be done to confirm the diagnosis and liver enzymes (a blood test) should be measured. Anti-HCV may not be present in the first four weeks of infection in about 30 percent of patients. HCV infection may be identified by the presence of anti-HCV in approximately 60 percent of people as early as five to eight weeks after exposure. In some individuals HCV antibodies may not be detected for five to twelve months. HCV-RNA and RT-PCR tests can determine HCV presence in as little as one to two weeks after infection.

About 55–85 percent of infections become chronic, which means liver inflammation persists for six months or more after the initial acute infection. The enzymes alanine aminotransferase (ALT) and aspartate aminotransferase (AST) are released when liver cells are injured or die, but they do not reliably predict the severity of the liver injury. Elevated ALT and AST levels may appear and disappear throughout the course of the infection. Current tests can indicate that the infection is chronic (infections that do not clear up within six months). High ALT and AST levels reveal ongoing liver damage but liver damage my progress even if these levels are normal. A liver biopsy can determine the severity of the disease. The disease may gradually progress over a period of ten to forty years.

Treatment for Hepatitis C

Currently, pegylated interferon combined with ribavirin is used to treat hepatitis C. Selection of patients for treatment may be determined by virologic, biochemical, and when necessary, liver biopsy findings, rather than presence or absence of symptoms. Interferon is given by injection, and may have a number of side effects including flu-like symptoms including headaches, fever, fatigue, loss of appetite, nausea, vomiting, depression, and thinning of hair. It may also interfere with the production of white blood cells and platelets by depressing the bone marrow. Periodic blood tests are required to monitor blood cells and platelets. Ribavirin can cause sudden, severe anemia, and birth defects so women should avoid pregnancy while taking it and for six months following treatment. The severity and type of side effects differ for each individual. Treatment of children with HCV is not currently approved but is under investigation.

Permanent clearance of HCV can be achieved in 45 to 85 percent of treated patients.

Currently, almost one half of all liver transplants in the United States are performed for end-stage hepatitis C. However, reinfection of the transplanted liver by HCV occurs at a high rate and progressive liver disease may recur.

Anyone with hepatitis C should be vaccinated against hepatitis A and B and should not drink alcohol.

Try to maintain as normal a life as possible by eating a well-balanced diet, drinking plenty of fluids, exercising, and keeping a positive attitude. Avoid depressing or overwhelming tasks and learn how to pace yourself. Rest when you feel tired. Plan physically exhausting tasks in the morning when your energy level is at its peak.

Hepatitis D (HDV)

A positive test for anti-HDV in a patient with acute hepatitis B indicates HBV/ HDV co-infection. Patients with chronic hepatitis B and a positive HDV test are super-infected.

Treatment for Hepatitis D

Interferon alfa-2b treatments may be beneficial to a small proportion of patients. Vaccination against HBV will prevent HDV.

Hepatitis E (HEV)

Testing for anti-HEV is usually reserved for returning travelers from the developing world in whom hepatitis is present but other hepatitis viruses cannot be detected. Currently there is no treatment for HEV. A vaccine for HEV is under development.

About Hepatitis Foundation International

Hepatitis Foundation International (HFI) provides educational materials and training to the public, patients, health educators, and medical professionals about the prevention, diagnosis, and treatment of viral hepatitis, and also provides support to hepatitis patients and researchers. HFI has a variety of materials available through its Liver Wellness/Hepatitis Education program, including the following:

- Videos for lending libraries
- Brochures on liver wellness and hepatitis
- Posters on hepatitis prevention
- Workplace programs
- Teacher and parent information
- Coloring books for children

For more information contact:

Hepatitis Foundation International
504 Blick Drive
Silver Spring, MD 20904-2901
Phone: 301-622-4200
Toll-Free Hotline: 800-891-0707
Fax: 301-622-4702
Website: http://www.HepFI.org

Section 12.2

Hepatitis Virus Test

Reprinted from "Hepatitis Virus Test or Panel," © 2005 A.D.A.M., Inc.
Reprinted with permission.

Alternative Names

Hepatitis A antibody test; Hepatitis B antibody test; Hepatitis C antibody test; Hepatitis D antibody test

Definition

Hepatitis virus blood tests detect the presence of antibodies to viruses that cause the disease hepatitis (inflammation of the liver). The tests are specific to Hepatitis A, Hepatitis B, or Hepatitis C viruses. A "panel" of tests can be used to screen blood samples for more than one kind of hepatitis virus at the same time.

How the Test Is Performed

Blood is drawn from a vein on the inside of the elbow or the back of the hand. The puncture site is cleaned with antiseptic, and an elastic band is placed around the upper arm to apply pressure and restrict blood flow through the vein. This causes veins below the band to fill with blood.

155

A needle is inserted into the vein, and the blood is collected in an airtight vial or a syringe. During the procedure, the band is removed to restore circulation. Once the blood has been collected, the needle is removed and the puncture site is covered to stop any bleeding.

For an infant or young child, the area is cleansed with antiseptic and punctured with a sharp needle or a lancet. The blood may be collected in a pipette (small glass tube), on a slide, onto a test strip, or into a small container. Cotton or a bandage may be applied to the puncture site if there is any continued bleeding.

How the Test Will Feel

When the needle is inserted to draw blood, some people feel moderate pain, while others feel only a prick or stinging sensation. Afterward, there may be some throbbing.

Why the Test Is Performed

These tests are performed to detect infection by hepatitis-causing viruses. Hepatitis is an inflammation of the liver. Three common viruses can cause hepatitis—the viruses are called Hepatitis A, Hepatitis B, and Hepatitis C.

Hepatitis A virus (HAV) is usually spread when something contaminated with infected stool is placed in the mouth. It has an incubation period of two to six weeks.

Hepatitis B virus (HBV) is most frequently transmitted by blood contact, but can also be transmitted through other body fluids. HBV can cause a severe and unrelenting form of hepatitis ending in liver failure and death. The incidence of HBV is higher among blood transfusion recipients, male homosexuals, dialysis patients, organ transplant patients, and IV drug users. It has a long incubation period (five weeks to six months).

The Hepatitis B virus is made up of an inner core surrounded by an outer capsule. The outer capsule contains a protein called HBsAg (Hep B surface antigen). The inner core contains HBcAg (Hep B core antigen). A third protein called HBeAg is also found within the core. In addition to detecting Hepatitis B virus itself, tests can detect antibodies a patient has made to these antigens. The antibodies are called HBsAb, HBcAb, and HBeAb.

Hepatitis C virus (HCV) is transmitted in a manner similar to Hepatitis B. The incubation period is two to twelve weeks after exposure. The symptoms and course of the illness are similar to HBV.

Hepatitis D only causes disease when Hepatitis B is also present. It is not routinely checked on a hepatitis antibody panel.

Normal Values

No presence of antibodies (a negative test) is normal.

What Abnormal Results Mean

Serology tests have been developed to detect the presence of antibodies to each of the hepatitis viruses in serum. IgM antibodies appear three to four weeks after exposure and usually return to normal in about eight weeks. IgG antibodies appear about two weeks after the IgM antibodies start to increase; such antibodies may persist forever.

If the IgM antibody is elevated in the absence of IgG antibody, acute hepatitis is suspected. If IgG antibody is increased, but not IgM antibody, a convalescent or chronic state is likely.

Positive tests may indicate:

- Hepatitis A
- Hepatitis B
- Hepatitis C
- chronic Hepatitis B or Hepatitis B carrier state
- Hepatitis D, when found in conjunction with Hepatitis B

Additional conditions under which the test may be performed:

- chronic persistent hepatitis
- delta agent (Hepatitis D)
- nephrotic syndrome

What the Risks Are

The risks associated with having blood drawn are:

- Excessive bleeding
- Fainting or feeling light-headed
- Hematoma (blood accumulating under the skin)
- Infection (a slight risk any time the skin is broken)

- Multiple punctures to locate veins

Special Considerations

Veins and arteries vary in size from one patient to another and from one side of the body to the other. Obtaining a blood sample from some people may be more difficult than from others.

Chapter 13

Hepatitis and Liver Cancer Risk

Why do cancers often form in the liver?

Because the liver filters blood from all parts of the body, cancer cells can lodge in the liver and develop into metastatic nodules. Cancers that begin in the gastrointestinal tract often spread to the liver. The immense regenerative capacity of the liver may also be linked to the development of liver cancers. Researchers have speculated that the repetitive divisions that result in liver regeneration may trigger the expression of cancer-promoting genes.

What causes liver cancer?

A gamut of carcinogens may play a role in the development of cancer in humans. Carcinogens bind covalently to DNA, linking the cancer development to the host's inability to repair the DNA or to be tolerant to the carcinogen. Certain toxins and chemicals may be specifically associated with cancer of the liver.

Aflatoxin, a poison produced by the mold *Aspergillus flavus*, can contaminate stored foods such as peanuts, grains, and cassava, especially in tropical areas. As well, prolonged exposure to polyvinyl chloride used in manufacturing plastics can give rise to a rare liver cancer called angiosarcoma, which involves the liver blood vessels. Viruses can also be carcinogenic. Hepatitis B virus can act as a co-carcinogen with aflatoxin in promoting liver cancer, and hepatitis C virus is becoming increasingly linked to liver cancer. Cirrhosis of the liver may also lead to liver cancer.

How are liver cancers classified?

Liver cancer classification is based on the cell of origin that becomes cancerous and whether the tumor resulting is benign (relatively harmless) or malignant (capable of spreading from the liver and thus more serious). The plethora of cancers found in the liver are either primary, arising from liver cells, or secondary, originating elsewhere in the body. Primary cancers can be benign or malignant. Secondary cancers are referred to as metastatic because the cancers metastasize or spread from their origin to the liver.

What is the incidence of primary and secondary tumors?

Primary liver cancers account for less than 1 percent of all cancers in North America whereas in Africa, Southeast Asia, and China, up to 50 percent of cancers are of this type. Higher incidence of people carrying the hepatitis B virus and having liver cirrhosis may account for this geographic discrepancy. Secondary liver cancers are thirty times more prevalent than primary liver cancers.

What common symptoms are associated with liver cancer?

Common symptoms of liver cancer include weight loss, appetite loss, lethargy, abdominal pain, jaundice, fluid in the abdomen, and health deterioration.

What are the risk factors associated with benign primary liver tumors?

The risk factors associated with benign primary liver tumors include, but are not limited to, the following:

- hepatitis B
- hepatitis C
- aflatoxin ingestion
- cirrhosis

What therapy is undertaken for benign primary tumors?

The majority of these tumors are asymptomatic and can be detected by ultrasound (US) or computed tomography (CT). Small tumors of this type may not require any specific therapy. If the tumors are large, there may be some abdominal pain due to blood clotting and pressure exerted on neighboring organs. In this case, resection of the liver is recommended. Cavernous hemangiomas, the most commonly occurring benign primary tumor, may enlarge in women taking hormone pills, such as contraceptives or menopause-regulating hormones. Women should be aware of the possibility of developing tumors with prolonged use of hormone pills and have abdominal examinations regularly.

What are the risk factors associated with malignant primary tumors?

The risk factors associated with malignant primary tumors of the liver include the following:

- chronic carriers of hepatitis B virus, especially those with chronic hepatitis B

- chronic hepatitis C virus infection (recent evidence suggests that it may be a more important contributing factor than hepatitis B)

- cirrhosis of the liver (although alcohol is perhaps not a direct carcinogen, cirrhosis resulting from alcoholism increases the incidence of hepatocellular carcinoma)

- aflatoxin ingestion

- hemochromatosis (iron overload) is a risk factor once cirrhosis has developed

- alpha-1-antitrypsin deficiency and tyrosinemia (congenital disorders)

- increased fatty acid oxidation by extramitochondrial pathways (increases hydrogen peroxide and thus oxidative stress)

- mutations in the p53 tumor suppressor gene (noted in tumors from Africa and Southeast Asia and linked to an increase in aflatoxin intake)

- sex (hepatocellular carcinomas are three times more prevalent in males than in females worldwide, perhaps due to an increase in hepatitis B incidence in males)

How are malignant tumors detected?

Common medical procedures for detecting malignant tumors of the liver include:

- periodic use of abdominal ultrasound (in high-risk patients)
- alpha-fetoprotein blood tumor test
- computer tomography scan (CT)
- magnetic resonance imaging (MRI)
- angiography
- needle liver biopsy
- high levels of serum vitamin B_{12}, ferritin, bilirubin, and sodium

Can malignant tumors be treated?

The prognosis for hepatocellular carcinoma depends on the stage and speed of tumor growth. Survival rates generally decrease as the tumor size increases. Most treatments are palliative. They attempt to maintain the patient's quality of life. Treatments may include chemotherapy, chemoembolization, radiotherapy, injection of absolute alcohol into the tumor, and resection or transplantation when possible.

What about secondary liver tumors?

The liver is involved in approximately one-third of all cancers and often those that begin in the gastrointestinal tract, colon, pancreas, stomach, breast, and lung. The risk factors involved in this type of liver cancer are numerous, given that the cancers originate elsewhere. Detection can be by ultrasound, CT, or MRI. The prognosis for patients with secondary liver tumors depends on the primary site of malignancy. In general, patients do not live longer than one year from the diagnosis of hepatic metastases. Chosen treatments are based on those that most slow the tumor growth with the least undesirable side effects. Treatments remain unsatisfactory but include chemotherapy, immunotherapy, and embolization.

What is the future for liver cancer treatment?

The available techniques that combat liver cancer serve to extend and maintain the patient's quality of life. Only when the tumor is small and limited to one lobe of the liver can surgical removal offer a cure. The success rate of liver transplantation for liver cancer, 20 to 30 percent, somewhat limits it as a viable treatment. Recent studies have shown that the combined therapies of transplantation and chemotherapy can offer 50 to 60 percent survival, but prevention is the best route of all. Control of viral hepatitis infection and better agricultural storage will help reduce the incidence of liver cancer.

Part Three

Hepatitis A Virus (HAV)

Chapter 14

HAV: What You Need to Know

What is hepatitis A?

Hepatitis A is a liver disease.
Hepatitis makes your liver swell and stops it from working right.
You need a healthy liver. The liver does many things to keep you alive. The liver fights infections and stops bleeding. It removes drugs and other poisons from your blood. The liver also stores energy for when you need it.

What causes hepatitis A?

Hepatitis A is caused by a virus. A virus is a germ that causes sickness. (For example, the flu is caused by a virus.) People can pass viruses to each other. The virus that causes hepatitis A is called the hepatitis A virus.

How could I get hepatitis A?

Hepatitis A is spread by close personal contact with someone else who has the infection.
You could also get hepatitis A by:

- eating food that has been prepared by someone with hepatitis A.

Reprinted from "What I Need to Know about Hepatitis A," National Institute of Diabetes and Digestive and Kidney Diseases, National Institutes of Health, NIH Publication No. 04-4244, December 2003.

- drinking water that has been contaminated by hepatitis A (in parts of the world with poor hygiene and sanitary conditions).

Who can get hepatitis A?

Anyone can get hepatitis A, but some people are more likely to than others:

- people who live with someone who has hepatitis A
- children who go to daycare
- people who work in a daycare center
- men who have sex with men
- people who travel to other countries where hepatitis A is common

What are the symptoms?

Hepatitis A can make you feel like you have the flu. You might:

- feel tired.
- feel sick to your stomach.
- have a fever.
- not want to eat.
- have stomach pain.
- have diarrhea.

Some people have:

- dark yellow urine.
- light-colored stools.
- yellowish eyes and skin.

Some people don't have any symptoms.

If you have symptoms or think you might have hepatitis A, go to a doctor. The doctor will test your blood.

How is hepatitis A treated?

Most people who have hepatitis A get well on their own after a few weeks.

You may need to rest in bed for several days or weeks, and you won't be able to drink alcohol until you are well. The doctor may give you medicine for your symptoms.

How can I protect myself?

You can get the hepatitis A vaccine.

A vaccine is a drug that you take when you are healthy that keeps you from getting sick. Vaccines teach your body to attack certain viruses, like the hepatitis A virus.

The hepatitis A vaccine is given through a shot. Children can get the vaccine after they turn two years old. Children aged two to eighteen will need three shots. The shots are spread out over a year. Adults get two or three shots over six to twelve months.

You need all of the shots to be protected. If you are traveling to other countries, make sure you get all the shots before you go. If you miss a shot, call your doctor or clinic right away to set up a new appointment.

You can protect yourself and others from hepatitis A in these ways, too:

- Always wash your hands after using the toilet and before fixing food or eating.

- Wear gloves if you have to touch other people's stool. Wash your hands afterward.

- Drink bottled water when you are in another country. (And don't use ice cubes or wash fruits and vegetables in tap water.)

Chapter 15

HAV Transmission by Food

Hepatitis A is caused by hepatitis A virus (HAV). Transmission occurs by the fecal oral route, either by direct contact with an HAV-infected person or by ingestion of HAV-contaminated food or water. Food-borne or waterborne hepatitis A outbreaks are relatively uncommon in the United States. However, food handlers with hepatitis A are frequently identified, and evaluation of the need for immunoprophylaxis and implementation of control measures are a considerable burden on public health resources. In addition, HAV-contaminated food may be the source of hepatitis A for an unknown proportion of persons whose source of infection is not identified.

Background

HAV is primarily transmitted by the fecal-oral route, either by person-to-person contact or by ingestion of contaminated food or water. Transmission also occurs after exposure to HAV-contaminated blood or blood products, but not by exposure to saliva or urine. Asymptomatic and nonjaundiced HAV-infected persons, especially children, are an important source of HAV transmission.

The incidence of hepatitis A in the United States varies in a cyclical pattern, with large increases approximately every ten years, followed

Excerpted from "Hepatitis A Transmitted by Food," Division of Viral Hepatitis, Centers for Disease Control and Prevention, March 2004. The full text of this document, including references, can be found online at http://www.cdc.gov/ncidod/diseases/hepatitis/a/fiore_ha_transmitted_by_food.pdf.

by decreases to less than the previous baseline incidence. Incidence rates in the western and southwestern United States have been consistently higher than in other regions of the United States. From 1980 through 2001, an average of 25,000 cases each year were reported to the Centers for Disease Control and Prevention (CDC), but when corrected for underreporting and asymptomatic infections, an estimated average of 263,000 HAV infections occurred per year. On the basis of surveillance data, children aged five to fourteen years historically have the highest incidence of hepatitis A, although the incidence of HAV infection is probably highest among those less than five years old. Approximately one-third of the United States population has been previously infected with HAV, with higher seroprevalence with increasing age and among persons with lower household incomes or of Hispanic ethnicity. Since 1999, the hepatitis A incidence has decreased to historic lows in the United States (CDC, unpublished data).

Risk factors for infection among reported cases are shown in Figure 15.1. Personal contact (usually among household contacts or sexual partners) is the most important reported risk factor. Relatively few reported cases (2 to 3 percent per year) are identified through

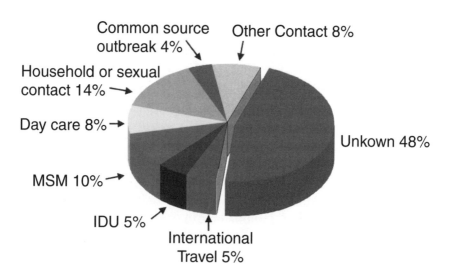

Figure 15.1. *Reported risk factors among persons with hepatitis A, United States, 1990–2000. Data are from the Viral Hepatitis Surveillance Program, Centers for Disease Control and Prevention. IDU: injection drug use; MSM: men who have sex with men.*

routine surveillance as part of common source outbreaks of disease transmitted by food or water. However, some hepatitis A transmission attributed to personal contact or other risk factors is likely to have been food-borne, occurring when an HAV-infected person contaminated food eaten by others. The proportion of sporadic cases that might be from food-borne sources is unknown but could be considerable; approximately 50 percent of reported patients with hepatitis A do not have an identified source of infection.

In developing countries, HAV transmission often is unrecognized, because most residents acquire HAV infection during early childhood. It is interesting to note that, as hygiene improves, the mean age of infected persons increases and the clinical manifestations of hepatitis A are more often recognized, leading to an increase in the hepatitis A incidence (i.e., symptomatic HAV infection), even as the incidence of HAV infection (which is commonly asymptomatic or does not cause jaundice in young children) may be decreasing. Food-borne outbreaks of infection are uncommon in developing countries because of high levels of immunity in the resident population, but food-borne transmission to nonimmune travelers might be an important source of travel-associated hepatitis A.

Characteristics of Food-Borne Transmission

HAV contamination of a food product can occur at any point during cultivation, harvesting, processing, distribution, or preparation. Recognizing food-borne transmission using routine surveillance data may be difficult because (1) case patients may have difficulty recalling food histories during the two to six weeks before illness, (2) cases may accrue gradually or not be reported, (3) a food item may be focally contaminated, (4) some exposed persons have unrecognized HAV infection, (5) some exposed persons have preexisting immunity (from a previous infection or previous vaccination), (6) persons who acquire infection through contaminated food are not recognized amid an ongoing high incidence in the community, and (7) cases are geographically scattered over several public health jurisdictions.

Transmission Due to Contamination of Food at the Point of Sale or Service

The source of most reported food-borne hepatitis A outbreaks has been HAV-infected food handlers present at the point of sale (such as in a restaurant) or who prepare food for social events (such as a wedding).

171

A single HAV-infected food handler can transmit HAV to dozens or even hundreds of persons and cause a substantial economic burden to public health. The societal cost of a single food-borne outbreak of hepatitis A in Denver involving forty-three cases was estimated to be more than $800,000, with more than 90 percent of these costs borne by the public health department and attributed to immunoglobulin administration. Table 15.1 lists selected food handler–associated outbreaks. Common themes of these outbreaks include (1) the presence of an HAV-infected food handler who worked while potentially infectious (two weeks before to one week after symptom onset) and had contact with uncooked food or food after it had been cooked, (2) secondary cases among other food handlers who ate food contaminated by the index case, and (3) relatively low attack rates among exposed patrons.

Food handlers are not at higher risk of hepatitis A because of their occupation. However, food handlers may belong to demographic groups, such as young persons and persons with lower socioeconomic status, who have a higher incidence of hepatitis A than does the rest of the population. Median hourly wages for food service workers are lower than the overall median hourly wage, and nearly two of three food counter attendants are aged sixteen to nineteen years. Among 38,881 adults with hepatitis A reported to the CDC during the period of 1992–2000 who had occupational data reported, 8 percent were identified as food handlers, including 13 percent of the 3,292 persons aged sixteen to nineteen years (CDC, unpublished data). The number of patients who were food handlers reflects the number of persons employed in the industry; there were 6.5 million food and beverage serving jobs in 2000, and the industry is the largest private employer in the United States.

Most food handlers with hepatitis A do not transmit HAV to consumers or restaurant patrons, as determined on the basis of surveillance data, but many hundreds of restaurant workers have hepatitis A every year. Evaluating HAV-infected food handlers is a common task for many public health departments, and assessing the need for postexposure immunoprophylaxis and implementing control measures consumes considerable time and resources at the state and local health department level. In a retrospective analysis of HAV-infected food handler investigations conducted during 1992–2000 in Seattle/ King County, Washington, and the state of Massachusetts, 230 HAV-infected food handlers were identified. Of these, 140 (59 percent) had worked during a time when they were potentially infectious, but only 12 (7 percent) were evaluated as representing an infection risk to those who ate food they had prepared; an average of 377 doses of immunoglobulin were dispensed by public health personnel in each episode.

Coworkers of the infected food handlers were given immunoglobulin in 121 investigations (51 percent; CDC, unpublished data).

Transmission Due to Contamination of Food during Growing, Harvesting, Processing, or Distribution

Hepatitis A outbreaks have been also associated with consumption of fresh produce contaminated with HAV during cultivation, harvesting, processing, or distribution (Table 15.2). Outbreaks involving a food item that was contaminated before distribution are particularly challenging to identify and might be widely distributed geographically. For example, HAV-contaminated frozen strawberries were implicated as the source of an outbreak involving at least 262 persons in five states. Low attack rates are common, probably because contamination is found in only a small portion of the distributed food. Additional cases might be prevented by rapid epidemiologic identification of the contaminated item, traceback, and product recall.

Experimental contamination studies suggest that the physical characteristics of some produce items might facilitate transmission. Lettuce, carrots, and fennel were immersed in HAV-contaminated water for twenty minutes followed by refrigerated storage; infectious HAV was recovered from lettuce for nine days after immersion, but it was recovered from carrots and fennel for only four to seven days. Washing reduced but did not eliminate detectable HAV. No investigation to date has determined the point in cultivation, harvesting, or processing at which contamination occurs. Produce might be contaminated by the hands of HAV-infected workers or children in the field, by contact with HAV-contaminated water during irrigation or rinsing after picking, or during the processing steps leading to packaging. Removal of stems by workers in the field during picking might be a potential mechanism for strawberry contamination. Green onions require extensive handling during harvesting and preparation for packing and receive no further processing until they reach the restaurant or the consumer's home, where they are often served raw or partially cooked. Recent large outbreaks associated with imported green onions that were contaminated before arrival in restaurants indicate a need for a better understanding of how contamination of fresh produce occurs and why certain produce items (e.g., strawberries and green onions) seem particularly prone to contamination.

HAV-contaminated shellfish have been the source of food-borne outbreaks of hepatitis A, including several outbreaks involving many thousands of cases (Table 15.3). Although reports of shellfish-related

Table 15.1. Characteristics of Selected Published Food-Borne Hepatitis A Outbreaks in the United States Associated with an Infected Food Handler

Year	Location	No. of Infected Persons	Contaminated Food	Symptoms while Working	Reason Ig Not Given[a]	Coworkers Infected	Identified Hepatitis A Risk Factor of Food Handler
1968	Bakery	61	Pastry icing	Vomiting, dark urine	Unknown	None	Not reported
1974	Cafeteria	133	Salad, fresh fruit	Diarrhea, vomiting	Food handling not initially reported	"Several"	Personal contact with another case patient
1973	Cafeteria	44	Sandwiches	None	Index case patient did not seek medical care	4	Household contact with another case patient
1974	Restaurant	107	Sandwiches	Malaise, vomiting	Diagnosis delayed	3	Household contact with another case patient
1975	Cafeteria	22	Multiple foods	Fatigue, nausea, vomiting	Unknown	5	Unknown
1975	Restaurant	33	Salads	None	Unknown	13	Unknown
1979	Cafeteria	30	Sandwiches	Back pain, "kidney infection"	Index case patient did not seek medical care	None	Not reported
1981	Cafeteria	37	Sandwiches	Jaundice, lethargy	Not reported to health department	None	Not reported
1986	Restaurant	103	Salad	Vomiting, dark urine	Index case patient did not seek medical care	5	MSM

Table 15.1. Characteristics of Selected Published Food-Borne Hepatitis A Outbreaks in the United States Associated with an Infected Food Handler (*continued*)

Year	Location	No. of Infected Persons	Contaminated Food	Symptoms while Working	Reason Ig Not Given[a]	Coworkers Infected	Identified Hepatitis A Risk Factor of Food Handler
1988	Restaurant	54	Multiple foods	Diarrhea	Unknown	None	Injection drug user
1990	Restaurant	110	Salads	Not reported	Food handling not initially reported	4	Not reported
1991	2 Restaurants	228	Sandwiches	None	Assessed as low risk	None	Not reported
1992	Restaurant	11	Sandwiches	Nausea, vomiting, diarrhea	Delayed diagnosis	None	Not reported
1992	Caterer	43	Multiple foods	None	Assessed as low risk	9	Not reported
1994	Caterer	91	Multiple foods	Gastroenteritis	Assessed as low risk	None	Not reported
1994	Bakery	64	Glazed baked goods	Diarrhea	Index case patient did not seek medical care	9	Not reported
2001	Restaurant	43	Sandwiches	None; food handler had a colostomy	Assessed as low risk	None	Not reported

Note: IG, immunoglobulin; MSM, man who has sex with men.

[a]To exposed persons within two weeks of last exposure.

Table 15.2. Characteristics of Selected Published Food-Borne Hepatitis A Outbreaks Associated with Produce Contaminated during Growing, Harvesting, or Processing

Year	No. of Infected Persons	Implicated Food	No. and Location of Sites	Source of Implicated Food
1983	24	Frozen raspberries	Aberdeen, United Kingdom	United Kingdom
1988	202	Iceberg lettuce	3 Restaurants in Kentucky	Unknown, probably Mexico
1990	35	Frozen strawberries	2 Schools in Georgia and Montana	California
1997	262	Frozen strawberries	5 States	Mexico
1998	43	Green onions	1 Restaurant in Ohio	Mexico or California
2000	31	Green onions or tomatoes	2 Restaurants in Kentucky and Florida	Green onions: Mexico or California; tomatoes: unknown
2003	>700	Green onions	4 States	Mexico

Table 15.3. Characteristics of Selected Food-Borne Hepatitis A Outbreaks Associated with Shellfish

Year	No. of Infected Persons	Implicated Food	Location of Cases	Source of Implicated Food	Suspected Cause of Contamination
1973	278	Oysters	Texas, Georgia	Louisiana	Untreated sewage from oil platforms and fishing boats
1981	132	Cockles	19 Boroughs in the United Kingdom	United Kingdom	Sewage discharged near shellfish beds
1988	61	Oysters	Alabama, Georgia, Florida, Tennessee, Hawaii	Florida	Harvest from unapproved oyster beds near sewage treatment plant
1988	292,301	Raw clams	Shanghai, China	Qi-Dong County, China	Untreated sewage discharged near shellfish beds
1996	5,889	Mussels and clams	Puglia	Italy	Unknown
1997	444	Oysters	New South Wales, Australia	Wallis Lake, Australia	Untreated sewage
1999	184	Coquina clams	Spain	Peru	Unknown

hepatitis A outbreaks continue to occur in some other countries, none have been reported recently in the United States. Factors contributing to contamination in shellfish-related outbreaks may include inappropriate or illegal shellfish harvesting near known sources of sewage, inappropriate discharge of sewage from fishing boats or oil platforms near shellfish beds, and use of fecally contaminated water to immerse harvested live shellfish. Identification of HAV in shellfish taken from approved areas in the United States has also been reported.

Transmission Due to Exposure to Contaminated Water

Waterborne outbreaks of hepatitis A are unusual in developed countries. Water treatment processes and dilution within municipal water systems are apparently sufficient to render HAV noninfectious, although no studies have demonstrated which specific treatment processes are the most effective. Outbreaks of hepatitis A among persons who use small private or community wells or swimming pools have been reported, and contamination by adjacent septic systems has been implicated as the source of contamination. Although the potential for hepatitis A outbreaks after flooding-related sewage contamination of potable water sources is recognized, no such incidents have been reported in the United States in several decades.

Prevention of Hepatitis A

Preexposure Prophylaxis

Hepatitis A is the only common vaccine-preventable food-borne disease in the United States. Hepatitis A vaccine is an inactivated preparation of a cell-culture-adapted virus and was licensed in 1995 for persons aged two years and older. More than 95 percent of adults and children have seroconversion after a single dose of hepatitis A vaccine, and long-term protection is provided by a second (booster) dose given at least six months later. Protective concentrations of anti-HAV are measurable in 54 to 62 percent of persons by two weeks and in greater than 90 percent by four weeks after receipt of a single dose of vaccine. The vaccine's efficacy is 94 to 100 percent, and protection is likely to last for at least twenty years after vaccination. Booster doses after the primary two-dose series are not currently recommended. Recent vaccination may confuse interpretation of diagnostic test results for hepatitis A, because IgM anti-HAV can be detected in some persons shortly after vaccination. However, when tested one month after vaccination, less than 1 percent of vaccinated persons had detectable IgM anti-HAV.

Hepatitis A vaccination is recommended for people at higher risk for hepatitis A, including men who have sex with men and illicit drug users (regardless of whether they inject the drugs or not). Because recent travel to countries where HAV infection is endemic is a commonly identified risk factor among patients in the United States, persons planning travel to developing countries for any reason, frequency, or duration who can receive the first dose of vaccine at least two to four weeks before departure should also be vaccinated. Persons with chronic liver disease are at risk for more severe hepatitis A and should receive vaccination also. Routine childhood vaccination is recommended in states and communities with a consistently high incidence of hepatitis A.

Routine vaccination of all food handlers is not recommended, because their profession does not put them at higher risk for infection. However, local regulations mandating proof of vaccination for food handlers or offering tax credits for food service operators who provide hepatitis A vaccine to employees have been implemented in some areas. One economic analysis concluded that routine vaccination of all food handlers would not be economical from a societal or restaurant owner's perspective. Costs in the economic model were driven by the turnover rate of employees and the small percentage of hepatitis A cases that are attributable to infected food service workers. Another analysis concluded that vaccination of one hundred thousand food handlers in the ten states with the highest incidence of hepatitis A would cost $13,969 per year-of-life saved.

Employers concerned about reducing the risk of hepatitis A among employees should focus on providing hepatitis A vaccination for those persons who have risk factors for infection, including men who have sex with men, illicit drug users, and persons who plan to travel to developing countries. Food handlers aged less than nineteen years who live in a state or community where routine childhood vaccination is recommended have both an indication for vaccine and a potential source for reimbursement for vaccination and for some administrative costs (i.e., the Vaccine for Children Fund).

Immunoglobulin provides short-term (one-to-two-month) protection from hepatitis A. Immunoglobulin is a sterile preparation of concentrated antibodies (immunoglobulins) made from pooled human plasma processed in a way that inactivates viruses. The intramuscular preparation (0.02 mL/kg) is often used in persons planning to travel within two to four weeks and who require immediate protection or for those with contraindications for vaccination. Immunoglobulin is also recommended for travelers aged less than two years, for whom the vaccine is not licensed. Although children of this age usually have mild infection, they commonly serve as a source of infection for contacts, and they occasionally have severe illness themselves.

Postexposure Prophylaxis

Postexposure prophylaxis with immunoglobulin is more than 85 percent effective in preventing hepatitis A if administered within two weeks after exposure to HAV, but the efficacy is highest when administered early in the incubation period. There are several specific circumstances in which the use of postexposure prophylaxis is indicated, including use for nonimmune persons who have had (1) household or sexual contact with an HAV-infected person during a time when the HAV-infected person was likely to be infectious (i.e., two weeks before to one week after onset of illness), and (2) whose last contact was within the previous two weeks. Postexposure prophylaxis consists of a single intramuscular dose of immunoglobulin (0.02 mL/kg). Persons who received a dose of hepatitis A vaccine more than one month previously or who have a history of laboratory-confirmed HAV infection should be considered immune and do not require immunoglobulin. Immunoglobulin is not necessary for persons whose only exposure to a person with hepatitis A occurred greater than one week after the onset of jaundice. Food service workers with hepatitis A can expose other food service workers, and immunoglobulin should be given to all other food service workers in the same establishment who do not have proof of previous vaccination or HAV infection.

CDC guidelines recommend that postexposure prophylaxis also be considered for persons who consume food prepared by an infected food handler if (1) the food handler had contact with food that was not cooked after contact, (2) the food handler had diarrhea or poor hygienic practices during the time when he or she was likely to be infectious, and (3) patrons can be identified and treated within two weeks after their last exposure. An algorithm for determining whether immunoprophylaxis is needed has been published (Figure 15.2). Although this algorithm is a useful framework for assessing the risk of transmission from an infected food handler, postexposure prophylaxis decisions are still largely based on retrospective hygiene assessments and other subjective information obtained during the case interview, as well as on the judgment and experience of public health officials. Interviews should include detailed, open-ended questions about job duties, work dates, clinical symptoms, and hygiene during the period of infectivity. Interviews with supervisors and coworkers and an inspection of restrooms and food preparation areas are also recommended. Opportunities for postexposure prophylaxis are often missed, either because the infected food handler did not receive a diagnosis of HAV infection until after transmission to patrons had occurred, the food handler with

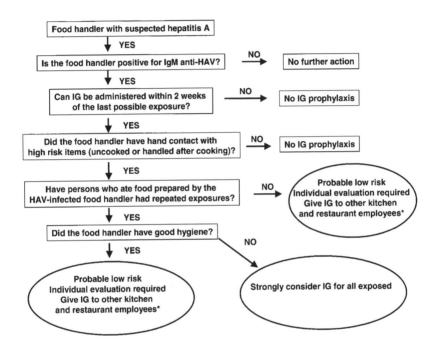

Figure 15.2. Algorithm for determining need for immunoprophylaxis after exposure to food prepared by a food handler with hepatitis A. Consider hepatitis A vaccine in addition to immunoglobulin (IG) for those with other risk factors for hepatitis A. Hygiene assessments are subjective; a visit to the food handling area and interviews with the infected food handler, coworkers, and supervisors are often helpful. Factors to consider include the food handler's self-assessment, assessments obtained from supervisors or coworkers, whether the food handler had bowel movements (especially diarrhea) while at work, presence of medical conditions that might make hygiene more difficult to maintain, glove use, availability of functioning hand washing facilities, hygiene training, and previous assessments of sanitation practices in the facility that employs the infected food handler. Anti-HAV: antibody to hepatitis A virus.

181

hepatitis A was not reported to the local public health authorities, or reported food handling practices incorrectly indicated that the risk of transmission to patrons was low. Postexposure prophylaxis should not be administered to exposed persons after cases have begun to occur, because the two-week period during which immunoglobulin is effective will have passed, unless other infected food handlers with later onsets have been identified.

Hepatitis A vaccine has also been used for postexposure prophylaxis. However, the effectiveness of postexposure prophylaxis using hepatitis A vaccine has not been directly compared with immunoglobulin in a controlled clinical trial, and immunoglobulin remains the recommended choice for postexposure prophylaxis in the United States. Hepatitis A vaccine can be given at the same time (but in a different anatomic site) as immunoglobulin, and exposed persons who have an indication for vaccination should receive both.

Hygiene Practices

The minimum infectious dose required for HAV infection in humans is unknown. In primate studies, HAV can remain infectious after one month on environmental surfaces at ambient temperatures, and it is more resistant than poliovirus (another picornavirus) to degradation over time while on environmental surfaces. Heating foods to 85°C (greater than 185°F) for one minute or disinfection with a 1:100 dilution of household bleach in water or cleaning solutions containing quaternary ammonium or HCl (including concentrations found in many toilet cleaners) is effective in inactivating HAV. HAV is resistant to disinfection by some organic solvents and by a pH as low as 3.

No specific food handler hygiene practice has been shown to reduce the likelihood of transmission. Experimental deposition of fecally suspended HAV onto hands indicates that infectious HAV remains present for more than four hours after application. In experimental settings, water rinsing alone reduces the amount of HAV that is transferred to lettuce by ten- to one hundred-fold.

Hygiene training for food handlers should include practical advice about the techniques of hand washing and education about the need to seek medical attention for postexposure prophylaxis after contact with a person with hepatitis A. Reducing bare hand contact with foods that are not subsequently cooked is also a reasonable preventative measure. Employers should provide access to hand washing stations and encourage ill food handlers to seek medical attention and to stay out of the workplace. Exclusion from duties that involve contact with food for at least one to two weeks after the onset of jaundice or until symptoms resolve is reasonable. Asymptomatic food handlers who are IgM anti-HAV positive are sometimes identified during investigations, and measurements of ALT levels, in combination with likely dates of exposure, might be used to estimate whether the food handler has had recent infection and is potentially still capable of transmission. However, the validity of this approach is unknown.

Providing sanitary facilities for field workers and discouraging the presence of children in areas where food is harvested reduces the potential for contamination of food during harvesting or processing. Chlorinated water or water from a source not likely to be contaminated by sewage should be used for rinsing produce or ice used for packing.

Disinfection of Potentially Contaminated Foods

Development of disinfection procedures for produce or shellfish has been hampered by the technical difficulties involved with detection of infectious HAV in food. Despite these challenges, methods are being developed to detect HAV on some types of produce, in shellfish, and in water.

The effectiveness of various disinfection methods in reducing HAV contamination of fresh fruits and vegetables is an area of active investigation. Preliminary results indicate that disinfection modalities that are potentially applicable to produce, including chlorinated water, hydrostatic pressure, and heat, are effective in reducing or eliminating HAV infectivity; however, adapting these techniques for use on commercially distributed produce will require further refinement.

Other than thorough cooking, no reliable disinfection method for shellfish exists. Shellfish are typically cooked until they open, which may occur at temperatures as low as 70°C. Steaming or boiling shellfish still in the shell for less than two minutes may not fully inactivate HAV. Shellfish have HAV concentrations as much as one hundred-fold that of surrounding water, and HAV has been detected in clams, mussels, and oysters harvested from areas linked to hepatitis A outbreaks. Depuration (placing harvested live shellfish in clean water to promote purging of gastrointestinal contents) for up to one week reduces but does not eliminate HAV that has been taken up by shellfish. If HAV-contaminated water is used during depuration, it may even introduce HAV into previously uncontaminated shellfish.

Reducing HAV contamination of foods should be possible using approaches, such as Hazard Analysis and Critical Control Point

(HACCP) systems, similar to those recommended for reducing contamination by other food-borne pathogens. Defining specific critical points for hepatitis A contamination will require a better understanding of how and when contamination occurs. The efficacy of various chemicals or washing processes in disinfecting fresh fruits, vegetables, and shellfish will have to be considered in the context of the need to preserve the marketability and quality (e.g., consistency, taste, and odor) of products.

Conclusion

Reducing food-borne transmission of hepatitis A can be achieved by improving food production and food handler hygiene and providing pre-exposure prophylaxis to persons at risk for infection. Food handlers acquire HAV infection from others within their communities, and reducing food-borne transmission of HAV will ultimately be achieved through routine vaccination of persons at risk for HAV infection within these communities.

Chapter 16

Testing for HAV

The Test Sample

What is being tested?

Hepatitis A antibody is produced in response to an infection with the hepatitis A virus or to the hepatitis A vaccine. The test detects the presence of this antibody.

How is the sample collected for testing?

A blood sample is taken by needle from the arm.

The Test

How is it used?

There are two versions of the test, and these detect antibodies. Antibodies are produced by the body to protect itself from antigens (foreign proteins). IgM (immunoglobulin M) is the first antibody produced by the body when it is exposed to a virus and is used for early detection of infection. IgM antibodies to HAV are used in a patient with evidence of acute hepatitis, such as jaundice, dark urine, pale-colored stools, fever, and loss of appetite. IgG (immunoglobulin G)

Reprinted from "Hepatitis A Virus," © 2005 American Association for Clinical Chemistry. Reprinted with permission. For additional information about clinical lab testing, visit the Lab Tests Online website at http://www.labtestsonline.org.

antibodies develop later and remain present for many years, protecting the person against further infection by the same virus. A total antibody test (which detects both IgM and IgG antibodies) detects both current and previous infection with HAV and also will be positive after receiving the hepatitis A vaccine.

When is it ordered?

Testing for the presence of IgM antibodies to hepatitis A is done if you have the symptoms or are likely to have been exposed to the virus. If you are being considered for the HAV vaccine, a total antibody test may be ordered before you are given the vaccine to see if you need it (if the antibodies are already present, the vaccine won't help you). Once you have completed the two doses of the vaccine, the total HAV antibody test can also be used to see if you have responded to the vaccine.

What does the test result mean?

If the test result is positive (or reactive) and you have not gotten the HAV vaccine, you have had a hepatitis A infection—even if you were not aware of it. About 30 percent of adults over age forty have antibodies to HAV. If you have been given the vaccine, a positive result means you are immune to HAV and cannot be infected by it.

Is there anything else I should know?

It is presumed that one infection with hepatitis A produces lasting immunity against further infections.

Chapter 17

Frequently Asked Questions about HAV Prevention

General Information

What is hepatitis A?

Hepatitis A is a liver disease caused by hepatitis A virus.

How is hepatitis A virus transmitted?

Hepatitis A virus is spread from person to person by putting something in the mouth that has been contaminated with the stool of a person with hepatitis A. This type of transmission is called "fecal-oral." For this reason, the virus is more easily spread in areas where there are poor sanitary conditions or where good personal hygiene is not observed.

Most infections result from contact with a household member or sex partner who has hepatitis A. Casual contact, as in the usual office, factory, or school setting, does not spread the virus.

What are the signs and symptoms of hepatitis A?

Persons with hepatitis A virus infection may not have any signs or symptoms of the disease. Older persons are more likely to have symptoms than children. If symptoms are present, they usually occur

Reprinted from "Frequently Asked Questions about Hepatitis A," National Center for Infectious Diseases, Centers for Disease Control and Prevention, December 2004.

abruptly and may include fever, tiredness, loss of appetite, nausea, abdominal discomfort, dark urine, and jaundice (yellowing of the skin and eyes). Symptoms usually last less than two months; a few persons are ill for as long as six months. The average incubation period for hepatitis A is twenty-eight days (range: fifteen to fifty days).

How do you know if you have hepatitis A?

A blood test (IgM anti-HAV) is needed to diagnose hepatitis A. Talk to your doctor or someone from your local health department if you suspect that you have been exposed to hepatitis A or any type of viral hepatitis.

How can you prevent hepatitis A?

Always wash your hands after using the bathroom, after changing a diaper, or before preparing or eating food.

Two products are used to prevent hepatitis A virus infection: immune globulin and hepatitis A vaccine.

Immune globulin is a preparation of antibodies that can be given before exposure for short-term protection against hepatitis A and for persons who have already been exposed to hepatitis A virus. Immune globulin must be given within two weeks after exposure to hepatitis A virus for maximum protection.

Hepatitis A vaccine has been licensed in the United States for use in persons two years of age and older. The vaccine is recommended (before exposure to hepatitis A virus) for persons who are more likely to get hepatitis A virus infection or are more likely to get seriously ill if they do get hepatitis A. The vaccines currently licensed in the United

Table 17.1. Recommended Dosages of HAVRIX®

Vaccinee's age (years)	Dose (EL.U.)[a]	Volume (mL)	No. doses	Schedule (mos.)[b]
2–18	720	0.5	2	0, 6–12
>18	1,440	1.0	2	0, 6–12

Note: HAVRIX: Hepatitis A vaccine, inactivated, GlaxoSmithKline.

[a]ELISA units.

[b]0 months represents timing of the initial dose; subsequent numbers represent months after the initial dose.

States are HAVRIX® (manufactured by GlaxoSmithKline) and VAQTA® (manufactured by Merck & Co., Inc).

Hepatitis A Vaccine

Can a patient receive the first dose of hepatitis A vaccine from one manufacturer and the second (last) dose from another manufacturer?

Yes. Although studies have not been done to look at this issue, there is no reason to believe that this would be a problem.

What should be done if the second (last) dose of hepatitis A vaccine is delayed?

The second dose should be administered as soon as possible. There is no need to repeat the first dose.

Can other vaccines be given at the same time that hepatitis A vaccine is given?

Yes. Hepatitis B, diphtheria, poliovirus (oral and inactivated), tetanus, oral typhoid, cholera, Japanese encephalitis, rabies, yellow fever vaccine, or immune globulin can be given at the same time that hepatitis A vaccine is given, but at a different injection site.

Is hepatitis A vaccine safe?

Yes, hepatitis A vaccine has an excellent safety profile. No serious adverse events have been attributed definitively to hepatitis A vaccine.

Table 17.2. Recommended dosages of VAQTA®

Vaccinee's age (years)	Dose (U)[a]	Volume (mL)	No. doses	Schedule (mos)[b]
2–18	25	0.5	2	0, 6–18
>18	50	1.0	2	0, 6–12

Note: VAQTA: Hepatitis A vaccine, inactivated, Merck & Co., Inc.

[a]Units.

[b]0 months represents timing of the initial dose; subsequent numbers represent months after the initial dose.

189

Soreness at the injection site is the most frequently reported side effect.

How are hepatitis A vaccines made?

There is no live virus in hepatitis A vaccines. The virus is inactivated during production of the vaccines, similar to Salk-type inactivated polio vaccine.

How long does hepatitis A vaccine protect you?

Although data on long-term protection are limited, estimates based on modeling techniques suggest that protection will last for at least twenty years.

When are persons protected after receiving hepatitis A vaccine?

Protection against hepatitis A begins four weeks after the first dose of hepatitis A vaccine.

Can hepatitis A vaccine be given after exposure to hepatitis A virus?

No, hepatitis A vaccine is not licensed for use after exposure to hepatitis A virus. In this situation, immune globulin should be used.

Should pre-vaccination testing be done?

Pre-vaccination testing is done only in specific instances to control cost (e.g., persons who were likely to have had hepatitis A in the past). This includes persons who were born in countries with high levels of hepatitis A virus infection, elderly persons, and persons who have clotting factor disorders and may have received factor concentrates in the past.

Should post-vaccination testing be done?

No.

Can hepatitis A vaccine be given during pregnancy or lactation?

We don't know for sure, but because vaccine is produced from inactivated hepatitis A virus, the theoretical risk to the developing fetus is expected to be low. The risk associated with vaccination, however, should be weighed against the risk for hepatitis A in women who may be at high risk for exposure to hepatitis A virus.

Can hepatitis A vaccine be given to immunocompromised persons (e.g., persons on hemodialysis or persons with AIDS)?

Yes.

What is Twinrix®?

It is a combined hepatitis A and hepatitis B vaccine for use in persons aged eighteen years and older. Primary vaccination consists of three doses, given on a zero-, one-, and six-month schedule, the same schedule as that used for hepatitis B vaccine alone.

Immune Globulin

What is immune globulin?

Immune globulin is a preparation of antibodies that can be given before exposure for short-term protection against hepatitis A and for persons who have already been exposed to hepatitis A virus. Immune globulin must be given within two weeks after exposure to hepatitis A virus for maximum protection.

Is immune globulin safe?

Yes. No instance of transmission of HIV (the virus that causes AIDS) or other virus has been observed with the use of immune globulin administered by the intramuscular route. Immune globulin can be administered during pregnancy and breast-feeding.

Need for Hepatitis A Vaccination

Who should get vaccinated against hepatitis A?

Hepatitis A vaccination provides protection before one is exposed to hepatitis A virus. Hepatitis A vaccination is recommended for the following groups who are at increased risk for infection and for any person wishing to obtain immunity.

- *Persons traveling to or working in countries that have high or intermediate rates of hepatitis A.* All susceptible persons traveling to or working in countries that have high or intermediate rates of hepatitis A should be vaccinated or receive immune globulin before traveling. Persons from developed countries who travel to developing countries are at high risk for hepatitis A. Such persons include tourists, military personnel, missionaries, and others who work or study abroad in countries that have high or intermediate levels of hepatitis A. The risk for hepatitis A exists even for travelers to urban areas, those who stay in luxury hotels, and those who report that they have good hygiene and that they are careful about what they drink and eat.

- *Children in states, counties, and communities where rates of hepatitis A were at least twice the national average during the baseline period of 1987–97.* Children living in states, counties, and communities where rates of hepatitis A are at least twice the national average (20 or more cases/1,000,000) in baseline period should be routinely vaccinated beginning at two years of age. High rates of hepatitis A have been found in these populations, both in urban and rural settings. In addition, to effectively prevent epidemics of hepatitis A, vaccination of previously unvaccinated older children is recommended within five years of initiation of routine childhood vaccination programs. Although rates differ among areas, available data indicate that a reasonable cutoff age in many areas is ten to fifteen years of age because older persons have often already had hepatitis A. Vaccination of children before they enter school should receive highest priority, followed by vaccination of older children who have not been vaccinated.

- *Men who have sex with men.* Sexually active men (both adolescents and adults) who have sex with men should be vaccinated. Hepatitis A outbreaks among men who have sex with men have been reported frequently. Recent outbreaks have occurred in urban areas in the United States, Canada, and Australia.

- *Illegal-drug users.* Vaccination is recommended for injecting and non-injecting illegal-drug users.

- *Persons who have occupational risk for infection.* Persons who work with hepatitis A virus-infected primates or with hepatitis A virus in a research laboratory setting should be vaccinated. No other groups have been shown to be at increased risk for hepatitis A virus infection because of occupational exposure. Outbreaks of hepatitis A have been reported among persons working with nonhuman primates that are susceptible to hepatitis A virus infection, including several Old World and New World species. Primates that were infected were those that had been born in the wild, not those that had been born and raised in captivity.

- *Persons who have chronic liver disease.* Persons with chronic liver disease who have never had hepatitis A should be vaccinated, as there is a higher rate of fulminant (rapid onset of liver failure, often leading to death) hepatitis A among persons with chronic liver disease. Persons who are either awaiting or have received liver transplants also should be vaccinated.

- *Persons who have clotting-factor disorders.* Persons who have never had hepatitis A and who are administered clotting-factor concentrates, especially solvent detergent-treated preparations, should be given hepatitis A vaccine.

- *Persons with hemophilia.* All persons with hemophilia (Factor VIII, Factor IX) who receive replacement therapy should be vaccinated because there appears to be an increased risk of transmission from clotting-factor concentrates that are not heat inactivated.

Which groups do not routinely need hepatitis A vaccine?

- *Food service workers.* Food-borne hepatitis A outbreaks are relatively uncommon in the United States; however, when they occur, intensive public health efforts are required for their control. Although persons who work as food handlers have a critical role in common-source food-borne outbreaks, they are not at increased risk for hepatitis A because of their occupation. Consideration may be given to vaccination of employees who work in areas where community-wide outbreaks are occurring and where state and local health authorities or private employers determine that such vaccination is cost-effective.

- *Sewerage workers.* In the United States, no work-related outbreaks of hepatitis A have been reported among workers exposed to sewage.

- *Health-care workers.* Health-care workers are not at increased risk for hepatitis A. If a patient with hepatitis A is admitted to the hospital, routine infection control precautions will prevent transmission to hospital staff.

- *Children under two years of age.* Because of the limited experience with hepatitis A vaccination among children under two years of age, the vaccine is not currently licensed for this age group.

- *Daycare attendees.* The frequency of outbreaks of hepatitis A is not high enough in this setting to warrant routine hepatitis A vaccination. In some communities, however, daycare centers play a role in sustaining community-wide outbreaks. In this situation, consideration should be given to adding hepatitis A vaccine to the prevention plan for children and staff in the involved center(s).

- *Residents of institutions for developmentally disabled persons.* Historically, hepatitis A virus infections were common among persons with developmental disabilities living in institutions. Currently, the occurrence of hepatitis A virus infections has diminished.

International Travel

Who should receive protection against hepatitis A before travel?

All susceptible persons traveling to or working in countries that have high or intermediate rates of hepatitis A should be vaccinated or receive immune globulin before traveling. Persons from developed countries who travel to developing countries are at high risk for hepatitis A. Such persons include tourists, military personnel, missionaries, and others who work or study abroad in countries that have high or intermediate levels of hepatitis A. The risk for hepatitis A exists even for travelers to urban areas, those who stay in luxury hotels, and those who report that they have good hygiene and that they are careful about what they drink and eat.

How soon before travel should the first dose of hepatitis A vaccine be given?

For optimal protection, at least four weeks prior to travel. Check with your doctor about when the next dose is due.

What should be done if a person cannot receive hepatitis A vaccine?

Travelers who are allergic to a vaccine component or who elect not to receive the vaccine should receive a single dose of immune globulin (0.02 mL/kg), which provides effective protection against hepatitis A

194

virus infection for up to three months. Travelers whose travel period exceeds two months should be administered immune globulin at 0.06 mL/kg; administration must be repeated if the travel period exceeds five months.

If travel starts sooner than four weeks prior to the first vaccine dose, what should be done?

Because protection might not be optimal until four weeks after vaccination, persons traveling to a high-risk area less than four weeks after the initial dose of hepatitis A vaccine should also be given immune globulin (0.02 mL/kg), but at a different injection site. Therefore, the first dose of hepatitis A vaccine should be administered as soon as travel to a high-risk area is planned.

What should be done for travelers who are younger than two years of age to protect them from hepatitis A virus infection?

Immune globulin is recommended for travelers younger than two years of age because the vaccine is currently not licensed for use in this age group.

Source: *MMWR*: Prevention of Hepatitis A Through Active or Passive Immunization

Chapter 18

The Search for a
Better HAV Vaccine

Researchers at the National Institute of Allergy and Infectious Diseases (NIAID) have located two genes that give hepatitis A virus (HAV) its virulent properties. The team, led by Suzanne Emerson, Ph.D., also has discovered that deliberately weakened HAV can quickly revert to its naturally occurring, infection-causing form. As published in the September 1, 2002, issue of *Journal of Virology*, these findings indicate that making an improved vaccine for HAV will be a very difficult task.

"As sanitation improves in developing countries, there will be an increased need for inexpensive and easy-to-administer vaccines to prevent hepatitis A, which is transmitted through contaminated food and water," notes Dr. Emerson. HAV is so common in developing countries that almost everyone is infected during childhood (often without becoming noticeably ill) and thereafter is immune to the virus. Improvements in sanitation and water quality, though, make such naturally acquired immunity less likely. Unfortunately, if HAV infection occurs for the first time later in life, it can result in dangerous illness, including severe liver damage.

A vaccine made from killed HAV does exist, but it requires multiple booster shots to be given intramuscularly—an expense and inconvenience that inhibits its use in less-developed countries. Scientists at NIAID have been attempting to develop a live, attenuated HAV

Reprinted from "Cause of Hepatitis A Virulence Pinpointed," Press Release, National Institute of Allergy and Infectious Diseases, August 8, 2002.

vaccine. An attenuated vaccine—one made from a deliberately weakened form of the virus—could be given orally in a single dose, a clear advantage to the existing vaccine.

To develop such a vaccine, Dr. Emerson and her co-workers first had to determine which genes give HAV its punch. They compared the genetic makeup of a virulent version of human HAV with that of an attenuated version of the same strain of virus by creating fourteen artificial "chimeric" viruses, each of which contained a different combination of genes taken from the parent strains. Monkeys exposed to a virus that contained either of two genes, 2C or VP1/2A, from the virulent parent developed symptoms of hepatitis. When both genes from the virulent parent were present, the disease was markedly more severe. Conversely, chimeras containing mutated forms of 2C and VP1/2A did not cause disease.

Weakening HAV by altering its two virulence-determining genes would seem to be a logical way to produce a hepatitis A vaccine. But when the researchers infected monkeys with just such an attenuated virus, it mutated within those animals, although it did not cause disease. Feces from the animals, however, contained infectious particles that could cause hepatitis in other monkeys.

"Although these results suggest that a live, attenuated HAV vaccine may be difficult to develop, they do help us better understand what controls HAV growth," notes Dr. Emerson. "Ultimately, this knowledge may provide us with a roadmap to a less expensive and more potent killed vaccine that could be used worldwide."

Reference

S. U. Emerson et al. "Identification of VP1/2A and 2C as Virulence Genes of Hepatitis A and Demonstration of Genetic Instability of 2C." *Journal of Virology* 76, no. 17 (2002): 8551–59.

Part Four

Hepatitis B Virus (HBV) and Hepatitis D Virus (HDV)

Chapter 19

Frequently Asked Questions about HBV

What is hepatitis B?

Hepatitis B is caused by a virus that attacks the liver. The virus, which is called hepatitis B virus (HBV), can cause lifelong infection, cirrhosis (scarring) of the liver, liver cancer, liver failure, and death.

What are the symptoms of viral hepatitis?

The symptoms of acute (newly acquired) hepatitis A, B, and C are the same. Symptoms occur more often in adults than in children. If symptoms occur, they might include:

- tiredness
- loss of appetite
- nausea
- abdominal discomfort
- dark urine
- clay-colored bowel movements
- yellowing of the skin and eyes (jaundice)

Reprinted from "Frequently Asked Questions about Hepatitis B," Centers for Disease Control, National Center for Infectious Diseases, December 2004.

How is hepatitis B virus spread?

HBV is spread when blood or body fluids from an infected person enters the body of a person who is not infected. For example, HBV is spread through having sex with an infected person without using a condom (the efficacy of latex condoms in preventing infection with HBV is unknown, but their proper use might reduce transmission); by sharing drugs, needles, or "works" when "shooting" drugs; through needlesticks or sharps exposures on the job; or from an infected mother to her baby during birth.

Can I donate blood if I have had any type of viral hepatitis?

If you have had any type of viral hepatitis since age eleven, you are not eligible to donate blood. In addition, if you have ever tested positive for hepatitis B or hepatitis C, at any age, you are not eligible to donate, even if you were never sick or jaundiced from the infection.

How long can HBV survive outside the body?

HBV can survive outside the body at least seven days and still be capable of transmitting infection.

For how long is hepatitis B vaccine effective?

Long-term studies of healthy adults and children indicate that hepatitis B vaccine protects against chronic HBV infection for at least fifteen years, even though antibody levels might decline below detectable levels.

Are booster doses of hepatitis B vaccine needed?

No, booster doses of hepatitis B vaccine are not recommended routinely. Data show that vaccine-induced hepatitis B surface antibody (anti-HBs) levels might decline over time; however, immune memory (anamnestic anti-HBs response) remains intact indefinitely following immunization. People with declining antibody levels are still protected against clinical illness and chronic disease.

What does the term "hepatitis B carrier" mean?

"Hepatitis B carrier" is a term that is sometimes used to indicate people who have chronic (long-term) infection with HBV. If infected,

2 to 6 percent of persons over five years of age, 30 percent of children one to five years of age, and up to 90 percent of infants develop chronic infection. Persons with chronic infection can infect others and are at increased risk of serious liver disease including cirrhosis and liver cancer. In the United States, an estimated 1.25 million people are chronically infected with HBV.

If my hepatitis B vaccination series is interrupted, do I have to start over?

No. If the vaccination series is interrupted, resume with the next dose in the series.

What is the treatment for chronic hepatitis B?

There are three drugs licensed for the treatment of persons with chronic hepatitis B: Adefovir dipivoxil, alpha interferon, and lamivudine.

Who is at risk?

In 2001, an estimated 78,000 persons in the United States were infected with HBV. People of all ages get hepatitis B and about 5,000 die per year of sickness caused by HBV.

How great is the risk for hepatitis B?

One out of twenty people in the United States will be infected with HBV some time during their lives. Your risk is higher if you:

- have sex with someone infected with HBV
- have sex with more than one partner
- shoot drugs
- are a man and have sex with a man
- live in the same house with someone who has lifelong HBV infection
- have a job that involves contact with human blood
- are a patient or work in a home for the developmentally disabled
- have hemophilia
- travel to areas where hepatitis B is common

Your risk is also higher if your parents were born in Southeast Asia, Africa, the Amazon Basin in South America, the Pacific Islands, or the Middle East.

If you are at risk for HBV infection, ask your health care provider about hepatitis B vaccine.

How do you get hepatitis B?

You get hepatitis B by direct contact with the blood or body fluids of an infected person; for example, you can become infected by having sex or sharing needles with an infected person. A baby can get hepatitis B from an infected mother during childbirth.

Hepatitis B is not spread through food or water or by casual contact.

How do you know if you have hepatitis B?

You may have hepatitis B (and be spreading the disease) and not know it; sometimes a person with HBV infection has no symptoms at all. Only a blood test can tell for sure.

If you have symptoms:

• your eyes or skin may turn yellow

• you may lose your appetite

• you may have nausea, vomiting, fever, or stomach or joint pain

• you may feel extremely tired and not be able to work for weeks or months

Is there a cure for hepatitis B?

There are medications available to treat long-lasting (chronic) HBV infection. These work for some people, but there is no cure for hepatitis B when you first get it. That is why prevention is so important. Hepatitis B vaccine is the best protection against HBV. Three doses are commonly needed for complete protection.

If you are pregnant, should you worry about hepatitis B?

If you have HBV in your blood, you can give hepatitis B to your baby. Babies who get HBV at birth may have the virus for the rest of their lives, can spread the disease, and can get cirrhosis of the liver or liver cancer.

All pregnant women should be tested for HBV early in their pregnancy. If the blood test is positive, the baby should receive the vaccine along with another shot, hepatitis B immune globulin (called HBIG), at birth. The second dose of the vaccine should be given at one to two months of age and the third dose at six months of age.

Who should get vaccinated?

- All babies, at birth
- All children zero to eighteen years of age who have not been vaccinated
- Persons of any age whose behavior puts them at high risk for HBV infection
- Persons whose jobs expose them to human blood

Chapter 20

HBV Transmission
and Symptoms

Transmission

Hepatitis B is transmitted through blood and infected bodily fluids. This can occur through:

- direct blood-to-blood contact

- unprotected sex

- unsterile needles

- from an infected woman to her newborn during the delivery process.

Other possible routes of infection include sharing sharp instruments such as razors, toothbrushes, or earrings. Body piercing, tattooing, and acupuncture are also possible routes of infection unless sterile needles are used

Hepatitis B is *not* transmitted casually. It cannot be spread through sneezing, coughing, hugging, or eating food prepared by someone who is infected with hepatitis B. Everyone is at some risk for a hepatitis B infection, but some groups are at higher risk because of their occupation or life choices.

Reprinted from "About Hepatitis B: Transmission and Symptoms." Reprinted with permission from the Hepatitis B Foundation, http://www.hepb .org. © 2003.

High-Risk Groups

- Health care workers and emergency personnel
- Infants born to mothers who are infected at the time of delivery
- Partners or individuals living in close household contact with an infected person
- Individuals with multiple sex partners, past or present
- Individuals who have been diagnosed with a sexually transmitted disease
- Illicit drug users (injecting, inhaling, snorting, popping pills)
- Men who have sex with men
- Individuals who received a blood transfusion prior to 1992
- Individuals who get tattoos or body piercing
- Individuals who travel to countries where hepatitis B is common (Asia, Africa, South America, the Pacific Islands, Eastern Europe, and the Middle East)
- Individuals emigrating from countries where hepatitis B is common, or born to parents who emigrated from these countries (see above)
- Families adopting children from countries where hepatitis B is common (see above)
- Individuals with early kidney disease or undergoing kidney dialysis
- Individuals who use blood products for medical conditions (i.e., hemophilia)
- Residents and staff of correctional facilities and group homes

Symptoms

Hepatitis B is called a "silent infection" because most people do not have noticeable symptoms when they are first infected. When a healthy adult is infected with the hepatitis B virus, his or her body can respond in different ways. People who do not know they are infected can unknowingly pass the virus to others.

- Hepatitis B causes no symptoms in about 69 percent of infected people.

- Approximately 30 percent of infected individuals will have some symptoms. Many will think they just have the flu and ignore the symptoms.

- About 1 percent of those infected will develop life-threatening "fulminant hepatitis." These people may go into liver failure and require immediate medical attention. Although this response is rare, fulminant hepatitis develops suddenly and can be fatal if left untreated.

Common symptoms of hepatitis B infection include:

- Fever, fatigue, muscle or joint pain
- Loss of appetite
- Mild nausea and vomiting

Serious symptoms that require immediate medical attention and maybe even hospitalization:

- Severe nausea and vomiting
- Yellow eyes and skin ("jaundice")
- Bloated or swollen stomach

It is always a good idea to talk to your doctor if you don't feel well or if you are uncertain about whether you have been infected with hepatitis B. A simple blood test can easily diagnose a hepatitis B infection.

Chapter 21

HBV Prevention

Chapter Contents

Section 21.1

HBV Vaccination

Reprinted from "Hepatitis B Vaccine Information." Reprinted with permission from the Hepatitis B Foundation, http://www.hepb.org. © 2003.

It takes only three shots to protect yourself and your loved ones against hepatitis B for a lifetime.

In 1981, the Food and Drug Administration approved the first vaccine for hepatitis B, which was plasma-derived (i.e., made from blood products). This vaccine was discontinued in 1990 and is no longer available in the United States.

The currently used hepatitis B vaccines are made synthetically (i.e., they do not contain blood products) and have been available in the United States since 1986. You cannot get hepatitis B from the vaccine.

This safe and effective vaccine is recommended for all infants at birth and for children up to eighteen years. Adults, especially those who fall into a high-risk group, should also seriously consider getting the hepatitis B vaccine.

Vaccine Side Effects and Safety

Common side effects include soreness, swelling, and redness at the injection site. The vaccine may not be recommended for those with documented yeast allergies or a history of an adverse reaction to the vaccine.

The Hepatitis B vaccine is considered one of the safest and most effective vaccines ever made. Numerous studies looking at the vaccine's safety have been conducted by the Centers for Disease Control, World Health Organization, and other professional medical associations. They have not found any evidence that the vaccine causes sudden infant deaths (SIDs), multiple sclerosis, or other neurological disorders.

Vaccine Recommendations

The hepatitis B vaccine is recommended specifically for all infants and children by the Centers for Disease Control and the American

Academy of Pediatrics. The CDC also recommends that adults in high-risk groups be vaccinated.

The following list is a general guide for vaccination, but since every person is at some risk for infection, these guidelines should be individualized for each situation.

- All infants at birth and all children up to eighteen years.
- Health care professionals and emergency personnel.
- Sexually active teens and adults
- Men who have sex with men.
- Sex partners or close family/household members living with an infected person.
- Families considering adoption, either domestic or international.
- Travelers to countries where hepatitis B is common (Asia, Africa, South America, the Pacific Islands, Eastern Europe, and the Middle East).
- Patients with kidney disease or undergoing dialysis.
- Residents and staff of correctional facilities and group homes.
- Any person who may fall into a high-risk group due to occupation or lifestyle choices.

Vaccine Schedule

The vaccine is readily available at your doctor's office or local health clinic. Three doses are generally required to complete the hepatitis B vaccine series, although there is an accelerated two-dose series for adolescents.

- First Injection: At any given time
- Second Injection: At least one month after the first dose
- Third Injection: Six months after the first dose

Cost of Vaccine

The three-shot vaccine series for children in the United States usually costs $75 to $165, but this can vary. Infants up to age eighteen months, and sometimes older children, can receive the vaccine free of charge from most local public health clinics.

213

Insurance companies will usually cover the cost of vaccines for infants and children. There is also a federal program to help cover the cost of children's vaccines. For more information, contact the Vaccines for Children Program.

The hepatitis B vaccine costs more for adults. If an adult is in a high-risk group, the cost may be also covered by insurance. Contact your insurance company for more information about the hepatitis B vaccine.

Approved Hepatitis B Vaccines

There are currently two commercial vaccines used to prevent hepatitis B infection among infants, children, and adults in the United States. They are both manufactured using recombinant technology and neither contains blood products. You cannot get hepatitis B from these vaccines.

- Engerix-B, produced by GlaxoSmithKline
- Recombivax HB, produced by Merck

There is also a combination vaccine for hepatitis A and B available for adults:

- Twinrix, produced by GlaxoSmithKline.

Section 21.2

HBV Immune Globulin

What is hepatitis B immune globulin?

Hepatitis B Immune Globulin (HBIG) is a sterile solution of ready-made antibodies against hepatitis B. Antibodies are proteins that our immune system makes to fight germs after we are exposed to them.

HBIG is prepared from human blood from selected donors who already have a high level of antibodies to hepatitis B. These antibodies are concentrated down to a small volume that can be given by (needle) injection.

Why is hepatitis B immune globulin needed?

Hepatitis B infection is a viral disease of the liver that can result in a mild to severe illness or even death. Some people are not able to get rid of the virus and carry the virus all their lives. These people can infect others with hepatitis B virus.

HBIG is recommended following exposure to hepatitis B virus because it provides immediate, short-term protection against the virus. A dose of hepatitis B vaccine is given at the same time. Two additional doses of hepatitis B vaccine are given to complete the series and ensure long-term protection.

When is hepatitis B immune globulin used?

HBIG is recommended for some people who have had a significant exposure to hepatitis B virus. This includes:

- people who have been exposed to blood (known or suspected to be) infected with hepatitis B by:
  - being poked with a used (injection) needle

215

- being splashed in the face or eyes with infected blood
- being bitten by someone infected with hepatitis B
- using the toothbrush, razor, or dental floss of someone infected with hepatitis B
- people who have had sexual contact with a person with hepatitis B;
- victims of sexual assault;
- newborns of mothers infected with hepatitis B;
- infants when mother, father, or primary caregiver is infected with hepatitis B; and
- newborns when mothers are intravenous drug users or sex trade workers.

In order to be effective, HBIG must be given as soon as possible after exposure to hepatitis B virus.

How is hepatitis B immune globulin given?

HBIG is given by injection. HBIG should be given into the buttock whenever possible, although it may be given in the arm. For children under five years of age it is given into the thigh muscle.

What are the possible vaccine reactions?

Some possible side effects include soreness, redness, and stiffness of muscles around the injection site lasting for several hours. Mild fever or just not feeling well may also occur.

With any vaccine or drug there is a possibility of a shock-like allergic reaction (anaphylaxis). This can be hives, wheezy breathing, or swelling of some part of the body. If this happens, particularly swelling around the throat, immediately get to your family doctor or hospital emergency.

It is suggested that persons stay in the clinic for at least fifteen minutes after receiving any type of immunization.

Report serious reactions to your local public health nurse or family doctor.

Note: Acetaminophen is recommended if there is fever or pain following immunization.

Acetylsalicylic acid (ASA or aspirin) must *not* be given to children.

Is hepatitis B immune globulin safe?

Yes, HBIG is safe. Human immune globulin products are among the safest blood-derived products available. No transmission of any viruses has been reported from receiving HBIG.

Why should you not get hepatitis B immune globulin?

You should *not* get HBIG if you have a history of shock-like allergic reaction (anaphylaxis) to a previous dose of HBIG or any of its components.

Chapter 22

Understanding
HBV Blood Tests

Basic HBV Blood Tests

Understanding your hepatitis B blood test results can be confusing. It is important to discuss your test results with your health care provider so that you can clearly understand whether you have a new infection, chronic infection, or have recovered from an infection. You may want to take this book with you to your appointment as a reference guide. In addition, it is helpful if you request a written copy of your blood tests so that you can be sure you know which tests are positive or negative.

Before explaining the tests, there are two basic medical terms that you should be familiar with:

- *Antigen:* A foreign substance in the body, such as the hepatitis B virus.

- *Antibody:* A protein that your immune system makes in response to a foreign substance. Antibodies can be produced in response to a vaccine or to a natural infection. Antibodies usually protect you against future infections.

The test that is used to help you understand your hepatitis B status is called the hepatitis B blood panel. This is a simple three-part blood test that your doctor can order. Your results can be returned within seven to ten days.

The three-part hepatitis B blood panel includes the following:

1. *Hepatitis B Surface Antigen (HBsAg):* The "surface antigen" is part of the hepatitis B virus that is found in the blood of someone who is infected. If this test is positive, then the hepatitis B virus is present.

2. *Hepatitis B Surface Antibody (HBsAb or anti-HBs):* The "surface antibody" is formed in response to the hepatitis B virus. Your body can make this antibody if you have been vaccinated, or if you have recovered from a hepatitis B infection. If this test is positive, then your immune system has successfully developed a protective antibody against the hepatitis B virus. This will provide long-term protection against future hepatitis B infection. Someone who is surface antibody positive is not infected, and cannot pass the virus on to others.

3. *Hepatitis B Core Antibody (HBcAb or anti-HBc):* This antibody does not provide any protection or immunity against the hepatitis B virus. A positive test indicates that a person may have been exposed to the hepatitis B virus. This test is often used by blood banks to screen blood donations. However, all three test results are needed to make a diagnosis.

Use the information in Table 22.1 to help you and your doctor interpret your blood panel results.

What Is Hepatitis B?

Hepatitis B is the world's most common serious liver infection. It is caused by the hepatitis B virus (HBV) that attacks liver cells and can lead to liver failure, cirrhosis (scarring), or cancer of the liver later in life. Approximately 90 percent of healthy adults who are exposed to the hepatitis B virus (HBV) recover on their own and develop the protective surface antibody. However, 10 percent of infected adults, 50 percent of infected children, and 90 percent of infected babies are unable to get rid of the virus and develop chronic infection. These people need further evaluation by a liver specialist or doctor knowledgeable about hepatitis B.

Who Should Be Tested?

HBV is transmitted through contact with blood or infected bodily fluids,
through unprotected sex, unsterile needles, and from an infected mother to her newborn during the delivery process. HBV is not transmitted casually, through the air, or from casual social contact (hugging, coughing, sneezing).

The following groups are especially at high risk for infection and should be tested:

- Health care workers and emergency personnel

- Partners or individuals living in close household contact with someone who is infected

- Individuals who have had multiple sex partners or who have been diagnosed with an STD

- Injection drug users

- Men who have sex with men

- Individuals who received a blood transfusion prior to 1972

- Individuals who have tattoos or body piercings

Table 22.1. Interpretation of Hepatitis B Blood Panel Tests

Tests	Results	Interpretation	Recommendation
HBsAg	Negative (-)	Not Immune—has not been	Get the vaccine
HBsAb	Negative (-)	infected but is still at risk for	
HBcAb	Negative (-)	possible future infection— needs vaccine	
HBsAg	Negative (-)	Immune—has been vacci-	Vaccine is not
HBsAb	Positive (+)	nated or recovered from	needed
HBcAb	Negative or positive (-/+)	previous infection—cannot infect others	
HBsAg	Positive (+)	Acute infection or chronic	Find a knowledge-
HBsAb	Negative (-)	infection—hepatitis B virus	able doctor for
HBcAb	Negative or positive (-/+)	is present—can spread the virus to others	further evaluation
HBsAg	Negative (-)	Unclear—several interpreta-	Find a knowledge-
HBsAb	Negative (-)	tions are possible—all three	able doctor for
HBcAb	Positive (+)	tests should be repeated	further evaluation

- Individuals who travel to countries where hepatitis B is common (Asia, Africa, South America, the Pacific Islands, Eastern Europe, and the Middle East)
- Individuals emigrating from countries where hepatitis B is common, or who are born to parents who emigrated from these countries (see above)
- *All* pregnant women should be tested for hepatitis B infection

Is There a Vaccine for Hepatitis B?

The good news is that there is a safe and effective vaccine for hepatitis B that lasts a lifetime. It is recommended in the United States and other countries for all infants and children up to age eighteen and adults at high risk for infection.

Additional Blood Tests

HBeAg (Hepatitis B e-Antigen)

This is a viral protein that is secreted by hepatitis B–infected cells. It is associated with chronic hepatitis B infections and is used as a marker of active viral disease and a patient's degree of infectiousness.

- A positive result indicates the person has high levels of virus and greater infectiousness.
- A negative result indicates low to zero levels of virus in the blood and a person is considered non-infectious.

This test is often used to monitor the effectiveness of some hepatitis B therapies, whose goal is to convert a chronically infected individual to "e-antigen negative."

The absence of e-antigen, however, does not necessarily exclude active viral replication. Some patient groups have mutant viruses that do not give rise to e-antigen. Patients with negative e-antigen, but detectable viral DNA, are traditionally thought to be more resistant to conventional treatment than those who have positive e-antigen levels.

HBeAb or anti-HBe (Hepatitis B e-Antibody)

This antibody is made in response to the e-antigen and is detected in patients who have recovered from hepatitis B infections as well as those who are chronically infected. Chronically infected individuals who stop producing e-antigen sometimes produce e-antibodies. The clinical significance of this result is unclear but it is generally considered to be a good thing. In rare cases, anti-HBe may be associated with active viral replication in patients with e-antigen-negative virus mutations.

Liver Function Tests (or Liver Enzymes)

Includes blood tests that assess the general health of the liver. When elevated above normal values, the ALT (alanine aminotransferase) and AST (aspartate aminotransferase) tests indicate liver

Table 22.2. A Guide to Common Blood Tests

Test	Normal Range	Abnormal Range (Mild to Moderate)	Abnormal Range (Severe)
Liver Enzymes			
Aspartate amino-transferase (AST)	<40 IU/L	40–200 IU/L	>200 IU/L
Alanine amino-transferase (ALT)	<40 IU/L	40–200 IU/L	>200 IU/L
Gamma-glutamyl transferase (GGT)	<60 IU/L	60–200 IU/L	>200 IU/L
Alkaline phosphatase	>112 IU/L	112–300 IU/L	>300 IU/L
Liver Function Tests			
Bilirubin	<1.2 mg/dL	1.2–2.5 mg/dL	>2.5 mg/dL
Albumin	3.5–4.5 g/dL	3.0–3.5 g/dL	<3.0 g/dL
Prothrombin time	<14 seconds	14–17 seconds	>17 seconds
Blood Count			
White blood count (WBC)	>6000	3000–6000	<3000
Hematocrit (HCT)	>40	35–40	<35
Platelets	>150,000	100,000–150,000	<100,000

Source: Hepatitis B Basics and Beyond, Bristol-Myers Squibb Company, Issue No. 2, October 2003.

Note: U= International Unit; L=liter; dL=deciliter; mg=milligrams

damage. They are enzymes located in liver cells that can leak out into the bloodstream when liver cells are injured.

ALT (alanine aminotransferase) is the liver enzyme marker that is followed most closely in those chronically infected with hepatitis B. This test is useful in deciding whether a patient would benefit from treatment, or for evaluating how well he or she is responding to therapy.

AFP (Alpha-Fetoprotein)

This is a normal protein produced in the developing fetus. Pregnant women will have elevated AFPs. Other adults, however, should not have elevated AFP in their blood. This test is used as a liver tumor marker for patients with chronic hepatitis B. Patients should have their AFP levels monitored routinely since high levels could indicate the possibility of liver cancer.

Ferritin

Iron is stored in the liver in the form of ferritin. Increased levels of ferritin mean a high level of iron is being stored. This could result from an increased iron intake in the diet (vitamin supplements, food cooked in iron pots, etc.), but it can also occur from a destruction of liver cells causing leakage of ferritin. More research is needed to understand the relationship between elevated ferritin and liver cancer.

Chapter 23

HBV Treatment: Approved and Experimental Treatments

Current Hepatitis B Treatment

The future looks bright for individuals living with chronic hepatitis B. There are three FDA-approved drugs for adults, two approved drugs for children, and many promising new drugs in development.

The approved drugs all appear to reduce or stop hepatitis B viral replication, which may also reduce the risk of progression to cirrhosis, liver failure, or liver cancer. Although none of the approved drugs appear to provide a complete cure (except in rare cases), they still offer a lot of hope to those living with chronic hepatitis B.

Approved Hepatitis B Treatments

Interferon-alpha (Intron A) is given by injection several times a week for six months up to a year, or longer. The drug can cause side effects such as flu-like symptoms, depression, and headaches. It was approved in 1991 and is available for children and adults.

Lamivudine (Epivir-HBV, Zeffix, or Heptodin) is a pill that is taken once a day for at least one year. The drug has few side effects, however, a primary concern is the possible development of hepatitis B

"Current Hepatitis B Treatment" is reprinted from "Approved Hepatitis B Treatment," © 2003 and "Experimental Hepatitis B Treatments" is reprinted from "Drug Watch: Compounds in Development for Chronic Hepatitis B," © 2004. Both reprinted with permission from the Hepatitis B Foundation, http://www.hepb.org.

Table 23.1. Compounds in Development for Chronic Hepatitis B

Family/Drug Name	Mechanism	Company	Status
Interferons: Mimic naturally occurring, infection-fighting immune substance produced in the body			
Intron A (Interferon alpha-2b)	Immunomodulator	Schering-Plough, Madison, NJ	**FDA Approved 1991**
Pegasys (Peginterferon alfa-2a)	Immunomodulator	Roche, Switzerland	Phase III outside USA
There are other brands of interferon approved for HCV treatment, but they have not been FDA-approved for HBV: Wellferon (Glaxo), Roferon (Hoffman-La Roche), and Infergen (Amgen).			
Nucleoside Analogues: Interfere with the viral DNA polymerase enzyme used for hepatitis B virus reproduction			
Epivir-HBV (Lamivudine)	Inhibits viral DNA polymerase	GlaxoSmithKline, Philadelphia, PA	**FDA Approved 1998**
Hepsera (Adefovir Dipivoxil)	Inhibits viral DNA polymerase	Gilead, Foster City, CA	**FDA Approved 2002**
Coviracil (FTC)	Inhibits viral DNA polymerase	Gilead, Foster City, CA	Phase III NDA Filed
Entecavir	Inhibits viral DNA polymerase	Bristol-Myers Squibb, Princeton, NJ	Phase III NDA Filed
Clevudine (L-FMAU)	Inhibits viral DNA polymerase	Bukwang, Seoul, Korea	Phase III, South Korea, Phase II, USA
Telbivudine (LdT)	Inhibits viral DNA polymerase	Idenix, Cambridge, MA	Phase III
Valtorcitabine (monoval LdC)	Inhibits viral DNA polymerase	Idenix, Cambridge, MA	Phase II
Amdoxovir (DAPD)	Inhibits viral DNA polymerase	Gilead, Foster City, CA	Phase II
Remofovir (Hepavir B)	Inhibits viral DNA polymerase	Valeant, Costa Mesa, CA	Phase II Europe, USA
Elvucitabine (ACH-126,443)	Inhibits viral DNA polymerase	Achillion, New Haven, CT	Phase II Central & Eastern Europe
Racivir	Inhibits viral DNA polymerase	Pharmasset, Tucker, GA	Phase II, Europe
MIV-210	Inhibits viral DNA polymerase	Medivir, Sweden	Phase I U.K.
Pentacept (L-3'-FD4C)	Inhibits viral DNA polymerase	Pharmasset, Tucker, GA	Preclinical
Robustaflavone (ALS-920)	Inhibits viral DNA polymerase	Advanced Life Sciences, Woodbridge, IL	Preclinical
LB80380	Inhibits viral DNA polymerase	LG Life Sciences, Seoul, Korea	Preclinical

Non-Nucleoside Anti-virals: Interfere with proteins involved in viral reproduction

Bam 205	"Small Molecule"	Novelos, Newton, MA	Phase II/III China
HepeX-B (XTL–001)	Human monoclonal antibodies	XTL Biopharm, Rehovot, Israel, and Cambridge, MA	Phase II Israel & USA (orphan drug approval in USA for liver transplants)
UT 231[a]	Small Molecule	United Therapeutics, Silver Spring, MD	Preclinical HBV (Phase II HCV)
HepBzyme	Nuclease-resistant ribozyme	Ribozyme, Boulder, CO	Preclinical
Bay 41-4109	Inhibits viral nucleocapsid	Bayer AG, Germany	Preclinical

Non-Interferon Immune Enhancers: Boost T-cell infection-fighting immune cells and natural interferon production

HE2000	Immune Stimulator	Hollis Eden, San Diego, CA	Phase II Singapore
Theradigm	Immune stimulator	Epimmune, San Diego, CA	Phase II
EHT899	Oral Viral Protein	Enzo Biochem, New York, NY	Phase II Israel
Zadaxin (Thymosin alpha-1)	Immune stimulator	SciClone, San Mateo, CA	Phase II with lamivudine; Orphan drug approval in USA for liver cancer
HBV DNA Vaccine	Immune stimulator	PowderJect, Oxford, U.K.	Phase I
SpecifEx-HepB	Immunological cell transfer	CellExSys, Seattle, WA	Preclinical/Phase I
eiRNA Technology	Expressed interfering RNA	Nucleonics, Horsham, PA	Preclinical

Post-Exposure and/or Post-Liver Transplant Treatment

BayHep B	HBV Immunoglobulin	Bayer U.S., Pittsburgh, PA	**FDA Approved 1977**
Nabi-HB	HBV Immunoglobulin	Nabi, Boca Raton, FL	**FDA Approved 1999**
Anti-hepatitis B	HBV Immunoglobulin	Cangene, Ontario, Canada	FDA Filing 2001

[a]Discovered by HBF Scientists.

227

virus mutants during and after treatment. It was approved in 1998 and is available for children and adults.

Adefovir (Hepsera) is a pill taken once a day for at least one year. The drug has few side effects, however, a primary concern is that kidney problems can develop, but they are generally reversible once treatment is stopped. It was approved in September 2002 and is available only for adults. Pediatric clinical trials are being planned.

Goal of Hepatitis B Treatment

The current goal of hepatitis B treatment is to halt disease progression by suppressing hepatitis B viral replication. A sustained virologic suppression will, hopefully, reduce the amount of hepatic inflammation, thereby decreasing the risk of progression to cirrhosis, liver failure, or liver cancer.

Evaluation of Treatment

Treatment responses are generally evaluated on the basis of normalization of ALT levels, clearance of HBe-antigen, and decreased or undetectable HBV DNA. If a liver biopsy is performed, histologic findings should show a decrease in liver inflammation, possibly even reversal of damage if compared to pretreatment biopsy results.

Chapter 24

Recent HBV Research

Chapter Contents

Section 24.1

Chinese Herbs Boost HBV Treatment

Reprinted from "Chinese Herbs Boost Hepatitis B Treatment," by Jennifer Warner, WebMD Medical News, October 1, 2002. © 2002 WebMD Inc. All rights reserved. Reprinted with permission.

Combining elements of Western and traditional Chinese herbal medicine may help rid the body of the hepatitis B virus, according to a new study.

If untreated, chronic hepatitis B infection increases the risk of liver cancer and liver failure. The drug interferon alpha is the mainstay of hepatitis B treatment, but many patients fail to respond. This has prompted a search for effective alternative therapies.

Researchers looked at results of twenty-seven studies on people with hepatitis B who took Chinese herbs alone or in combination with interferon and compared them with others who took only interferon. They saw the best results with the combination of herbs and interferon.

Overall, researchers found the combination of Chinese herbal medicine and interferon was up to two times more effective at reducing the level of the hepatitis B virus to nearly undetectable levels.

In particular, researcher Michael McCulloch says in a news release, herbs with the active ingredients bufotoxin or kurorinone showed the most promise and merit more study. The study appears in the October 1, 2002, issue of the *American Journal of Public Health*.

"The results are encouraging enough, that if I had hepatitis B and had previously failed interferon treatment, I would talk to my doctor about combining interferon with Chinese herbal medicine," says McCulloch, a doctoral student in epidemiology at the school of public health at the University of California, Berkeley.

According to the World Health Organization, more than 350 million people have the chronic form of hepatitis B, and about 75 percent of those live in Asia.

"There is a wealth of information about hepatitis B from researchers in Asia because the disease is endemic in that part of the world, but accessing that information has been—and still is—difficult because few of these studies are published in English-language journals," says McCulloch.

Although the quality of many of these studies was poor, researchers say more clinical trials on the subject are justified due to the need for effective, alternative treatments for hepatitis B.

Section 24.2

New HBV Drug Better Than Others

Reprinted from "New Hepatitis B Drug Better Than Others," by Salynn Boyles, WebMD Medical News, February 26, 2003. © 2003 WebMD Inc. All rights reserved. Reprinted with permission.

A new drug appears to be giving patients with chronic hepatitis B something they have not had before—effective suppression of their virus without the acquired resistance and hard-to-live-with side effects that have plagued current treatments.

An international team of researchers is reporting that Hepsera, approved by the FDA in September 2002, is as effective as the two standard therapies now used to treat chronic hepatitis B virus infections. But unlike with the oldest hepatitis B drug, interferon alfa, patients in the study groups experienced few treatment-related side effects. Even more surprising is that none of the patients developed resistance to the treatment during the forty-eight-week study period. Patients on lamivudine—the most widely used hepatitis B drug—develop resistance at a rate of about 15 percent a year. Resistance has been reported in up to 65 percent of patients.

The studies are published in the February 27, 2003, issue of the *New England Journal of Medicine*. In an accompanying editorial viral hepatitis experts Mark E. Mailliard, M.D., and John Gollan, M.D., PhD, wrote that the new drug is ushering in a new era in the treatment of hepatitis B.

"[Hepsera] is the first of a large group of [drugs] that [is] coming out for the treatment of hepatitis B," Mailliard tells WebMD. "As more drugs become available we are likely to see a combination approach to therapy similar to AIDS and hepatitis C treatment. By combining

231

drugs you make it more difficult for nature to find ways to develop resistance."

Worldwide, more than 350 million people, including 1.25 million Americans, are chronically infected with hepatitis B. The virus is transmitted through body fluids and is one hundred times more contagious than HIV. It can lead to cirrhosis, liver cancer, and liver failure in about 40 percent of people with chronic infection but symptoms typically do not occur until decades after infection.

Hepsera was originally developed as an HIV drug, but was rejected because high doses caused kidney damage. In the new studies, researchers concluded that a relatively low dose (10 mg per day) was as effective as higher doses, and no kidney problems were reported.

The drug elicited good responses among patients who were positive for hepatitis B e antigen (HBeAg), a marker of infectiousness, and also harder-to-treat patients who were HBeAg-negative. HBeAg-negative hepatitis B infection is common in southern Europe and Asia, but a continued suppression of the virus with treatment is rare in this group.

In the two studies, 53 percent of the patients with HBeAg-positive virus and 64 percent with HBeAg-negative virus showed improvement in liver function after forty-eight weeks of 10 mg of Hepsera per day. The patients tolerated the drug well and no drug resistance was seen.

Most of the patients in the study are still taking the drug, and Patrick Marcellin, M.D., tells WebMD that they continue to show very little resistance two years into treatment.

"We are seeing that the rate of response among these patients is continuing to increase the longer they stay on [Hepsera], and so far the rate of resistance is still close to zero," he says. "And patients who responded during the first year of therapy have maintained that response."

While most of the patients had not been treated for hepatitis B prior to the study, Marcellin says the drug shows great promise for those who have failed therapy with lamivudine. Hepatitis specialist Eugene Schiff, M.D., says it is this group of patients that can benefit most from the new drug. Schiff is chief of hepatology at the University of Miami School of Medicine.

"We started using [Hepsera] on a compassionate-use basis in these patients," he tells WebMD. "Many of them had jaundice and some were not far from needing a transplant. We saw some dramatic improvements with some of them."

Schiff says the drug has definite advantages for patients who need to stay on treatment indefinitely, but adds there is still a place for lamivudine and interferon alfa in hepatitis B treatment.

"This gives us more options, and in the future we will have even more drugs," he says. "We still aren't talking about a cure for hepatitis B, but we have come a long way."

Sources

New England Journal of Medicine, February 27, 2003. Patrick Marcellin, M.D., head of the viral hepatitis research unit, Hopital Beaujon, Clichy, France; professor, University of Paris. Mark E. Mailliard, M.D., associate professor of medicine, University of Nebraska Medical Center, Omaha, Nebraska. Eugene Schiff, M.D., chief of hepatology, University of Miami School of Medicine.

Section 24.3

More Effective HBV Treatment

Reprinted from "More Effective Hepatitis B Treatment," by Salynn Boyles, WebMD Medical News, July 2, 2003. © 2003 WebMD Inc. All rights reserved. Reprinted with permission.

A new form of an old hepatitis drug appears to be a more effective hepatitis B treatment. Twice as many patients taking a longer-acting version of the drug interferon—called pegylated interferon—had effective results as patients on standard interferon.

This first trial comparing the two hepatitis B treatments is published in the July 2003 issue of the *Journal of Viral Hepatitis*.

In 2002, the FDA approved pegylated interferon for patients with hepatitis C virus infection. Standard interferon has been around for many years. But the pegylated form of interferon has been altered to allow the treatment to stay in the bloodstream longer. As a result, hepatitis C patients get pegylated interferon once a week—compared with three injections a week for standard interferon. Hepatitis B patients often get daily injections.

The hepatitis B virus is transmitted through body fluids and is one hundred times more contagious than HIV, but the infection goes away on its own in most patients. But when the infection does take hold, treatment is needed to prevent life-threatening liver failure.

Approved hepatitis B treatments for those who become chronically infected include standard interferon and the drugs lamivudine and adefovir. Lamivudine and adefovir are more easily tolerated than interferon, but most patients do not achieve long-term responses.

In this study, 194 patients with chronic hepatitis B were randomly chosen to receive either standard interferon, three times a week, or three different doses of the pegylated interferon PEGASYS once a week for six months. All the patients were then followed for an additional six months.

PEGASYS is manufactured by Roche Pharmaceuticals, a WebMD sponsor.

At the end of the follow-up, 24 percent of the patients on pegylated interferon had measurable responses to the hepatitis B treatment, compared with 12 percent on standard interferon.

Of those on the middle dose of PEGASYS, 33 percent had sustained suppression of the hepatitis B virus six months after the end of hepatitis B treatment, compared with 25 percent of patients on standard interferon.

"The viral reduction achieved with PEGASYS is substantially more pronounced than what's achieved with conventional interferon," lead researcher Graham Cooksley, M.D., said in a news release.

But Howard J. Worman, M.D., who has written several books on hepatitis treatment, says he's not convinced that pegylated interferon represents a significant advance over standard interferon for the treatment of chronic hepatitis B.

The Columbia University professor tells WebMD that new drugs are being tested for hepatitis B treatment, but they are not very different from the already approved drugs lamivudine and adefovir.

"With hepatitis C there are bigger drugs on the horizon with different mechanisms of action than those now on the market," he says. "But I don't see that with hepatitis B."

Sources

Journal of Viral Hepatitis, July 2003. Graham Cooksley, M.D., FRACP, Royal Brisbane Hospital, Herston, Australia. Howard J. Worman, M.D., associate professor of medicine and anatomy and cell biology, College of Physicians and Surgeons, Columbia University, New York.

Section 24.4

HBV Vaccine May Be Linked to Multiple Sclerosis

Reprinted from "Hepatitis B Vaccine May Be Linked to MS," by Salynn Boyles, WebMD Medical News, September 13, 2004. © 2004 WebMD Inc. All rights reserved. Reprinted with permission.

The hepatitis B vaccine series has been administered to more than twenty million people in the United States and more than five hundred million people in the world. It is more than 95 percent effective in preventing an infection that kills millions annually. However anecdotal evidence has linked the vaccine to an increased risk for multiple sclerosis.

Now a new study in the September 14, 2004, issue of the journal *Neurology* offers some of the strongest evidence supporting the link.

In the study, researchers report that vaccination with the recombinant hepatitis B vaccine is associated with a threefold increased risk of multiple sclerosis.

They concluded that the benefits of the vaccine still appear to outweigh the risks, but added that the findings "challenge the idea that the relation between hepatitis B vaccination and the risk of MS is well understood."

"We aren't policy makers, but it is important to recognize that many lives are saved by this vaccine," researcher Susan Jick, DSc, tells WebMD. "We certainly aren't suggesting that people stop getting vaccinated. But this study raises important questions."

The actual cause of MS is still unknown but MS is believed to be an autoimmune disease in genetically susceptible persons. Reports of hepatitis B vaccination and MS were from anecdotal case reports, not scientifically controlled studies.

A Billion Doses

Approximately 350 million people worldwide are infected with hepatitis B virus, and as many as 65 million will die from liver cancer or cirrhosis of the liver as a result. The hepatitis B vaccine has generally been considered one of the safest vaccines ever produced, and more than a billion doses have been given since it was first made available in the early 1980s.

Reports in the mid-1990s pointing to a link between the vaccine and MS led the French government to temporarily suspend the routine immunization of pre-adolescents in schools, but most clinical trials have not supported the association.

Two years ago an immunization safety committee guided by the Centers for Disease Control and Prevention and the Institutes of Health reported that the clinical evidence "favors rejection of a causal relationship between hepatitis B vaccine and multiple sclerosis."

In the newly published study, researcher Miguel Hernan, M.D., used a national health database from the U.K. to identify MS patients and people who had gotten the hepatitis B vaccine. Roughly three million Britons were registered in the database, and the researchers included only 163 of more than 700 cases of MS patients and ten times as many people who did not have MS in the analysis.

The researchers estimated that immunization was associated with a threefold increase in MS risk within the three years following vaccination.

Most with MS Weren't Vaccinated

While conceding that the new study was well designed and well executed, University of Washington neurology professor Anne H. Cross, M.D., argues that the exclusion of so many MS patients in the analysis could have been a factor in the outcome. Of 713 MS cases identified, the researchers included only 163 in their study and just 11 of these developed first symptoms of MS within three years of vaccination.

"One must consider whether this selection process, which was deemed necessary to properly perform the study, might have led to some unrecognized bias," Cross wrote in an editorial she co-authored.

It makes little sense, she says, that the hepatitis B vaccine causes MS when there is no evidence linking the virus to the disease.

"The vaccine is just a peptide (a small protein) of the virus, so it stands to reason that if there is a link between the vaccine and MS there would also be a link between hepatitis B virus infection and MS," she tells WebMD.

She also pointed out that more than 90 percent of the multiple sclerosis patients in the database had not been vaccinated against hepatitis B.

The hepatitis B vaccine is now routinely given to infants in the United States as a series of shots, and CDC spokesman Eric Mast, M.D., MPH, noted that there is no evidence linking the vaccine to MS or any other neurological disease in children.

Mast, who is acting director of the division of viral hepatitis, tells WebMD that even with the addition of the newest study, the clinical evidence does not support a link between the hepatitis B vaccine and MS.

"This has certainly been on our radar screen, and we need to continue to look at it," he says. "But the preponderance of evidence suggests no association."

Sources

Hernan, M. *Neurology*, September 14, 2004; vol 63: pp 772–73. Susan Jick, DSc, associate professor of epidemiology, Boston School of Public Health. Anne H. Cross, M.D., professor of neurology, Washington University, St. Louis. Eric Mast, M.D., MPH, acting director, division of viral hepatitis, CDC.

Chapter 25

HBV: Pregnancy Concerns

Chapter Contents

Section 25.1

HBV Guidelines for Pregnant Women

Reprinted from "Hepatitis B Guidelines for Pregnant Women."
Reprinted with permission from the Hepatitis B Foundation, http://
www.hepb.org. © 2005.

What is hepatitis B?

Hepatitis B is the most common serious liver infection in the world. It is caused by the hepatitis B virus (HBV) that attacks liver cells and can lead to liver failure, cirrhosis (scarring) or cancer of the liver later in life. The virus is transmitted through contact with infected blood and bodily fluids.

If I am pregnant, should I be tested for hepatitis B?

Yes! Pregnant women who are infected with hepatitis B can transmit the virus to their newborns during delivery. 90 percent of these babies will become chronically infected with hepatitis B at birth if there is no prevention.

All pregnant women should be tested for hepatitis B to prevent infection.

What if I test positive for hepatitis B while I am pregnant?

If a pregnant woman tests positive for hepatitis B, then she should be referred to a liver specialist for further evaluation. Although most women do not have any pregnancy complications as a result of HBV infection, it is still a good idea to be seen by a specialist.

How can I protect my newborn from hepatitis B?

If a pregnant woman tests positive for hepatitis B, Her newborn must be given two shots in the delivery room—the first dose of hepatitis B vaccine and one dose of hepatitis B immune globulin (HBIG). If these two medications are given correctly within the first twelve hours of life, a newborn has a 95 percent chance of being protected against a lifelong hepatitis B infection. The infant will need additional doses of hepatitis B vaccine at one and six months of age to provide complete protection. If a woman knows that she is infected, it is important that she tell her doctor to have these two drugs available when she is ready to deliver. If a baby does not receive these drugs in time, then there is a greater than 90 percent chance that he or she will become chronically infected. There is no second chance!

It is vitally important that all newborns be vaccinated at birth against hepatitis B!

Can I breastfeed my baby if I am infected with hepatitis B?

According to the Centers for Disease Control and Prevention (CDC) and the World Health Organization (WHO), it is safe for an infected woman to breastfeed her child. All women with hepatitis B are encouraged to breastfeed their babies since the benefits of breastfeeding outweigh the potential risk of transmitting the virus through breast milk. In addition, since all newborns should receive the hepatitis B vaccine at birth, the risk of transmission is reduced even further.

How will I know if I am infected with hepatitis B?

The test that is used to help you understand your hepatitis B status is called the hepatitis B blood panel, a simple three-part blood test that your doctor can order. All pregnant women should be tested for hepatitis B.

The three-part hepatitis B blood panel includes the following:

1. Hepatitis B Surface Antigen (HBsAg): The "surface antigen" is part of the hepatitis B virus that is found in the blood of someone who is infected. If this test is positive, then the hepatitis B virus is present.

2. Hepatitis B Surface Antibody (HBsAb or anti-HBs): The "surface antibody" is formed in response to the hepatitis B virus. Your body can make this antibody if you have been vaccinated, or if you have recovered from a hepatitis B infection. If this test is positive, then your immune system has successfully developed a protective antibody against the hepatitis B virus. This will provide long-term protection against future hepatitis B infection.

3. Hepatitis B Core Antibody (HBcAb or anti-HBc): This antibody does not provide any protection or immunity against the hepatitis B virus. A positive test indicates that a person may have

been exposed to the hepatitis B virus. This test is often used by blood banks to screen blood donations. However, all three test results are needed to make a diagnosis.

How do I protect my child if another family member is infected with hepatitis B?

Babies and children can be exposed to HBV from an infected dad, sibling, or other family member living in the same household. This can occur through contact with infected blood and bodily fluids. Vaccination is the best prevention against spreading the hepatitis B virus!

How can I prevent getting hepatitis B if someone in my household is infected?

We recommend that anyone living in a household with an infected family member should be vaccinated. This is especially important for babies and children since they are at greatest risk for developing a chronic infection if exposed to HBV at an early age. The vaccine is a series of three shots given over a six-month period that will provide a lifetime of protection.

Until your vaccine series is complete, it is important to avoid sharing any sharp instruments such as razors, toothbrushes, or earrings, and the like, since small amounts of blood can be exchanged through these items. Also, infected individuals should be careful to keep all cuts properly covered. Blood spills should be cleaned with gloves and a 10 percent bleach/water solution. Hepatitis B is not transmitted casually and it cannot be spread through sneezing, coughing, hugging, or eating food prepared by someone who is infected with Hepatitis B.

Remember that the best protection for you and your loved ones is the hepatitis B vaccine. Over one billion doses of the vaccine have been given worldwide, making it the most widely used vaccine in the world!

Section 25.2

Preventing Perinatal HBV Transmission

"Labor & Delivery and Nursery Unit Guidelines to Prevent Hepatitis B Virus Transmission," reprinted with permission from the Immunization Action Coalition, http://www.immunize.org. © 2005.

The following guidelines may be used to help your hospital establish standing orders for preventing perinatal hepatitis B virus (HBV) transmission in your Labor & Delivery and Nursery Units. They have been reviewed for technical accuracy by the Centers for Disease Control and Prevention (CDC).

Note: Procedures must be in place to (1) review the hepatitis B surface antigen (HBsAg) test results of all pregnant women at the time of hospital admission and (2) give immunoprophylaxis within twelve hours after birth to infants of HBsAg-positive mothers and infants of mothers who do not have documentation of HBsAg test results in their charts. Administration of hepatitis B (HepB) vaccine at birth to all infants is recommended by CDC's Advisory Committee on Immunization Practices, the American Academy of Pediatrics, the American Academy of Family Physicians, and the American College of Obstetricians and Gynecologists.

Labor and Delivery Unit Guidelines

1. Upon admission, review the HBsAg[1] lab report and copy the test result onto (1) the labor and delivery record and (2) the infant's delivery record. It is essential to examine a copy of the original lab report instead of relying only on the handwritten prenatal record due to the possibility of transcription error, misinterpretation of test results, or misordering of the test.

2. If the HBsAg result is not available, order the test ASAP. Instruct the lab to call the nursery with the result ASAP.

3. Alert the nursery if the mother is HBsAg positive or if the mother's HBsAg result is unknown. These infants require immunoprophylaxis within twelve hours of birth with HepB vaccine (and HBIG if the mother is HBsAg positive).

243

4. If the woman's HBsAg test result is positive or unknown at the time of admission, notify her of the need to give immuno-prophylaxis to her infant within twelve hours of birth.

Nursery Unit Guidelines

Infants Born to HBsAg-Negative Mothers

1. Give HepB vaccine (0.5 mL, IM) before discharge from the nursery.[2,3]

2. Give the mother an immunization record that includes the HepB vaccination date. Remind the mother to bring this personal record card with her each time she brings her baby to the doctor or clinic.

3. Instruct the mother about the importance of her baby's completing the entire HepB vaccination series.

4. Make sure that the infant's hospital record clearly indicates the date of HepB vaccine administration and that the hospital record is always forwarded to the infant's primary care provider.

Infants Born to Mothers with Unknown HBsAg Status

1. Give HepB vaccine (0.5 mL, IM) within twelve hours of birth.[2] Do not wait for test results before giving vaccine. (For infants weighing less than 2 kg, see special recommendations in item 6 of this section.)

2. Give the mother an immunization record card noting HepB vaccine date and explain the need for further doses to complete the series.

3. Confirm that the lab has drawn a serum specimen from the mother for an HBsAg test, and verify when the result will be available and that it will be reported to the nursery ASAP. If the nursery does not receive the report at the expected time, call the lab for the result.

4. If the mother's HBsAg report is positive:

   • Give HBIG (0.5 ml, IM) to the infant ASAP and alert the mother's and infant's physician(s) of the test result. There is little benefit in giving HBIG if more than seven days have elapsed since birth.

- Follow instructions in the section "Infants Born to HBsAg-Positive Mothers."

5. If infant must be discharged before mother's HBsAg result is known:

   - Clearly document how to reach the parents (addresses, telephone numbers, emergency contacts) as well as the infant's primary care provider, in case further treatment is needed.

   - Notify the mother's and infant's doctor(s) that the HBsAg result is pending.

6. For infants weighing less than 2 kg, administer HepB vaccine and HBIG within twelve hours of birth. Do not count this as the first dose. Then initiate the full HepB vaccine series at one to two months of age.

Infants Born to HBsAg-Positive Mothers

1. Give HBIG (0.5 mL, IM) and HepB vaccine (0.5 mL, IM) at separate sites within twelve hours of birth.[2] (For infants weighing less than 2 kg, see special recommendations in item 7 of this section.)

2. Give the mother an immunization record that includes the dates of the HepB vaccine and HBIG, and instruct her to bring this personal record card with her each time her baby sees a provider.

3. Encourage mothers who wish to breastfeed to do so, including immediately following delivery, even if the infant has not yet been vaccinated.

4. Provide the mother with educational and written materials regarding:

   - the importance of having her baby complete the HepB vaccination schedule on time (one to two months and 6 months for monovalent vaccine, and two, four, and twelve months for Comvax);

   - the importance of postvaccination testing for the infant following the HepB series to assure immunity;

   - the mother's need for ongoing medical follow-up for her chronic HBV infection; and

- the importance of testing household members for hepatitis B and then vaccinating if susceptible.

5. Notify your local or state health department that the infant has been born and has received postexposure prophylaxis (include dates of receipt of HBIG and HepB vaccine).

6. Obtain the name, address, and phone number of the infant's primary care clinic and doctor. Notify them of the infant's birth, the receipt of postexposure prophylaxis, and the importance of additional on-time vaccination and postvaccination testing.

7. For infants weighing less than 2 kg, administer HepB vaccine and HBIG within twelve hours of birth. Do not count this dose as the first dose. Then initiate the hepatitis B vaccine series at one to two months of age.

Notes

1. Do not confuse the HBsAg test result with any of the following tests:

   - HBsAb or anti-HBs = antibody to hepatitis B surface antigen

   - HBcAb or anti-HBc = antibody to hepatitis B core antigen

   Make sure you order the hepatitis B surface antigen (HBsAg) test for your patient, and that this test result is accurately recorded on the labor and delivery record and on the infant's delivery summary sheet.

2. Federal law requires that you give parents a HepB Vaccine Information Statement (VIS) prior to vaccine administration. To obtain VISs, call CDC's Immunization Information Hotline at 800-232-4636, call your state health department, or download them from Immunization Action Coalition's website at: www .immunize.org/vis

3. Delaying the initial HepB vaccination until up to two months of age may be considered only for infants of mothers whose HBsAg test is assured to be negative. As of October 17, 2001, the CDC's recommendation is now consistent with the American Academy of Pediatrics (AAP) policy. Since 1992, AAP has recommended a birth dose for all infants and has referred to an alternative schedule beginning with a dose at two months as "acceptable."

Chapter 26

Children and HBV

Hepatitis B does not usually affect a child's normal growth and development. Most children with chronic hepatitis B infections will enjoy long and healthy lives. Unlike other chronic medical conditions, there are generally no physical disabilities associated with hepatitis B, nor are there usually any physical restrictions for these children.

As a parent, you can take comfort from the fact that every child presents unique challenges. Therefore, your child with hepatitis B is just like any other child. The challenges of raising a child with hepatitis B are manageable if you are well informed and use common sense.

Adoption

The key to successful adoption of a child with hepatitis B is to be prepared with accurate information about the disease, and to protect yourself and other members of your household with the hepatitis B vaccine prior to the child's arrival.

International and Domestic Adoption

Many people wish to adopt children from countries where hepatitis B infections are common: Asia, South America, Eastern Europe, and some parts of Africa. Children from these regions are often infected with the virus from their birth mothers who have hepatitis B

Reprinted with permission from the Hepatitis B Foundation, http://www .hepb.org, © 2003.

and unknowingly pass the disease on to their children during delivery. In addition, many of these countries re-use needles for medications or blood tests, a practice that places children at risk if they have not already been infected at birth.

Domestic adoptions also present some risk to potential adoptive families. Children born to women in high-risk groups (e.g., illicit drug users, multiple sexual partners, etc.) could have been infected with hepatitis B at birth. In addition, children from group homes are at increased risk for hepatitis B infection.

Hepatitis B Testing

Your agency should be able to tell you if a child has been tested for hepatitis B. With an international adoption, it is advised that you do not request that your child be tested since the blood test itself could be a source of infection. If you are concerned about the results of these tests, please contact the Hepatitis B Foundation. They can also refer you to a parent who has adopted a child with hepatitis B.

Reassurance for Adoptive Parents

Finding out that the child you wish to adopt has chronic hepatitis B can be upsetting, but should not be cause for alarm or stopping an adoption. We hope that a hepatitis B diagnosis will not change your decision to adopt a child. You can be reassured that most children will enjoy a long and healthy life. Hepatitis B does not usually affect a child's normal growth and development, and there are generally no physical disabilities or restrictions associated with this diagnosis.

Advice for Parents

Parents face a whole host of issues when making the decision to raise children. A child with hepatitis B presents new challenges, but they are manageable if you are well informed and use common sense.

The Hepatitis B Foundation has compiled a list of useful guidelines that may be helpful. Since each family is unique, and each community is different, please adjust your decisions accordingly.

Avoid the Spread of Hepatitis B

All parents, siblings, and other household members should be vaccinated. Extended family members, childcare providers, family, friends, and others should consider vaccination if they have frequent and close contact with your child.

Know the Facts

If people are unfamiliar with hepatitis B, there is a possibility they will become alarmed when told your child has chronic hepatitis B. The key to reducing people's anxiety is to give them clear, simple facts.

- Hepatitis B is not transmitted casually. It cannot be spread through the sharing of toys, sneezing, coughing, spitting, or hugging.

- Hepatitis B is spread through blood and infected bodily fluids. Therefore, it could be spread through bites and scratches that result in broken skin.

- Inform people that there is a safe hepatitis B vaccine and that the American Academy of Pediatrics recommends that all infants and children up to age eighteen years be vaccinated.

Know the Risk

In making the decision about telling others, be sure to consider whether your child is at high or low risk for exposing others to his or her blood (e.g., consider age, frequency of accidents, nosebleeds, biting, etc.). Consider the degree of risk a person has for exposure (frequent vs. occasional contact), and whether a person or child may have already been vaccinated.

Although there is no specific law that addresses hepatitis B, the Americans with Disabilities Act (1991) is a federal law that may protect children and adults with hepatitis B from discrimination.

Telling Others

Use common sense in deciding who you should tell about your child's hepatitis B. Once you tell, you can't take it back. So take your time and choose wisely as you decide who can be trusted with this information.

Fortunately, most children are now vaccinated against hepatitis B, so the risk of your child infecting others is reduced. Most states also require the hepatitis B vaccine for school entry. Although you do not necessarily have a "duty" to inform people of your child's hepatitis B, there may be situations where it is wise to disclose your child's diagnosis.

If possible, give literature to reinforce your facts. The Hepatitis B Foundation publishes free educational literature that you can request to give other parents, teachers, or school nurses.

What Should You Say?

Know your facts, use simple explanations, and remain calm. Emphasize that your child is healthy and poses no risk if blood accidents are handled carefully. Remind people (and health care providers) that blood is a two-way street. Other children may have unknown infections that can be spread to your child; therefore, the blood of all children should be handled carefully.

In addition, the hepatitis B vaccine is recommended for all infants and children up to eighteen years. Therefore, most children should already be vaccinated and protected against hepatitis B.

Universal Precautions

The Centers for Disease Control (CDC) recommends that everyone use "universal precautions" for any accident. This means that the blood and bodily fluids of all adults and children should be treated as if it is potentially infectious.

Universal precautions (or "standard precautions") should be followed for *all* accidents, not just the blood of those with known chronic hepatitis B infection.

Cleaning Up Blood Spills

Avoid direct contact with blood, vomit, diarrhea, and other bodily secretions, and ensure that others will not come into contact with them either.

- Clean all spills with a diluted solution of bleach (mix one part fresh household bleach with nine parts water).
- Discard cleaning materials into a plastic bag and tie securely. Dispose of properly in the garbage can.
- Wash your hands thoroughly with soap and warm water.

Treatment for Children

Chronic hepatitis B is normally a mild disease in children and teens. Most children can expect to live full, healthy lives unmarked by visible symptoms. In some children, however, the virus can cause serious liver damage. These children will need medical intervention and treatment.

All children with chronic hepatitis B should be seen regularly by a pediatric liver specialist or knowledgeable doctor, whether they are on treatment or not. Visits may be every six months or once a year, depending on your child's situation. A physical exam, blood tests, and possible ultrasounds of the liver are part of the usual visit.

Approved Treatments

There are currently two approved treatment options available in the United States for children with chronic hepatitis B.

- Interferon alpha (Intron A) is an injection usually given three times a week for six months to a year. Children generally experience fewer side effects than adults, but they can include flu-like symptoms.

- Lamivudine (Epivir-HBV, Zeffix, Heptodin) is a pill that is taken once a day for at least one year. There are almost no side effects.

Not every child (or adult) with chronic hepatitis B needs to be treated. A pediatric liver specialist should evaluate your child to see if she or he is a candidate for treatment based on a physical exam, blood tests, and other test results. Treatment appears to be of greatest benefit to those who show signs of active liver disease.

Hepatitis B and the School

As more states require the hepatitis B vaccine for school entry, parents are increasingly asking whether they need to inform the school of their child's diagnosis. This is a gray area where parents must use their personal discretion since there is no perfect answer.

Disclosing Your Child's Diagnosis

If you decide to disclose your child's hepatitis B, remain calm, provide literature to reinforce the facts, and give the school a letter from your child's doctor stating that he or she is healthy and poses no risk to the other children if appropriate precautions are maintained. Most states require hepatitis B vaccination prior to school entry, so this reduces any potential risk to other students.

We recommend the following when disclosing your child's hepatitis B to school officials:

- Stress the importance of confidentiality and universal precautions to protect your child from social discrimination.

251

- Remind school officials that hepatitis B is transmitted through exposure to blood; it is not transmitted casually.

- Explain that hepatitis B is not the only blood-borne disease that puts children at risk.

- Consider saying, "Treat my child as you should treat every child—with care. You know what risk my child poses, but you don't know the risk that other children might present."

Americans with Disabilities Act

The Americans with Disabilities Act (1991) is a federal law that may protect against discrimination related to chronic hepatitis B. Many states have clauses written into their AIDS disclosure laws, which may also protect persons with hepatitis B.

State Hepatitis B Vaccine Laws

A list of the Hepatitis B Prevention Mandates for all states is published by the Immunization Action Coalition. This organization will help you find out each state's laws regarding hepatitis B vaccine requirements for daycare, elementary school, and middle school.

Chapter 27

Living with Hepatitis:
Chronic HBV Infection

Will I recover from a hepatitis B infection?

The answer depends on whether you are infected as an adult, a child, or a baby. Most infected adults will recover without any problems, but unfortunately, most infected babies and children will develop chronic hepatitis B infections.

- *Adults:* 90 percent will get rid of the virus and recover without any problems; 10 percent will develop chronic hepatitis B.

- *Young Children:* 40 percent will get rid of the virus and recover without problems; 60 percent will develop a chronic hepatitis B infection.

- *Infants:* 90 percent will become chronically infected; only 10 percent will be able to get rid of the virus.

What is the difference between an "acute" and a "chronic" hepatitis B infection?

A hepatitis B infection is considered to be "acute" during the first six months after being exposed. This is the average period of time it takes to recover from a hepatitis B infection. If you still test positive for the hepatitis B virus (HBsAg+) after six months, you are considered to have a "chronic" hepatitis B infection, which can last a lifetime.

Reprinted from "FAQ: Living with Hepatitis B." Reprinted with permission from the Hepatitis B Foundation, http://www.hepb.org, © 2003.

Will I become sick if I have acute hepatitis B?

Hepatitis B is considered a "silent infection" because it often does not cause any symptoms. Most people feel healthy and do not know they have been infected, which means they can unknowingly pass the virus on to others. Other people may have mild symptoms such as fever, fatigue, joint or muscle pain, or loss of appetite that are mistaken for the flu. Less common but more serious symptoms include severe nausea and vomiting, yellow eyes and skin (called "jaundice"), and a swollen stomach—these symptoms require immediate medical attention and a person may need to be hospitalized.

How will I know when I have recovered from an "acute" hepatitis B infection?

Once your doctor has confirmed through a blood test that you have successfully cleared the virus from your system and developed the protective antibodies (HBsAb+), you will be protected from any future hepatitis B infection and are no longer contagious to others.

What should I do if I am diagnosed with chronic hepatitis B?

If you test positive for the hepatitis B virus for longer than six months, this indicates that you have a chronic hepatitis B infection. You should make an appointment with a hepatologist (liver specialist) or gastroenterologist familiar with hepatitis B. This specialist will order blood tests and possibly a liver ultrasound to evaluate your hepatitis B status and the health of your liver. Your doctor will probably want to see you at least once or twice a year to monitor your hepatitis B and determine if you would benefit from treatment.

Most people chronically infected with hepatitis B can expect to live long, healthy lives. Once you are diagnosed with chronic hepatitis B, the virus may stay in your blood and liver for a lifetime. It is important to know that you can pass the virus along to others, even if you don't feel sick. This is why it's so important that you make sure that all close household contacts and sex partners are vaccinated against hepatitis B.

What tests will be used to monitor my hepatitis B?

Common tests used by doctors to monitor your hepatitis B include the hepatitis B blood panel, liver function tests (ALT), hepatitis B e-Antigen (HBeAg), hepatitis B e-Antibody (HBeAb), ultrasound and imaging, and possibly liver biopsy before starting treatment.

Is there a cure for chronic hepatitis B?

Right now, there is no cure for chronic hepatitis B, but the good news is there are new treatments that can help slow the progression of liver disease in chronically infected persons by slowing down the virus. If there is less hepatitis B virus being produced, then there is less damage being done to the liver. Sometimes these drugs can even get rid of the virus, although this is not common.

With all of the new exciting research, there is great hope that a complete cure will be found for chronic hepatitis B in the near future.

Are there any approved drugs to treat chronic hepatitis B?

Yes, there are currently three approved treatments for hepatitis B in the United States. They are:

- Intron A (interferon alpha) is given by injection several times a week for six months to a year, or sometimes longer. The drug can cause side effects such as flu-like symptoms, depression, and headaches.

- Epivir-HBV (lamivudine) is a pill that is taken once a day, with almost no side effects, for at least one year. A primary concern is the possible development of hepatitis B virus mutants during and after treatment.

- Hepsera (adefovir-dipivoxil) is a pill taken once a day, with few side effects, for at least one year. The primary concern is that kidney problems can occur while taking the drug.

Although they do not provide a complete cure, except in rare cases (a "cure" means that a person loses the hepatitis B virus and develops protective surface antibodies), they do slow down the virus and decrease the risk of more serious liver disease later in life.

If I have a chronic hepatitis B infection, should I be on medication?

It is important to understand that not every person with chronic hepatitis B needs to be on medication. You should talk to your doctor about whether you are a good candidate for drug therapy or a clinical trial. Be sure that you understand the pros and cons of each treatment option. Whether you decide to start treatment or not, you should be seen regularly by a liver specialist or a doctor knowledgeable about hepatitis B.

What advice do you have for those living with chronic hepatitis B?

We strongly recommend avoiding alcohol, as it can be extremely harmful to a liver already infected with the hepatitis B virus. Additionally, you should avoid smoking for the same reason. You should be sure to talk to your doctor before taking any prescription, over-the-counter medication, or herbal remedies.

Although there is no special diet for people who have chronic hepatitis B, a healthy, well-balanced diet that is low in fat and includes plenty of vegetables is recommended. You may want to avoid eating raw shellfish, since they can contain bacteria that are harmful to your liver.

Can I donate blood if I have hepatitis B?

No. The blood bank will not accept any blood that has been exposed to hepatitis B, even if you have recovered from an acute infection.

Chapter 28

HDV: A Risk for People with HBV Infection

What is hepatitis D (HDV)?

Hepatitis D (HDV) is a viral infection of the liver that can only be acquired if a person has active hepatitis B (HBV).

How common is hepatitis D?

Hepatitis D is linked directly to hepatitis B, particularly to chronic HBV infection. There are particular pockets worldwide where chronic HBV infection is high, but HDV infection is low or uncommon, such as Southeast Asia and China.

How can I get hepatitis D?

- The modes of HDV transmission are similar to those for HBV. However, sexual transmission of HDV is less efficient than for HBV.

- Hepatitis D can only infect people with active HBV infection.

- HDV is passed most often through sharing IV drug needles with an infected person.

- People receiving clotting factor concentrates may also be at a higher risk.
- Transmission of HDV from mother to child during birth is rare.

What are the signs or symptoms of hepatitis D?

- Many with both HBV and HDV may or may not develop symptoms. When present, symptoms are similar to those of HBV.
- People with both HBV and HDV are more likely to have sudden, severe symptoms, called fulminant hepatitis.
- Those who are infected with both HBV and HDV are at greater risk for developing serious complications associated with chronic liver disease.
- People infected with HBV and HDV may become chronically infected and may be contagious from time to time for the rest of their lives.

How can I find out if I have hepatitis D?

Your health care provider can test for hepatitis D through blood tests that identify HDV antigen or HDV antibodies.

What can I do to reduce my risk of getting hepatitis D?

- Get vaccinated against hepatitis B. This also provides protection against HDV since hepatitis B must be present in order for HDV infection to occur.
- If you inject drugs and can't stop, avoid sharing your works— needles, syringes, cotton, water, spoons, pots (cookers)—or any other drug paraphernalia. If you choose to share your works, clean them with water and bleach to reduce your risk of getting hepatitis C, filling syringes for at least thirty seconds.
- Use latex condoms the right way every time you have vaginal, anal, or oral sex. Even though HDV is not commonly transmitted through sex, hepatitis B is, and having hepatitis B makes it possible to get HDV.

What is the treatment for hepatitis D?

- Most people with acute viral hepatitis experience a self-limited illness (one that runs a defined, limited course) and go on to recover completely. There is no accepted therapy, nor restrictions on diet or activity.

- People with chronic hepatitis B and D can be treated with interferon. Your health care provider can help you make decisions about your care needs based upon your medical history and liver condition.

- In most cases, hospitalization should be considered for patients who are severely ill for supportive care.

Why worry about hepatitis D?

- Hepatitis D can cause a more severe acute disease than an HBV infection alone. The severity of the diseases together can result in death.

- When hepatitis D is acquired and HBV infection already exists, chronic liver diseases with cirrhosis are more likely to occur than with an HBV infection alone.

- People with chronic HBV and HDV have a greater chance of developing chronic liver disease and cirrhosis.

Do I need to talk to my partner about hepatitis D?

Yes. When you and your partner understand how hepatitis D is passed, you can both agree to protect your health. Remember:

- Hepatitis D is very rarely sexually transmitted, but using latex condoms the right way every time for vaginal, oral, and anal sex greatly reduces the risk of passing or getting an STD, like hepatitis B.

- If your partner uses injecting drugs, talk to them about stopping.

- If you inject drugs and can't stop, avoid sharing your works—needles, syringes, cotton, water, spoons, pots (cookers)—or any other drug paraphernalia. If you choose to share your works, clean them with water and bleach to reduce your risk of getting hepatitis C, filling syringes for at least thirty seconds.

Should I talk to my health care provider about hepatitis D?

You should talk to your health care provider about hepatitis D if:

- You use injecting drugs and share your needles or works.
- You have received clotting factor concentrates.
- You have hepatitis B.

Remember: Getting vaccinated against hepatitis B helps prevent an HDV infection as well.

Where can I get more information?

If you have additional questions about hepatitis D, call the National STD and AIDS Hotlines at 800-342-2437 or 800-227-8922. The hotlines are open twenty-four hours a day, seven days a week. For information in Spanish call 800-344-7432, 8:00 a.m. to 2:00 a.m. Eastern Time, seven days a week. For the deaf and hard-of-hearing call 800-243-7889, 10:00 a.m. to 10:00 p.m. Eastern Time, Monday through Friday. The hotlines provide referrals and more answers to your questions.

For more information about the hepatitis B vaccine, call the National Immunization Information Hotline at 800-232-2522 or 800-232-0233 for information in Spanish. The hotline is open Monday through Friday from 8:00 a.m. to 11:00 P.m., Eastern Time. For the Deaf and Hard-of-Hearing call 800-243-7889, 10:00 a.m. to 10:00 p.m. Eastern Time, Monday through Friday.

Part Five

Hepatitis C Virus (HCV)

Chapter 29

HCV: An Overview

Introduction

The hepatitis C virus (HCV) is one of the most important causes of chronic liver disease in the United States. It accounts for about 15 percent of acute viral hepatitis, 60 to 70 percent of chronic hepatitis, and up to 50 percent of cirrhosis, end-stage liver disease, and liver cancer. Almost four million Americans, or 1.8 percent of the U.S. population, have antibody to HCV (anti-HCV), indicating ongoing or previous infection with the virus. Hepatitis C causes an estimated ten thousand to twelve thousand deaths annually in the United States.

A distinct and major characteristic of hepatitis C is its tendency to cause chronic liver disease. At least 75 percent of patients with acute hepatitis C ultimately develop chronic infection, and most of these patients have accompanying chronic liver disease.

Chronic hepatitis C varies greatly in its course and outcome. At one end of the spectrum are patients who have no signs or symptoms of liver disease and completely normal levels of serum liver enzymes. Liver biopsy usually shows some degree of chronic hepatitis, but the degree of injury is usually mild, and the overall prognosis may be good. At the other end of the spectrum are patients with severe hepatitis C who have symptoms, HCV RNA in serum, and elevated serum liver enzymes, and who ultimately develop cirrhosis and end-stage liver

Reprinted from "Chronic Hepatitis C: Current Disease Management," National Institute of Diabetes and Digestive and Kidney Diseases (NIDDK), National Institutes of Health, NIH Publication No. 03-4230, February 2003.

disease. In the middle of the spectrum are many patients who have few or no symptoms, mild to moderate elevations in liver enzymes, and an uncertain prognosis.

Chronic hepatitis C can cause cirrhosis, liver failure, and liver cancer. Researchers estimate that at least 20 percent of patients with chronic hepatitis C develop cirrhosis, a process that takes at least ten to twenty years. After twenty to forty years, a smaller percentage of patients with chronic disease develop liver cancer. Liver failure from chronic hepatitis C is one of the most common reasons for liver transplants in the United States. Hepatitis C is the cause of about half of the cases of primary liver cancer in the developed world. Men, alcoholics, patients with cirrhosis, people over age forty, and those infected for twenty to forty years are more likely to develop HCV-related liver cancer.

Risk Factors and Transmission

HCV is spread primarily by contact with blood and blood products. Blood transfusions and the use of shared, unsterilized, or poorly sterilized needles and syringes have been the main causes of the spread of HCV in the United States. With the introduction in 1991 of routine blood screening for HCV antibody and improvements in the test in mid-1992, transfusion-related hepatitis C has virtually disappeared. At present, injection drug use is the most common risk factor for contracting the disease. However, many patients acquire hepatitis C without any known exposure to blood or to drug use.

The major high-risk groups for hepatitis C are:

• Injection drug users, including those who used drugs briefly many years ago.

• People who had blood transfusions before June 1992, when sensitive tests for anti-HCV were introduced for blood screening.

• People who have frequent exposure to blood products. These include patients with hemophilia, solid-organ transplants, chronic renal failure, or cancer requiring chemotherapy.

• Infants born to HCV-infected mothers.

• Health care workers who suffer needle-stick accidents.

Other groups who appear to be at slightly increased risk for hepatitis C are:

- people with high-risk sexual behavior, multiple partners, and sexually transmitted diseases.

- people who use cocaine, particularly with intranasal administration, using shared equipment.

Maternal-Infant Transmission

Maternal-infant transmission is not common. In most studies, only 5 percent of infants born to infected women become infected. The disease in newborns is usually mild and free of symptoms. The risk of maternal-infant spread rises with the amount of virus in the mother's blood and with complications of delivery such as early rupture of membranes and fetal monitoring. Breast-feeding has not been linked to spread of HCV.

Sexual Transmission

Sexual transmission of hepatitis C between monogamous partners appears to be uncommon. Surveys of spouses and monogamous sexual partners of patients with hepatitis C show that less than 5 percent are infected with HCV, and many of these have other risk factors for this infection. Spread of hepatitis C to a spouse or partner in stable, monogamous relationships occurs in less than 1 percent of partners per year. For these reasons, changes in sexual practices are not recommended for monogamous patients. Testing sexual partners for anti-HCV can help with patient counseling. People with multiple sex partners should be advised to follow safe sex practices, which should protect against hepatitis C as well as hepatitis B and HIV.

Sporadic Transmission

Sporadic transmission, when the source of infection is unknown, occurs in about 10 percent of acute hepatitis C cases and in 30 percent of chronic hepatitis C cases. These cases are usually referred to as sporadic or community-acquired infections. These infections may have come from exposure to the virus from cuts, wounds, or medical injections or procedures.

Unsafe Injection Practices

In many areas of the world, unsafe injection practices are an important and common cause of hepatitis C (and hepatitis B as well).

Use of inadequately sterilized equipment, lack of disposable needles and syringes, and inadvertent contamination of medical infusions are unfortunately well-documented causes of transmission of hepatitis C. Careful attention to universal precautions and injection techniques should prevent this type of spread. In the United States, multiple-use vials are a frequent culprit in leading to nosocomial spread of hepatitis C.

The Hepatitis C Virus

HCV is a small (40 to 60 nanometers in diameter), enveloped, single-stranded RNA virus of the family Flaviviridae and genus *Hepacivirus* (see Figure 29.1). Because the virus mutates rapidly, changes in the envelope proteins may help it evade the immune system. There are at least six major genotypes and more than fifty subtypes of HCV. The different genotypes have different geographic distributions. Genotypes 1a and 1b are the most common in the United States (about 75 percent of cases). Genotypes 2 and 3 are present in only 10 to 20 percent of patients. There is little difference in the severity of disease or outcome of patients infected with different genotypes. However, patients with genotypes 2 and 3 are more likely to respond to interferon treatment.

Clinical Symptoms and Signs

Many people with chronic hepatitis C have no symptoms of liver disease. If symptoms are present, they are usually mild, nonspecific, and intermittent. They may include:

- fatigue
- mild right-upper-quadrant discomfort or tenderness ("liver pain")
- nausea
- poor appetite
- muscle and joint pains

Similarly, the physical exam is likely to be normal or show only mild enlargement of the liver or tenderness. Some patients have vascular spiders or palmar erythema.

Clinical Features of Cirrhosis

Once a patient develops cirrhosis or if the patient has severe disease, symptoms and signs are more prominent. In addition to fatigue,

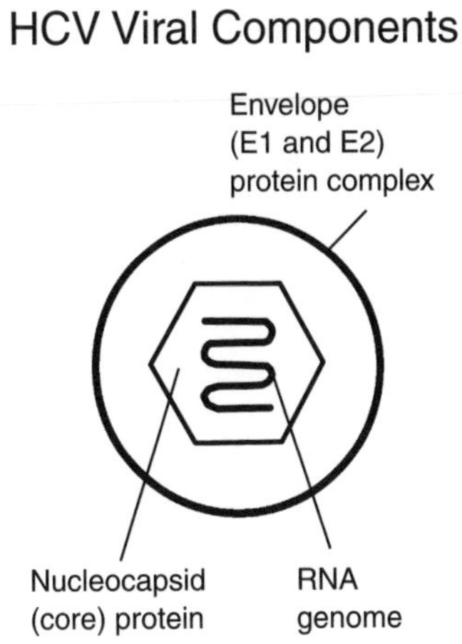

HCV Viral Components

Envelope
(E1 and E2)
protein complex

Figure 29.1. Hepatitis C Virus

Nucleocapsid   RNA
(core) protein   genome

the patient may complain of muscle weakness, poor appetite, nausea, weight loss, itching, dark urine, fluid retention, and abdominal swelling.

Physical findings of cirrhosis may include the following:

- enlarged liver
- enlarged spleen
- jaundice
- muscle wasting
- excoriations
- ascites
- ankle swelling

Extrahepatic Manifestations

Complications that do not involve the liver develop in 1 to 2 percent of people with hepatitis C. The most common is cryoglobulinemia, which is marked by the following:

- skin rashes, such as purpura, vasculitis, or urticaria
- joint and muscle aches
- kidney disease
- neuropathy
- cryoglobulins, rheumatoid factor, and low complement levels in serum

These are other complications of chronic hepatitis C:

- glomerulonephritis
- porphyria cutanea tarda

Diseases that are less well documented to be related to hepatitis C are the following:

- seronegative arthritis
- keratoconjunctivitis sicca (Sjögren syndrome)
- non-Hodgkin's type, B-cell lymphomas
- fibromyalgia
- lichen planus

Serologic Tests

Enzyme Immunoassay

Anti-HCV is detected by enzyme immunoassay (EIA). The third-generation test (EIA-3) used today is more sensitive and specific than previous ones. However, as with all enzyme immunoassays, false-positive results are occasionally a problem with the EIA-3. Additional or confirmatory testing is often helpful.

The best approach to confirm the diagnosis of hepatitis C is to test for HCV RNA using a sensitive assay such as polymerase chain reaction (PCR) or transcription mediated amplification (TMA). The presence of HCV RNA in serum indicates an active infection.

Testing for HCV RNA is also helpful in patients in whom EIA tests for anti-HCV are unreliable. For instance, immunocompromised patients may test negative for anti-HCV despite having HCV infection because they may not produce enough antibodies for detection with EIA. Likewise, patients with acute hepatitis may test negative for anti-HCV when first tested. Antibody is present in almost all patients by one month after onset of acute illness; thus, patients with acute hepatitis who initially test negative may need follow-up testing. In these situations, HCV RNA is usually present and confirms the diagnosis.

Recombinant Immunoblot Assay

Immunoblot assays can be used to confirm anti-HCV reactivity as well. These tests are also called "Western blots"; serum is incubated on nitrocellulose strips on which four recombinant viral proteins are blotted. Color changes indicate that antibodies are adhering to the proteins. An immunoblot is considered positive if two or more proteins react and is considered indeterminate if only one positive band is detected. In some clinical situations, confirmatory testing by immuno-blotting is helpful, such as for the person with anti-HCV detected by EIA who tests negative for HCV RNA. The EIA anti-HCV reactivity could represent a false-positive reaction, recovery from hepatitis C, or continued virus infection with levels of virus too low to be detected (the last occurs only rarely when sensitive PCR or TMA assays are used). If the immunoblot test for anti-HCV is positive, the patient has most likely recovered from hepatitis C and has persistent antibody. If the immuno-blot test is negative, the EIA result was probably a false positive.

Immunoblot tests are routine in blood banks when an anti-HCV-positive sample is found by EIA. Immunoblot assays are highly specific and valuable in verifying anti-HCV reactivity. Indeterminate tests require further follow-up testing, including attempts to confirm the specificity by repeat testing for HCV RNA.

Direct Assays for HCV RNA

PCR and TMA amplification can detect low levels of HCV RNA in serum. Testing for HCV RNA is a reliable way of demonstrating that hepatitis C infection is present and is the most specific test for infection. Testing for HCV RNA is particularly useful when aminotransferases are normal or only slightly elevated, when anti-HCV is not present, or when several causes of liver disease are possible. This method also helps diagnose hepatitis C in people who are immunosuppressed, have recently had an organ transplant, or have chronic renal failure. A PCR assay has now been approved by the Food and Drug Administration for general use. This assay will detect HCV RNA in serum down to a lower limit of 50 to 100 copies per milliliter (mL), which is equivalent to 25 to 50 international units (IU). A slightly more sensitive TMA test is currently under evaluation and may soon become available. Almost all patients with chronic hepatitis C will test positive by these assays.

Quantification of HCV RNA in Serum

Several methods are available for measuring the concentration or level of virus in serum, which is an indirect assessment of viral load. These methods include a quantitative PCR and a branched DNA (bDNA) test. Unfortunately, these assays are not well standardized, and different methods from different laboratories can provide different results

269

on the same specimen. In addition, serum levels of HCV RNA can vary spontaneously by three- to tenfold over time. Nevertheless, when performed carefully, quantitative assays provide important insights into the nature of hepatitis C. Most patients with chronic hepatitis C have levels of HCV RNA (viral load) between 100,000 (105) and 10,000,000 (107) copies per mL. Expressed as IU, these averages are 50,000 to 5 million IU.

Viral levels as measured by HCV RNA do not correlate with the severity of the hepatitis or with a poor prognosis (as in HIV infection); but viral load does correlate with the likelihood of a response to antiviral therapy. Rates of response to a course of alpha interferon and ribavirin are higher in patients with low levels of HCV RNA. There are several definitions of a "low level" of HCV RNA, but the usual definition is below 1 million IU (2 million copies) per mL.

In addition, monitoring HCV RNA levels during the early phases of treatment may provide early information on the likelihood of a response. Yet because of the shortcomings of the current assays for HCV RNA level, these tests are not always reliable guides to therapy.

Genotyping and Serotyping of HCV

There are six known genotypes and more than fifty subtypes of hepatitis C. The genotype of infection is helpful in defining the epidemiology of hepatitis C. More important, knowing the genotype or serotype (genotype-specific antibodies) of HCV is helpful in making recommendations and counseling regarding therapy. Patients with genotypes 2 and 3 are two to three times more likely to respond to interferon-based therapy than patients with genotype 1. Furthermore, when using combination therapy, the recommended dose and duration of treatment depend on the genotype. For patients with genotypes 2 and 3, a twenty-four-week course of combination treatment using interferon and 800 milligrams (mg) of ribavirin daily is adequate, whereas for patients with genotype 1, a forty-eight-week course and full dose of ribavirin (1,000 to 1,200 mg daily) is recommended. For these reasons, testing for HCV genotype is often clinically helpful. Once the genotype is identified, it need not be tested again; genotypes do not change during the course of infection.

Biochemical Indicators of Hepatitis C Virus Infection

- In chronic hepatitis C, increases in the alanine and aspartate aminotransferases range from zero to twenty times (but usually less than five times) the upper limit of normal.

270

- Alanine aminotransferase (ALT) levels are usually higher than aspartate aminotransferase (AST) levels, but that finding may be reversed in patients who have cirrhosis.

- Alkaline phosphatase and gamma glutamyl transpeptidase are usually normal. If elevated, they may indicate cirrhosis.

- Rheumatoid factor and low platelet and white blood cell counts are frequent in patients with severe fibrosis or cirrhosis, providing clues to the presence of advanced disease.

- The enzymes lactate dehydrogenase and creatine kinase are usually normal.

- Albumin levels and prothrombin time are normal until late-stage disease.

- Iron and ferritin levels may be slightly elevated.

Normal Serum ALT Levels

Some patients with chronic hepatitis C have normal serum alanine aminotransferase (ALT) levels, even when tested on multiple occasions. In this and other situations in which the diagnosis of chronic hepatitis C may be questioned, the diagnosis should be confirmed by testing for HCV RNA. The presence of HCV RNA indicates that the patient has ongoing viral infection despite normal ALT levels.

Liver Biopsy

Liver biopsy is not necessary for diagnosis but is helpful for grading the severity of disease and staging the degree of fibrosis and permanent architectural damage. Hematoxylin and eosin stains and Masson's trichrome stain are used to grade the amount of necrosis and inflammation and to stage the degree of fibrosis. Specific immunohistochemical stains for HCV have not been developed for routine use. Liver biopsy is also helpful in ruling out other causes of liver disease, such as alcoholic liver injury or iron overload.

HCV causes the following changes in liver tissue:

- Necrosis and inflammation around the portal areas, so-called piecemeal necrosis or interface hepatitis.

- Necrosis of hepatocytes and focal inflammation in the liver parenchyma.

- Inflammatory cells in the portal areas ("portal inflammation").

- Fibrosis, with early stages being confined to the portal tracts, intermediate stages being expansion of the portal tracts and bridging between portal areas or to the central area, and late stages being frank cirrhosis characterized by architectural disruption of the liver with fibrosis and regeneration. Several scales are used to stage fibrosis, most commonly a scale from 0 to 4 where 0 indicates none and 4 indicates cirrhosis. Stage 1 and 2 fibrosis is limited to the portal and periportal areas. Stage 3 fibrosis is characterized by bridges of fibrosis bands linking up portal and central areas.

Grading and staging of hepatitis by assigning scores for severity are helpful in managing patients with chronic hepatitis. The degree of inflammation and necrosis can be assessed as none, minimal, mild, moderate, or severe. The degree of fibrosis can be similarly assessed. Scoring systems are particularly helpful in clinical studies on chronic hepatitis.

Serum Markers of Hepatic Fibrosis

Liver biopsy is an invasive procedure that is expensive and not without complications. At least 20 percent of patients have pain requiring medications after liver biopsy. More uncommon complications include puncture of another organ, infection, and bleeding. Significant bleeding after liver biopsy occurs in 1/100 to 1/1,000 cases, and deaths are reported in 1/5,000 to 1/10,000 cases. Obviously, noninvasive means of grading and staging liver disease would be very helpful.

ALT levels, particularly if tested over an extended period, are reasonably accurate reflections of disease activity. Thus, patients with repeatedly normal ALT levels usually have mild necroinflammatory activity on liver biopsy. Furthermore, patients who maintain ALT levels above five times the upper limit of normal usually have marked necroinflammatory activity. But for the majority of patients with mild to moderate ALT elevations, the actual level is not very predictive of liver biopsy findings.

More important is a means to stage liver disease short of liver biopsy. Unfortunately, serum tests are not reliable in predicting fibrosis, particularly earlier stages (0, 1, and 2). When patients develop bridging (stage 3) fibrosis and cirrhosis (stage 4), serum tests may be helpful. The "danger signals" that suggest the presence of advanced fibrosis include an aspartate aminotransferase (AST) that is higher than ALT (reversal of the ALT/AST ratio), a high gamma glutamyl transpeptidase or alkaline phosphatase, a low platelet count (which is perhaps the earliest change), rheumatoid factor, elevations in globulins, and, of course, abnormal bilirubin, albumin, or prothrombin time. Physical findings of a firm liver, enlarged spleen, prominent spider angiomata, or palmar erythema, are also danger signals. While none of these findings are perfect, their presence should raise the suspicion of significant fibrosis and lead to evaluation for treatment earlier rather than later.

Diagnosis

Hepatitis C is most readily diagnosed when serum aminotransferases are elevated and anti-HCV is present in serum. The diagnosis is confirmed by the finding of HCV RNA in serum.

Acute Hepatitis C

Acute hepatitis C is diagnosed on the basis of symptoms such as jaundice, fatigue, and nausea, along with marked increases in serum ALT (usually greater than tenfold elevation), and presence of anti-HCV or de novo development of anti-HCV.

Diagnosis of acute disease can be problematic because anti-HCV is not always present when the patient develops symptoms and sees the physician. In 30 to 40 percent of patients, anti-HCV is not detected until two to eight weeks after onset of symptoms. In this situation, testing for HCV RNA is helpful, as this marker is present even before the onset of symptoms and lasts through the acute illness. Another approach to diagnosis of acute hepatitis C is to repeat the anti-HCV testing a month after onset of illness. Of course, a history of an acute exposure is also helpful in establishing the diagnosis.

Chronic Hepatitis C

Chronic hepatitis C is diagnosed when anti-HCV is present and serum aminotransferase levels remain elevated for more than six months. Testing for HCV RNA (by PCR) confirms the diagnosis and documents that viremia is present; almost all patients with chronic infection will have the viral genome detectable in serum by PCR.

Diagnosis is problematic in patients who cannot produce anti-HCV because they are immunosuppressed or immunoincompetent. Thus, HCV RNA testing may be required for patients who have a solid-organ transplant, are on dialysis, are taking corticosteroids, or have agammaglobulinemia. Diagnosis is also difficult in patients with anti-HCV who have another form of liver disease that might be responsible for the liver injury, such as alcoholism, iron overload, or autoimmunity. In these situations, the anti-HCV may represent a false-positive reaction, previous HCV infection, or mild hepatitis C occurring on top of another liver condition. HCV RNA testing in these situations helps confirm that hepatitis C is contributing to the liver problem.

Differential Diagnosis

The major conditions that can be confused clinically with chronic hepatitis C include the following:

- autoimmune hepatitis
- chronic hepatitis B and D
- alcoholic hepatitis
- nonalcoholic steatohepatitis (fatty liver)
- sclerosing cholangitis
- Wilson disease
- alpha-1-antitrypsin-deficiency-related liver disease
- drug-induced liver disease

Treatment

The therapy for chronic hepatitis C has evolved steadily since alpha interferon was first approved for use in this disease more than ten years ago. At the present time, the optimal regimen appears to be a twenty-four- or forty-eight-week course of the combination of pegylated alpha interferon and ribavirin.

Alpha interferon is a host protein that is made in response to viral infections and has natural antiviral activity. Recombinant forms of alpha interferon have been produced, and several formulations (alfa-2a, alfa-2b, consensus interferon) are available as therapy for hepatitis C. These standard forms of interferon, however, are now being replaced by pegylated interferons (peginterferons). Peginterferon is alpha interferon that has been modified chemically by the addition of a large inert molecule of polyethylene glycol. Pegylation changes the uptake, distribution, and excretion of interferon, prolonging its half-life. Peginterferon can be given once weekly and provides a constant level of interferon in the blood, whereas standard interferon must be given several times weekly and provides intermittent and fluctuating levels. In addition, peginterferon is more active than standard interferon in inhibiting HCV and yields higher sustained response rates with similar side effects. Because of its ease of administration and better efficacy, peginterferon has been replacing standard interferon both as monotherapy and as combination therapy for hepatitis C.

Ribavirin is an oral antiviral agent that has activity against a broad range of viruses. By itself, ribavirin has little effect on HCV, but adding it to interferon increases the sustained response rate by two- to threefold. For these reasons, combination therapy is now recommended for hepatitis C, and interferon monotherapy is applied only when there are specific reasons not to use ribavirin.

Two forms of peginterferon have been developed and studied in large clinical trials: peginterferon alfa-2a (Pegasys: Hoffman La Roche: Nutley, NJ) and peginterferon alfa-2b (Pegintron: Schering-Plough Corporation, Kenilworth, NJ). These two products are roughly equivalent in efficacy and safety, but have different dosing regimens. Peginterferon alfa-2a is given subcutaneously in a fixed dose of 180 micrograms (mcg) per week. Peginterferon alfa-2b is given subcutaneously weekly in a weight-based dose of 1.5 mcg per kilogram per week (thus in the range of 75 to 150 mcg per week).

Ribavirin is an oral medication, given twice a day in 200-mg capsules for a total daily dose based upon body weight. The standard dose of ribavirin is 1,000 mg for patients who weigh less than 75 kilograms (165 pounds) and 1,200 mg for those who weigh more than 75 kilograms. In certain situations, an 800-mg dose (400 mg twice daily) is recommended (see following).

Combination therapy leads to rapid improvements in serum ALT levels and disappearance of detectable HCV RNA in up to 70 percent of patients. However, long-term improvement in hepatitis C occurs only if HCV RNA disappears during therapy and stays undetectable once therapy is stopped. Among patients who become HCV RNA negative during treatment, a proportion relapse when therapy is stopped. The relapse rate is lower in patients treated with combination therapy compared with monotherapy. Thus, a forty-eight-week course of combination therapy using peginterferon and ribavirin yields a sustained response rate of approximately 55 percent. A similar course of peginterferon monotherapy yields a sustained response rate of only 35 percent. A response is considered "sustained" if HCV RNA remains undetectable for six months or more after stopping therapy.

The optimal duration of treatment varies depending on whether interferon monotherapy or combination therapy is used, as well as by HCV genotype. For patients treated with peginterferon monotherapy, a forty-eight-week course is recommended, regardless of genotype. For patients treated with combination therapy, the optimal duration of treatment depends on viral genotype. Patients with genotypes 2 and 3 have a high rate of response to combination treatment (70 to 80 percent), and a twenty-four-week course of combination therapy yields results equivalent to those of a forty-eight-week course. In contrast, patients with genotype 1 have a lower rate of response to combination therapy (40 to 45 percent), and a forty-eight-week course yields a significantly better sustained response rate. Again, because of the variable responses to treatment, testing for HCV genotype is clinically useful when using combination therapy.

In addition, the optimal dose of ribavirin appears to vary depending on genotype. For patients with genotypes 2 or 3, a dose of 800 mg daily appears adequate. For patients with genotype 1, the full dose of ribavirin (1,000 or 1,200 mg daily depending on body weight) appears to be needed for an optimal response.

Who Should Be Treated?

Patients with anti-HCV, HCV RNA, elevated serum aminotransferase levels, and evidence of chronic hepatitis on liver biopsy, and with no contraindications, should be offered therapy with the combination of alpha interferon and ribavirin. The National Institutes of Health Consensus Development Conference Panel recommended that therapy for hepatitis C be limited to those patients who have histological evidence of progressive disease. Thus, the panel recommended that all patients with fibrosis or moderate to severe degrees of inflammation and necrosis on liver biopsy should be treated and that patients with less severe histological disease be managed on an individual basis. Patient selection should not be based on the presence or absence of symptoms, the mode of acquisition, the genotype of HCV RNA, or serum HCV RNA levels.

Patients with cirrhosis found through liver biopsy can be offered therapy if they do not have signs of decompensation, such as ascites, persistent jaundice, wasting, variceal hemorrhage, or hepatic encephalopathy. However, interferon and combination therapy have not been shown to improve survival or the ultimate outcome in patients with preexisting cirrhosis.

Patients older than sixty years also should be managed on an individual basis, since the benefit of treatment in these patients has not been well documented and side effects appear to be worse in older patients. However, even patients in their late seventies have been successfully treated for hepatitis C.

The role of interferon therapy in children with hepatitis C remains uncertain. Ribavirin has yet to be evaluated adequately in children, and pediatric doses and safety have not been established. Thus, if children with hepatitis C are treated, monotherapy is recommended, and ribavirin should not be used outside of controlled clinical trials.

People with both HCV and HIV infection should be offered therapy for hepatitis C as long as there are no contraindications. Indeed, hepatitis C tends to be more rapidly progressive in patients with HIV co-infection, and end-stage liver disease has become an increasingly common cause of death in HIV-positive persons. For these reasons, therapy for hepatitis C should be recommended even in HIV-infected patients with early and mild disease. Once HIV infection becomes advanced, complications of therapy are more difficult and response rates are lower. The decision to treat people co-infected with HIV must take into consideration the concurrent medications and medical conditions. The efficacy of peginterferon and ribavirin in HIV-infected people has been tested in only a small number of patients. Ribavirin may still have significant interactions with other antiretroviral drugs.

In many of these indefinite situations, the indications for therapy should be reassessed at regular intervals. In view of the rapid developments in hepatitis C today, better therapies may become available within the next few years, at which point expanded indications for therapy would be appropriate.

Patients with acute hepatitis C are a major challenge to management and therapy. Because such a high proportion of patients with acute infection develop chronic hepatitis C, prevention of chronicity has become a focus of attention. In small studies, 83 to 100 percent of persons treated within one to four months of onset have had resolution of the infection. What is unclear is what dose, duration, and regimen of treatment to use. A practical regimen is peginterferon monotherapy for twenty-four weeks. The possible role for ribavirin, for short courses of therapy, and for lower doses of peginterferon are under evaluation.

In patients with clinically significant extrahepatic manifestations, such as cryoglobulinemia and glomerulonephritis, therapy with alpha interferon can result in remission of the clinical symptoms and signs. However, relapse after stopping therapy is common. In some patients, long-term or maintenance alpha interferon therapy can be used despite persistence of HCV RNA in serum if clinical symptoms and signs resolve on therapy.

Who Should Not Be Treated?

Therapy is inadvisable outside of controlled trials for patients who have

- clinically decompensated cirrhosis because of hepatitis C
- normal aminotransferase levels
- a kidney, liver, heart, or other solid-organ transplant
- specific contraindications to either monotherapy or combination therapy

Contraindications to alpha interferon therapy include severe depression or other neuropsychiatric syndromes, active substance or alcohol abuse, autoimmune disease (such as rheumatoid arthritis, lupus erythematosus, or psoriasis) that is not well controlled, bone marrow compromise, and inability to practice birth control. Contraindications to ribavirin and thus combination therapy include marked anemia, renal dysfunction, and coronary artery or cerebrovascular disease, and, again, inability to practice birth control.

Alpha interferon has multiple neuropsychiatric effects. Prolonged therapy can cause marked irritability, anxiety, personality changes, depression, and even suicide or acute psychosis. Patients particularly susceptible to these side effects are those with preexisting serious psychiatric conditions and patients with neurological disease.

Strict abstinence from alcohol is recommended during therapy with interferon. Interferon therapy can be associated with relapse in people with a previous history of drug or alcohol abuse. Therefore, alpha interferon should be given with caution to a patient who has only recently stopped alcohol or substance abuse. Typically a six-month abstinence is recommended before starting therapy, but this should be applied only to patients with a history of alcohol abuse, not to social drinkers. Patients with continuing alcohol or substance abuse problems should be treated only in collaboration with alcohol or substance abuse specialists or counselors. Patients can be successfully treated while on methadone or in an active substance abuse program. Indeed, the rigor and regular monitoring that accompany methadone treatment provide a structured format for combination therapy. The dose of methadone may need to be modified during interferon-based therapy for hepatitis.

Alpha interferon therapy can induce autoantibodies, and a twenty-four- to forty-eight-week course triggers an autoimmune condition in about 2 percent of patients, particularly if they have an underlying susceptibility to autoimmunity (high titers of antinuclear or antithyroid antibodies, for instance). Exacerbation of a known autoimmune disease (such as rheumatoid arthritis or psoriasis) occurs commonly during interferon therapy.

Alpha interferon has bone marrow suppressive effects. Therefore, patients with bone marrow compromise or cytopenias, such as low platelet count (< 75,000 cells/mm^3) or neutropenia (< 1,000 cells/mm^3) should be treated cautiously and with frequent monitoring of cell counts. These side effects appear to be more common with peginterferon than standard interferon.

Ribavirin causes red cell hemolysis to a variable degree in almost all patients. Therefore, patients with a preexisting hemolysis or anemia (hemoglobin < 11 grams [g] or hematocrit < 33 percent) should not receive ribavirin. similarly, patients who have significant coronary or cerebral vascular disease should not receive ribavirin, as the anemia caused by treatment can trigger significant ischemia. Fatal myocardial infarctions and strokes have been reported during combination therapy with alpha interferon and ribavirin.

Growth factors such as erythropoietin to raise red blood cell counts or granulocyte stimulating factor to raise neutrophil counts have been used successfully to treat patients with cytopenias during combination therapy. The proper role, dose, and side effects of these adjunctive therapies have yet to be defined.

Ribavirin is excreted largely by the kidneys. Patients with renal disease can develop hemolysis that is severe and even life threatening. Patients who have elevations in serum creatinine above 2.0 mg per deciliter (dL) should not be treated with ribavirin.

Finally, ribavirin causes birth defects in animal studies and should not be used in women or men who are not practicing adequate means of birth control. Alpha interferon also should not be used in pregnant women, as it has direct antigrowth and antiproliferative effects.

Combination therapy should therefore be used with caution. Patients should be fully informed of the potential side effects before starting therapy.

Side Effects of Treatment

Common side effects of alpha interferon and peginterferon (occurring in more than 10 percent of patients) include the following:

- fatigue
- muscle aches
- headaches

- nausea and vomiting
- skin irritation at the injection site
- low-grade fever
- weight loss
- irritability
- depression
- mild bone marrow suppression
- hair loss (reversible)

Most of these side effects are mild to moderate in severity and can be managed. They are worse during the first few weeks of treatment, especially with the first injection. Thereafter, side effects diminish. Acetaminophen may be helpful for the muscle aches and low-grade fever. Fatigue and depression are occasionally so troublesome that the dose of interferon should be decreased or therapy stopped early. Depression and personality changes can occur on interferon therapy and be quite subtle and not readily admitted by the patient. These side effects need careful monitoring. Patients with depression may benefit from antidepressant therapy using selective serotonin reuptake inhibitors. Generally, the psychiatric side effects resolve within two to four weeks of stopping combination therapy.

Ribavirin also causes side effects, and the combination is generally less well tolerated than interferon monotherapy. These are the most common side effects of ribavirin:

- anemia
- fatigue and irritability
- itching
- skin rash
- nasal stuffiness, sinusitis, and cough

Ribavirin causes a dose-related hemolysis of red cells; with combination therapy, hemoglobin usually decreases by 2 to 3 g/dL and the hematocrit by 5 to 10 percent. The amount of decrease in hemoglobin is highly variable. The decrease starts between weeks one and four of therapy and can be precipitous. Some patients develop symptoms of anemia, including fatigue, shortness of breath, palpitations, and headache.

The sudden drop in hemoglobin can precipitate angina pectoris in susceptible people, and fatalities from acute myocardial infarction and stroke have been reported in patients receiving combination therapy

Figure 29.2. Algorithm for Treatment

Make the diagnosis based on aminotransferase elevations, anti-HCV and HCV RNA in serum, and chronic hepatitis shown by liver biopsy.

↓

Assess for suitability of therapy and contraindications. Discuss side effects and possible treatment outcomes.

↓

Test for HCV genotype.

↓

Genotype 1: Test for HCV RNA level immediately before starting therapy (baseline level).

↓

Genotype 1: Start therapy with peginterferon alfa-2a in a dose of 180 mg weekly or peginterferon alfa-2b in a dose of 1.5 mg/kg weekly in combination with oral ribavirin in two divided doses of 1,000 mg daily if body weight is < 75 kilograms (165 lbs.) or 1,200 mg daily if body weight is > 75 kilograms.

↓

Genotype 2 or 3: Start therapy with peginterferon alfa-2a in a dose of 180 mcg weekly or with alfa-2b in a dose of 1.5 mcg per kilogram weekly and oral ribavirin 800 mg daily in two divided doses.

↓

All patients: At weeks 1, 2, and 4 and then at intervals of every four to eight weeks thereafter, assess side effects, symptoms, blood counts, and aminotransferases.

↓

Genotype 1: At week 12, retest for HCV RNA level. If HCV RNA is negative or has decreased by at least two $\log_{10}$ units (such as from 2 million IU to 20,000 IU or from 500,000 IU to 5,000 IU or less), continue therapy for a full forty-eight weeks, monitoring symptoms, blood counts, and ALT at four- to eight-week intervals. If HCV RNA has not fallen by two $\log_{10}$ units, stop therapy.

↓

Genotype 2 or 3: At twenty-four weeks, assess aminotransferase levels and HCV RNA and stop therapy.

↓

All patients: After therapy, assess aminotransferases at two- to six-month intervals. In responders, repeat HCV RNA testing six months after stopping.

for hepatitis C. For these important reasons, ribavirin should not be used in patients with preexisting anemia or with significant coronary or cerebral vascular disease. If such patients require therapy for hepatitis C, they should receive alpha interferon monotherapy.

Ribavirin has also been found to cause itching and nasal stuffiness. These are histamine-like side effects; they occur in 10 to 20 percent of patients and are usually mild to moderate in severity. In some patients, however, sinusitis, recurrent bronchitis, or asthma-like symptoms become prominent. It is important that these symptoms be recognized as attributable to ribavirin, because dose modification (by 200 mg per day) or early discontinuation of treatment may be necessary.

Uncommon side effects of alpha interferon, peginterferon, and combination therapy (occurring in less than 2 percent of patients) include the following:

- autoimmune disease (especially thyroid disease)
- severe bacterial infections
- marked thrombocytopenia
- marked neutropenia
- seizures
- depression and suicidal ideation or attempts
- retinopathy (microhemorrhages)
- hearing loss and tinnitus

Rare side effects include acute congestive heart failure, renal failure, vision loss, pulmonary fibrosis or pneumonitis, and sepsis. Deaths have been reported from acute myocardial infarction, stroke, suicide, and sepsis.

A unique but rare side effect is paradoxical worsening of the disease. This is assumed to be caused by induction of autoimmune hepatitis, but its cause is really unknown. Because of this possibility, aminotransferases should be monitored. If ALT levels rise to greater than twice the baseline values, therapy should be stopped and the patient monitored. Some patients with this complication have required corticosteroid therapy to control the hepatitis.

Options for Patients Who Do Not Respond to Treatment

Few options exist for patients who either do not respond to therapy or who respond and later relapse. Patients who relapse after a course of interferon monotherapy may respond to a course of combination therapy, particularly if they became and remained HCV RNA negative during the period of monotherapy. The response rates and optimal dose (800 vs. 1,000 mg to 1,200 mg of ribavirin) and duration (twenty-four or forty-eight weeks) of peginterferon and ribavirin for relapse or previous nonresponder patients have not been defined. The algorithm for treatment given here is for treatment of naive patients.

An experimental approach to treatment of nonresponders is the use of long-term or maintenance interferon, which is feasible only if the peginterferon is well tolerated and has a clear-cut effect on serum aminotransferases or liver histology, despite lack of clearance of HCV RNA. This approach is now under evaluation in long-term clinical trials in the United States. New medications and approaches to treatment are needed. Most promising for the future are the use of other cytokines and the development of newer antivirals, such as RNA polymerase, helicase, or protease inhibitors.

Hope Through Research

Basic Research

A major focus of hepatitis C research is developing a tissue culture system that will enable researchers to study HCV outside the human body. Animal models and molecular approaches to the study of HCV are also important. Understanding how the virus replicates and how it injures cells would be helpful in developing a means of controlling it and in screening for new drugs that would block it.

Diagnostic Tests

More sensitive and less expensive assays for measuring HCV RNA and antigens in the blood and liver are needed. Although current tests for anti-HCV are quite sensitive, a small percentage of patients with hepatitis C test negative for anti-HCV (false-negative reaction), and a percentage of patients who test positive are not infected (false-positive reaction). Also, there are patients who have resolved the infection but still test positive for anti-HCV. Convenient tests to measure HCV in serum and to detect HCV antigens in liver tissue would be helpful. Clinically, noninvasive tests that would reliably predict liver fibrosis would be a very valuable advance.

New Treatments

Most critical for the future is the development of new antiviral agents for hepatitis C. Most interesting will be specific inhibitors of

Figure 29.3. Considerations: Before, During and After Therapy

Before Starting Therapy

• Do a liver biopsy to confirm the diagnosis of HCV, assess the grade and stage of disease, and rule out other diagnoses. In situations where a liver biopsy is contraindicated, such as clotting disorders, combination therapy can be given without a pretreatment liver biopsy.

• Test for serum HCV RNA to document that viremia is present.

• Test for HCV genotype (or serotype) to help determine the duration of therapy and dose of ribavirin.

• Measure blood counts and aminotransferases to establish a baseline for these values.

• Counsel the patient about the relative risks and benefits of treatment. Side effects should be thoroughly discussed.

During Therapy

• Measure blood counts and aminotransferases at weeks 1, 2, and 4 and at four- to eight-week intervals thereafter.

• Adjust the dose of ribavirin downward (by 200 mg at a time) if significant anemia occurs (hemoglobin less than 10 g/dL or hematocrit < 30 percent) and stop ribavirin if severe anemia occurs (hemoglobin < 8.5 g/dl or hematocrit < 26 percent).

• Adjust the dose of peginterferon downward if there are intolerable side effects such as severe fatigue, depression, irritability, or marked decreases in white blood cell counts (absolute neutrophil count below 500 cells/mm^3) or platelet counts (decrease below 30,000 cells/mm^3). When using peginterferon alfa-2a, the dose can be reduced from 180 to 135 and then to 90 mcg per week. When using peginterferon alfa-2b, the dose can be reduced from 1.5 to 1.0 and then to 0.5 mcg per kilogram per week.

Figure 29.3. Considerations: Before, During and After Therapy,
continued

During Therapy, *continued*

• In patients with genotype 1, measure HCV RNA level immediately
before therapy and again (by the same method) at week 12.
Therapy can be stopped early if HCV RNA levels have not
decreased by at least two $\log_{10}$ units, as studies have shown that
genotype 1 patients without this amount of decrease in HCV RNA
are unlikely to have a sustained response (likelihood is < 1
percent). In situations where HCV RNA levels are not obtainable,
repeat testing for HCV RNA by PCR (or TMA) should be done at
twenty-four weeks and therapy stopped if HCV RNA is still
present, as a sustained response is unlikely.

• Reinforce the need to practice strict birth control during therapy
and for six months thereafter.

• Measure thyroid-stimulating hormone levels every three to six
months during therapy. Patients with genotypes 2 or 3 can stop
therapy at twenty-four weeks. Patients with genotype 1 and a drop
in HCV RNA by twelve weeks should continue therapy for forty-
eight weeks.

• At the end of therapy, test HCV RNA by PCR to assess whether
there is an end-of-treatment response.

After Therapy

• Measure aminotransferases every two months for six months.

• Six months after stopping therapy, test for HCV RNA by PCR. If
HCV RNA is still negative, the chance for a long-term "cure" is
excellent; relapses have rarely been reported after this point.

HCV-derived enzymes such as protease, helicase, and polymerase inhibitors. Drugs that inhibit other steps in HCV replication may also be helpful in treating this disease, by blocking production of HCV antigens from the RNA (IRES [internal ribosome entry site] inhibitors), preventing the normal processing of HCV proteins (inhibitors of glycosylation), or blocking entry of HCV into cells (by blocking its receptor). In addition, nonspecific cytoprotective agents might be helpful for hepatitis C by blocking the cell injury caused by the virus infection. Further, molecular approaches to treating hepatitis C are worthy of investigation; these consist of using ribozymes, which are enzymes that break down specific viral RNA molecules, and antisense oligonucleotides, which are small complementary segments of DNA that bind to viral RNA and inhibit viral replication. All of these approaches remain experimental and few have been applied to humans. The serious nature and the frequency of hepatitis C in the population make the search for new therapies of prime importance.

Prevention

At present, the only means of preventing new cases of hepatitis C are to screen the blood supply, encourage health professionals to take precautions when handling blood and body fluids, and inform people about high-risk behaviors. Programs to promote needle exchange offer some hope of decreasing the spread of hepatitis C among injection drug users. Furthermore, all drug users should receive instruction in safer injection techniques, simple interventions that can be lifesaving. Vaccines and immunoglobulin products do not exist for hepatitis C, and development seems unlikely in the near future because these products would require antibodies to all the genotypes and variants of hepatitis C. Nevertheless, advances in immunology and innovative approaches to immunization make it likely that some form of vaccine for hepatitis C will eventually be developed.

Selected Review Articles and References

Alter HJ, Seeff LB. Recovery, persistence, and sequelae in hepatitis C virus infection: a perspective on long-term outcome. *Seminars in Liver Disease*. 2000; 20(1): 17–35.

Centers for Disease Control and Prevention. Hepatitis A to E. Available at: www.cdc.gov/ncidod/diseases/hepatitis/slideset/httoc.htm (accessed Nov. 25, 1996).

Centers for Disease Control and Prevention. Recommendations for prevention and control of hepatitis C virus (HVC) infection and HVC-related chronic disease. *Morbidity and Mortality Weekly Report.* 1998; 47:1–39.

Fried MW, Shiffman ML, Reddy KR, et al. Peginterferon alfa-2a plus ribavirin for chronic hepatitis C infection. *New England Journal of Medicine.* 2002; 347:972–82.

Lauer GM, Walker BD. Hepatitis C virus infection. *New England Journal of Medicine.* 2001; 345:41–52.

Liang TJ, Reherman B, Seeff LB, Hoofnagle JH. Pathogenesis, natural history, treatment, and prevention of hepatitis C. *Annals of Internal Medicine.* 2000; 132:296–305.

Manns MP, McHutchison JG, Gordon SC, Rustgi VK, Shiffman M, Reindollar R, Goodman ZD, Koury K, Ling M, Albrecht JK. Peginterferon alfa-2b plus ribavirin compared with interferon alfa-2b plus ribavirin for initial treatment of chronic hepatitis C: a randomised trial. *Lancet.* 2001; 358:958–65.

McHutchison JG, Gordon SC, Schiff ER, Shiffman ML, Lee WM, Rustgi VK, Goodman ZD, Ling M-H, Cort S, Albrecht JK. Interferon alfa-2b alone or in combination with ribavirin as initial treatment for chronic hepatitis C. *New England Journal of Medicine.* 1998; 339(21): 1485–92.

Proceedings of the June 10-12 "Management of Hepatitis C: 2002. National Institutes of Health Consensus Development Conference Update." *Hepatology.* 2002; 36 (5, part 2).

Zeuzem S, Feinman SV, Rasenack J, Heathcote EJ, Lai M-Y, Gane E, O'Grady J, Reichen J, Diago M, Lin A, Hoffman J, Brunda MJ. Peginterferon alfa-2a in patients with chronic hepatitis C. *New England Journal of Medicine.* 2000; 343:1666–72.

Chapter 30

Frequently Asked Questions about HCV

Diagnosis and Testing

What is hepatitis C?

Hepatitis C is a liver disease caused by the hepatitis C virus (HCV), which is found in the blood of persons who have this disease. HCV is spread by contact with the blood of an infected person.

Is there a vaccine for the prevention of HCV infection?

No.

What blood tests are available to check for hepatitis C?

There are several blood tests that can be done to determine if you have been infected with HCV. Your doctor may order just one or a combination of these tests. The following are the types of tests your doctor may order and the purpose for each:

- Anti-HCV (antibody to HCV): Anti-HCV does not tell whether the infection is new (acute), chronic (long-term) or is no longer present.

  - EIA (enzyme immunoassay) or CIA (enhanced chemiluminescence immunoassay): This test is usually done first. If positive, it should be confirmed

Reprinted from "Frequently Asked Questions about Hepatitis C," Centers for Disease Control, National Center for Infectious Diseases, December 2004.

- RIBA (recombinant immunoblot assay): A supplemental test used to confirm a positive EIA test
- Qualitative tests to detect presence or absence of virus (HCV RNA)
- Quantitative tests to detect amount (titer) of virus (HCV RNA)

A single positive PCR (polymerase chain reaction) test indicates infection with HCV. A single negative test does not prove that a person is not infected. Virus may be present in the blood and just not found by PCR. Also, a person infected in the past who has recovered may have a negative test. When hepatitis C is suspected and PCR is negative, PCR should be repeated.

Can you have a "false positive" anti-HCV test result?

Yes. A false positive test means the test looks as if it is positive, but it is really negative. This happens more often in persons who have a low risk for the disease for which they are being tested. For example, false positive anti-HCV tests happen more often in persons such as blood donors who are at low risk for hepatitis C. Therefore, it is important to confirm a positive anti-HCV test with a supplemental test as most false positive anti-HCV tests are reported as negative on supplemental testing.

Can you have a "false negative" anti-HCV test result?

Yes. Persons with early infection may not as yet have developed antibody levels high enough that the test can measure. In addition, some persons may lack the (immune) response necessary for the test to work well. In these persons, research-based tests such as PCR may be considered.

How long after exposure to HCV does it take to test positive for anti-HCV?

Anti-HCV can be found in seven out of ten persons when symptoms begin and in about nine out of ten persons within three months after symptoms begin. However, it is important to note that many persons who have hepatitis C have no symptoms.

How long after exposure to HCV does it take to test positive with PCR?

It is possible to find HCV within one to two weeks after being infected with the virus.

Who should get tested for hepatitis C?

- persons who ever injected illegal drugs, including those who injected once or a few times many years ago

- persons who were treated for clotting problems with a blood product made before 1987 when more advanced methods for manufacturing the products were developed

- persons who were notified that they received blood from a donor who later tested positive for hepatitis C

- persons who received a blood transfusion or solid organ transplant before July 1992 when better testing of blood donors became available

- long-term hemodialysis patients

- persons who have signs or symptoms of liver disease (e.g., abnormal liver enzyme tests)

- healthcare workers after exposures (e.g., needle sticks or splashes to the eye) to HCV-positive blood on the job

- children born to HCV-positive women

What is the next step if you have a confirmed positive anti-HCV test?

Measure the level of ALT (alanine aminotransferase, a liver enzyme) in the blood. An elevated ALT indicates inflammation of the liver and you should be checked further for chronic (long-term) liver disease and possible treatment. The evaluation should be done by a healthcare professional familiar with chronic hepatitis C.

Can you have a normal liver enzyme (e.g., ALT) level and still have chronic hepatitis C?

Yes. It is common for persons with chronic hepatitis C to have a liver enzyme level that goes up and down, with periodic returns to normal or near normal. Some persons have a liver enzyme level that is normal for over a year but they still have chronic liver disease. If the liver enzyme level is normal, persons should have their enzyme level re-checked several times over a six- to twelve-month period. If the liver enzyme level remains normal, your doctor may check it less frequently, such as once a year.

Spread of HCV from One Person to Another

How could a person have gotten hepatitis C?

HCV is spread primarily by direct contact with human blood. For example, you may have gotten infected with HCV if:

• you ever injected street drugs, as the needles and other drug "works" used to prepare or inject the drug(s) may have had someone else's blood that contained HCV on them.

• you received blood, blood products, or solid organs from a donor whose blood contained HCV.

• you were ever on long-term kidney dialysis, as you may have unknowingly shared supplies or equipment that had someone else's blood on them.

• you were ever a healthcare worker and had frequent contact with blood on the job, especially accidental needlesticks.

• your mother had hepatitis C at the time she gave birth to you. During the birth her blood may have gotten into your body.

• you ever had sex with a person infected with HCV.

• you lived with someone who was infected with HCV and shared items such as razors or toothbrushes that might have had that person's blood on them.

How long can HCV live outside the body and transmit infection?

Recent studies suggest that HCV may survive on environmental surfaces at room temperature at least sixteen hours, but no longer than four days.

Is there any evidence that HCV has been spread during medical or dental procedures done in the United States?

Medical and dental procedures done in the United States generally do not pose a risk for the spread of HCV. However, there have been a few situations in which HCV has been spread between patients when supplies or equipment were shared between them.

Can HCV be spread by sexual activity?

Yes, but this does not occur very often. See following section on counseling for more information on hepatitis C and sexual activity.

Can HCV be spread by oral sex?

There is no evidence that HCV has been spread by oral sex. See section on counseling for more information on hepatitis C and sexual activity.

Can HCV be spread within a household?

Yes, but this does not occur very often. If HCV is spread within a household, it is most likely due to direct exposure to the blood of an infected household member.

Since more advanced tests have been developed for use in blood banks, what is the chance now that a person can get HCV infection from transfused blood or blood products?

Less than one chance per million units transfused.

Pregnancy and Breastfeeding

Should pregnant women be routinely tested for anti-HCV?

No. Pregnant women have no greater risk of being infected with HCV then nonpregnant women. If pregnant women have risk factors for hepatitis C, they should be tested for anti-HCV.

What is the risk that HCV-infected women will spread HCV to their newborn infants?

About five out of every one hundred infants born to HCV-infected women become infected. This occurs at the time of birth, and there is no treatment that can prevent this from happening. Most infants infected with HCV at the time of birth have no symptoms and do well during childhood. More studies are needed to find out if these children will have problems from the infection as they grow older. There are no licensed treatments or guidelines for the treatment of infants or children infected with HCV. Children with elevated ALT (liver enzyme) levels should be referred for evaluation to a specialist familiar with the management of children with HCV-related disease.

Should a woman with hepatitis C be advised against breastfeeding?

No. There is no evidence that breastfeeding spreads HCV. HCV-positive mothers should consider abstaining from breastfeeding if their nipples are cracked or bleeding.

When should babies born to mothers with hepatitis C be tested to see if they were infected at birth?

Children should not be tested for anti-HCV before eighteen months of age, as anti-HCV from the mother might last until this age. If diagnosis is desired prior to eighteen months of age, testing for HCV RNA could be performed at or after an infant's first well-child visit at age one to two months. HCV RNA testing should then be repeated at a subsequent visit independent of the initial HCV RNA test result.

Counseling

How can persons infected with HCV prevent spreading HCV to others?

- Do not donate blood, body organs, other tissue, or semen.

- Do not share personal items that might have your blood on them, such as toothbrushes, dental appliances, nail-grooming equipment, or razors.

- Cover your cuts and skin sores to keep from spreading HCV.

How can people protect themselves from getting hepatitis C and other diseases spread by contact with human blood?

- Don't ever shoot drugs. If you shoot drugs, stop and get into a treatment program. If you can't stop, never reuse or share syringes, water, or drug works, and get vaccinated against hepatitis A and hepatitis B.

- Do not share toothbrushes, razors, or other personal care articles. They might have blood on them.

- If you are a healthcare worker, always follow routine barrier precautions and safely handle needles and other sharps. Get vaccinated against hepatitis B

- Consider the health risks if you are thinking about getting a tattoo or body piercing: You can get infected if:

- the tools that are used have someone else's blood on them.

- the artist or piercer doesn't follow good health practices, such as washing hands and using disposable gloves.

HCV can be spread by sex, but this does not occur very often. If you are having sex, but not with one steady partner:

- You and your partners can get other diseases spread by having sex (e.g., AIDS, hepatitis B, gonorrhea, or chlamydia).

- You should use latex condoms correctly and every time. The efficacy of latex condoms in preventing infection with HCV is unknown, but their proper use may reduce transmission.

- You should get vaccinated against hepatitis B.

Should patients with hepatitis C change their sexual practices if they have only one long-term steady sex partner?

No. There is a very low chance of spreading HCV to that partner through sexual activity. If you want to lower the small chance of spreading HCV to your sex partner, you may decide to use barrier precautions such as latex condoms. The efficacy of latex condoms in preventing infection with HCV is unknown, but their proper use may reduce transmission. Ask your doctor about having your sex partner tested.

What can persons with HCV infection do to protect their liver?

- Stop using alcohol.

- See your doctor regularly.

- Don't start any new medicines or use over-the-counter, herbal, and other medicines without a physician's knowledge.

- Get vaccinated against hepatitis A if liver damage is present.

What other information should patients with hepatitis C be aware of?

- HCV is not spread by sneezing, hugging, coughing, food or water, sharing eating utensils or drinking glasses, or casual contact.

- Persons should not be excluded from work, school, play, child-care or other settings on the basis of their HCV infection status.

- Involvement with a support group may help patients cope with hepatitis C.

Should persons with chronic hepatitis C be vaccinated against hepatitis B?

If persons are in risk groups for whom hepatitis B vaccine is recommended, they should be vaccinated.

Long-Term Consequences of HCV Infection

What are the chances of persons with HCV infection developing long-term infection, chronic liver disease, cirrhosis, or liver cancer, or dying as a result of hepatitis C?

Of every one hundred persons infected with HCV, about:

- Fifty-five to eighty-five persons might develop long-term infection
- Seventy persons might develop chronic liver disease
- Five to twenty persons might develop cirrhosis over a period of twenty to thirty years
- One to five persons might die from the consequences of long-term infection (liver cancer or cirrhosis)

Hepatitis C is a leading indication for liver transplants.

Do medical conditions outside the liver occur in persons with chronic hepatitis C?

A small percentage of persons with chronic hepatitis C develop medical conditions outside the liver (this is called extrahepatic). These conditions are thought to occur due to the body's natural immune system fighting against itself. Such conditions include: glomerulonephritis, essential mixed cryoglobulinemia, and porphyria cutanea tarda.

Management and Treatment of Chronic Hepatitis C

When might a specialist (gastroenterologist, infectious disease physician, or hepatologist) be consulted in the management of HCV-infected persons?

A referral to or consultation with a specialist for further evaluation and possible treatment may be considered if a person is anti-HCV positive and has elevated liver enzyme levels. Any physician who manages a person with hepatitis C should be knowledgeable and current on all aspects of the care of a person with hepatitis C.

What is the treatment for chronic hepatitis C?

Combination therapy with pegylated interferon and ribavirin is the treatment of choice resulting in sustained response rates of 40 to 80 percent (up to 50 percent for patients infected with the most common genotype found in the United States [genotype 1] and up to 80 percent for patients infected with genotypes 2 or 3). Interferon monotherapy is generally reserved for patients in whom ribavirin is contraindicated. Ribavirin, when used alone, does not work. Combination therapy using interferon and ribavirin is now FDA approved for the use in children aged three to seventeen years.

What are the side effects of interferon therapy?

Most persons have flu-like symptoms (fever, chills, headache, muscle and joint aches, fast heart rate) early in treatment, but these lessen with continued treatment. Later side effects may include tiredness, hair loss, low blood count, trouble with thinking, moodiness, and depression. Severe side effects are rare (seen in less than two out of one hundred persons). These include thyroid disease, depression with suicidal thoughts, seizures, acute heart or kidney failure, eye and lung problems, hearing loss, and blood infection. Although rare, deaths have occurred due to liver failure or blood infection, mostly in persons with cirrhosis. An important side effect of interferon is worsening of liver disease with treatment, which can be severe and even fatal. Interferon dosage must be reduced in up to forty out of one hundred persons because of severity of side effects, and treatment must be stopped in up to fifteen out of one hundred persons. Pregnant women should not be treated with interferon.

What are the side effects of combination (ribavirin + interferon) treatment?

In addition to the side effects due to interferon described previously, ribavirin can cause serious anemia (low red blood cell count) and can be a serious problem for persons with conditions that cause anemia, such as kidney failure. In these persons, combination therapy should be avoided or attempts should be made to correct the anemia. Anemia caused by ribavirin can be life-threatening for persons with certain types of heart or blood vessel disease. Ribavirin causes birth defects and pregnancy should be avoided during treatment. Patients and their healthcare providers should carefully review the product manufacturer information prior to treatment.

Can anything be done to reduce symptoms or side effects due to antiviral treatment?

You should report what you are feeling to your doctor. Some side effects may be reduced by giving interferon at night or lowering the dosage of the drug. In addition, flu-like symptoms can be reduced by taking acetaminophen before treatment.

Can children receive interferon therapy for chronic hepatitis C?

The Food and Drug Administration has approved the use of the combination antiviral therapy for the treatment of hepatitis C in children three to seventeen years old.

Genotype

What does the term genotype mean?

Genotype refers to the genetic make-up of an organism or a virus. There are at least six distinct HCV genotypes identified. Genotype 1 is the most common genotype seen in the United States.

Is it necessary to do genotyping when managing a person with chronic hepatitis C?

Yes, as there are six known genotypes and more than fifty subtypes of HCV, and genotype information is helpful in defining the epidemiology of hepatitis C. Knowing the genotype or serotype (genotype-specific antibodies) of HCV is helpful in making recommendations and counseling regarding therapy. Patients with genotypes 2 and 3 are almost three times more likely than patients with genotype 1 to respond to therapy with alpha interferon or the combination of alpha interferon and ribavirin. Furthermore, when using combination therapy, the recommended duration of treatment depends on the genotype. For patients with genotypes 2 and 3, a twenty-four-week course of combination treatment is adequate, whereas for patients with genotype 1, a forty-eight-week course is recommended. For these reasons, testing for HCV genotype is often clinically helpful. Once the genotype is identified, it need not be tested again; genotypes do not change during the course of infection.

Why do most persons remain infected?

Persons infected with HCV mount an antibody response to parts of the virus, but changes in the virus during infection result in changes that are not recognized by preexisting antibodies. This appears to be how the virus establishes and maintains long-lasting infection.

Can persons become infected with different genotypes?

Yes. Because of the ineffective immune response described previously, prior infection does not protect against reinfection with the same or different genotypes of the virus. For the same reason, there is no effective pre- or postexposure prophylaxis (i.e., immune globulin) available.

Hepatitis C and Healthcare Workers

What is the risk for HCV infection from a needlestick exposure to HCV-contaminated blood?

After needlestick or sharps exposure to HCV-positive blood, about two (1.8 percent) healthcare workers out of one hundred will get infected with HCV (range 0 percent to 10 percent).

What are the recommendations for follow-up of healthcare workers after exposure to HCV-positive blood?

Anti-viral agents (e.g., interferon) or immune globulin should not be used for postexposure prophylaxis.

1. For the source, baseline testing for anti-HCV.

2. For the person exposed to an HCV-positive source, baseline and follow-up testing including

   - baseline testing for anti-HCV and ALT activity; and

   - follow-up testing for anti-HCV (e.g., at four to six months) and ALT activity. (If earlier diagnosis of HCV infection is desired, testing for HCV RNA may be performed at four to six weeks.)

3. Confirmation by supplemental anti-HCV testing of all anti-HCV results reported as positive by enzyme immunoassay.

Should HCV-infected healthcare workers be restricted in their work?

No, there are no recommendations to restrict a healthcare worker who is infected with HCV. The risk of transmission from an infected healthcare worker to a patient appears to be very low. As recommended for all healthcare workers, those who are HCV positive should follow strict aseptic technique and standard precautions, including appropriate use of hand washing, protective barriers, and care in the use and disposal of needles and other sharp instruments.

Chapter 31

HCV Transmission

Chapter Contents

Section 31.1

Facts about HCV Transmission

Reprinted from "Hepatitis C Virus Transmission," VA National Hepatitis
C Program, Department of Veterans Affairs (VA), November 2004.

Some modes of transmission of hepatitis C virus are well documented and widely accepted; others are less well defined and require
further study. It is clear that HCV is most frequently transmitted
through large or repeated direct percutaneous exposures to infected
blood. The two most common exposures associated with transmission
of HCV are blood transfusion and injection drug use.

Blood Transfusion or Receipt of Blood Products

Early case-control studies of patients with newly acquired, symptomatic non-A, non-B hepatitis found a significant association between
disease acquisition and a history six months prior to illness of blood
transfusions, injection drug use, health care employment with frequent exposure to blood, personal contact with others who had hepatitis, multiple sexual partners, or low socioeconomic status.[1,2] Today,
HCV is rarely transmitted by blood transfusion or transplantation of
organs due to thorough screening of the blood supply for the presence
of the virus and inactivation procedures that destroy blood-borne viruses. In the last several years, blood banks have instituted techniques
that utilize nucleic acid amplification of the hepatitis C virus, which
will detect the presence of virus even in newly infected patients who
are still hepatitis C antibody-negative. These techniques are estimated
to have prevented fifty-six transfusion-associated HCV infections per
year in the United States since 1999, and have lowered the current risk
of acquiring HCV via transfused blood products to one in two million.[3]

Injection Drug Use

Injection drug use has been the principal mode of transmission of
HCV since the 1970s. In comparison to other viral infections, HCV is
more rapidly acquired after initiation of intravenous drug use.[4] In

addition, rates of HCV among young injecting drug-users are four times higher than HIV infection.[5] Studies of injection drug users have demonstrated that the prevalence of HCV infection in them is extremely high, with up to 90 percent having been exposed.[6] In addition, the incidence of new infections is also high, with seroconversion rates of 10 to 20 percent per year of injecting.[7,8] Duration of injecting is the strongest single predictor of risk of HCV infection among injection drug users.[9]

Sexual Transmission

Sexual transmission of HCV has been controversial. It is believed that HCV can be transmitted sexually, but that such transmission is inefficient. The likelihood of HCV infection increases with the number of lifetime sexual partners. A history of a sexually transmitted disease, sex with a prostitute, more than five sexual partners per year, or a combination of these has been independently associated with positive HCV serology.[10] Distinction appears to exist between the specific sexual behaviors listed previously and stable, monogamous sexual activity, which is rarely associated with HCV transmission. The frequency of HCV transmission between monogamous sexual partners is very low according to most studies.[11,12]

Other Modes of Transmission

Household Transmission

The prevalence of HCV among household contacts of people with HCV infection is low. Moreover, the study of HCV transmission among household contacts is complicated by the difficulty in ruling out other possible modes of acquisition. Many of the studies include a small number of nonsexual contacts, and often include children born to mothers with HCV infection.[13] Therefore, it is difficult to determine whether nonsexual, nonblood contact is a route of transmission for HCV.

Occupational Exposures

Healthcare workers who have exposure to blood are at risk of infection with HCV and other blood-borne pathogens. The prevalence of HCV infection, however, is no greater in healthcare workers, including surgeons, than for the general population. According to the CDC, the average rate of anti-HCV seroconversion after unintentional needlesticks or sharps exposure from an HCV-positive source is 1.8 percent (range 0 to 7 percent). An Italian study of 4,403 needlesticks among healthcare workers found fourteen seroconversions (0.31 percent).[14] There is an emerging body of literature, however, that close follow-up of healthcare workers after a needlestick from a patient with chronic HCV, with early interferon and ribavirin therapy for the healthcare worker if he or she develops HCV viremia but fails to clear within three to six months, can be a beneficial management strategy.[15]

No Identifiable Source of Infection

According to the Centers for Disease Control and Prevention, injection drug use accounts for approximately 60 percent of all HCV infections in the United States, while other known exposures account for 20 to 30 percent.[5] Approximately 10 percent of patients in most epidemiological studies, however, have no identifiable source of infection.[16] HCV exposure in these patients may be from a number of uncommon modes of transmission, including vertical transmission and parenteral transmission from medical or dental procedures prior to the availability of HCV testing. There are no conclusive data to show that persons with a history of exposures such as intranasal cocaine use, tattooing, or body piercing are at an increased risk for HCV infection based on these exposures solely. It is believed, however, that these are potential modes of HCV acquisition in the absence of adequate sterilization techniques.

References

1. Alter MJ, et al. Sporadic non-A, non-B hepatitis: frequency and epidemiology in an urban United States population. *J Infect Dis* 1982; 145:886–93.

2. Alter MJ, et al. Importance of heterosexual activity in the transmission of hepatitis B and non-A, non-B hepatitis. *JAMA* 1989; 262:1201–5.

3. Stramer SL, et al. Detection of HIV-1 and HCV infections among antibody-negative blood donors by nucleic acid-amplification testing. *N Engl J Med* 2004; 351:760–68.

4. Garfein RS, et al. Viral infections in short-term injection drug users: the prevalence of the hepatitis C, hepatitis B, human immunodeficiency, and human T-lymphotropic viruses.. *Am J Public Health* 1996; 86:655–71.

5. Centers for Disease Control and Prevention. Recommendations for prevention and control of hepatitis C virus (HCV) infection and HCV-related chronic disease. *MMWR* 1998; 47 (RR-19): 1–39.

6. Patrick DM et al. Public health and hepatitis C. *Can J Public Health* 2000; 91 (suppl 1): S18–S23.

7. Hahn JA, et al. Hepatitis C virus infection and needle exchange use among young injection drug users in San Francisco. *Hepatology* 2001; 34:180–87.

8. Thorpe LE, et al. Risk of hepatitis C virus infection among young injection drug users who share injection equipment. *Am J Epidemiol* 2002; 155:645–53.

9. Conry-Cantilena C, et al. Routes of infection, viremia, and liver disease in blood donors found to have hepatitis C virus infection. *N Engl J Med* 1996; 334:1691–6.

10. Gross JB. Hepatitis C: A sexually transmitted disease? *Am J Gastroenterol* 2001; 96:3051–53.

11. Vandelli C, Renzo F, Romano L, Tisminetzky S, De Palma M, et al. Lack of evidence of sexual transmission of hepatitis C among monogamous couples: results of a 10-year prospective follow-up study.. *Am J Gastroenterol* 2004; 99:855–59.

12. Terrault NA. Sexual activity as a risk factor for hepatitis C. *Hepatol* 2002; 36:S99–105.

13. Ackerman Z, Ackerman E, Paltiel O. Intrafamilial transmission of hepatitis C virus: a systematic review. *J Viral Hepatitis* 2000; 7:93–103.

14. De Carli G, Puro V, Ippolito G, et al. Risk of hepatitis C virus transmission following percutaneous exposure in healthcare workers.. *Infection* 2003; 31-suppl 2: 22–27.

15. Sulkowski MS, Ray SC, Thomas DL. Needlestick transmission of hepatitis C. *JAMA* 2002; 287:2406–13.

16. Flamm SL, Parker RA, Chopra S. Risk factors associated with chronic hepatitis C virus infection: limited frequency of an unidentified source of transmission. *Am J Gastroenterol* 1998; 93:597–600.

Section 31.2

Needlestick Exposure and HCV

Hepatitis C virus (HCV) is a hepatitis virus transmitted through blood-to-blood exposure. Hepatitis C is commonly acquired through blood product transfusions (primarily before 1992), needle sharing (including acupuncture), tattooing, body-piercing, and even through sharing personal hygiene items. In as many as 10 percent of individuals transmission route cannot be explained.

What is my risk of acquiring hepatitis C from a needlestick?

Unlike hepatitis B virus, hepatitis C is not efficiently transmitted from a needlestick. The average rate of seroconversion (changing from hepatitis C antibody negative to hepatitis C antibody positive) after an occupational exposure to HCV positive blood is about 1.8 percent, but has ranged as high as 7 to 10 percent in some studies. This risk is highest with hollow-bore needles.

What can be done to prevent the transmission of hepatitis C?

There is currently no vaccine or immunoglobulin (IG) to protect against HCV transmission. Several studies evaluating the response to passive immunoglobulin found that high anti-HCV titer IG did not prevent transmission. This makes sense given that the rapid mutation rate of HCV allows the virus to escape from any protective antibody that may form during infection. Postexposure treatment with interferon, with or without ribavirin, is also confusing and controversial. At present, however, there is no recommendation for the use of antiviral therapy following needlestick exposure to an HCV-positive source.

What should I do if I'm exposed to HCV-positive blood?

Currently, the best recommendation is to carefully monitor for laboratory abnormalities, signs, and symptoms of acute hepatitis C infection. Acute hepatitis C is a difficult disease to study. This is due to the declining incidence of acute hepatitis C and the fact that most patients are not initially symptomatic. Given these limitations, a noncontrolled study evaluating the response to a twenty-four-week course of interferon alfa (Jaeckel et al.,: Treatment of Acute Hepatitis C with Interferon Alfa-2b. *NEJM* 2001; 345:1452–57) found that 98 percent of treated patients exhibited a sustained biochemical and virologic response twenty-four weeks after treatment of acute hepatitis C. These are exciting results, especially given that previous studies suggested that only 15 to 30 percent of individuals with acute infection recover without treatment.

Should we treat everyone with acute hepatitis C or exposure to hepatitis C?

Before recommending any treatment, we should be sure that it is the best thing for the patient. Interferon is expensive and has many side effects, some of which could be life-threatening. The study was not controlled (i.e., there was not a group with acute hepatitis C that did not receive treatment). We know that 15 to 30 percent of patients exposed to hepatitis C will recover without any treatment. In addition, the patients in the study were symptomatic and often had jaundice. Previous investigations suggest that progression to chronic hepatitis C is much lower in young patients with jaundice, making it more likely that these individuals could have spontaneous clearance. The individuals in the study were not treated immediately after exposure, but rather months after they had symptoms. This would suggest that therapy could be delayed without adverse affects, allowing patients to spontaneously recover before prescribing an expensive and difficult-to-tolerate medication. But the number one reason that interferon therapy is not standard in acute infection is that we need more data to ensure that this is the most beneficial treatment to offer. Currently, the U.S. public health service guidelines for management of HCV exposures include:

1. Baseline testing for anti-HCV and ALT activity

2. Follow-up testing at four to six months for anti-HCV and ALT activity or HCV RNA at four to six weeks

3. Exposed individuals should not donate blood, plasma, organs, tissue, or semen

4. Exposed person does not need to modify sexual practices or refrain from pregnancy or discontinue breast-feeding

5. When HCV infection is confirmed early, the person should be referred for medical management to a specialist in this area

6. IG and anti-viral agents are not recommended

The 2002 NIH Consensus conference recommended that patients with acute hepatitis C were potential candidates for interferon therapy, but realized many questions remained unanswered, particularly: which patients with acute HCV should be treated, and when is the ideal time to start therapy?

Section 31.3

HCV Infection in Cocaine Users

Reprinted from "Hepatitis C Virus Infection in Cocaine Users: A Silent Epidemic," October 2000. © 2000 Medical College of Wisconsin. Reprinted with permission of Medical College of Wisconsin HealthLink, www.health link.mcw.edu.

Researchers at the Medical College of Wisconsin have found that up to one-third of cocaine users who thought they were healthy may be infected with hepatitis C. Hepatitis C can lead to chronic hepatitis, cirrhosis of the liver, and even liver cancer. There is no cure or vaccine.

It has been suggested by some researchers that hepatitis C infection may be the major cause of liver disease in the United States. The use of alcohol may make the effects of hepatitis C on the liver more severe.

"Our observations suggest a significant epidemic in an unsuspecting population with little regular access to health care," notes study author Harold H. Harsch, M.D., associate professor of psychiatry at the Medical College. "These individuals also form a large pool for the continued transmission of hepatitis C to the general population. As this reservoir of virus increases, even what may be minor transmission channels, such as sexual activity, ear piercing, and tattooing will become more significant."

The study screened cocaine users who volunteered for a study of how the brain reacts to cocaine. Of the 144 people screened, 47 were found to have hepatitis C, while only seven tested positive for hepatitis B and only two for HIV. Of the 144, 56 percent were African American, 81 percent were male, 75 percent were never married, and 55 percent were unemployed. The average age was thirty-six. None of the subjects had ever received a blood transfusion.

Twenty-nine percent who tested negative for hepatitis C reported intravenous drug use, while 77 percent of those testing positive for the disease reported IV drug use. Those who tested positive for hepatitis C tended to be three to four years older than hepatitis C-free patients.

One of the most surprising findings was that about 14 percent of those with hepatitis C said they had never used intravenous drugs. This suggests that there are other ways for the spread of the disease among cocaine users, such as sharing straws to snort cocaine, particularly if nosebleeds occur. For hepatitis C to be spread, the virus generally must enter the bloodstream through the skin or mucous membranes. Hepatitis C does not spread as easily through sexual contact as hepatitis B or HIV.

A recent study of blood donors who tested positive for hepatitis C found that intranasal cocaine use, sexual promiscuity, intravenous drug use, history of transfusion, and ear piercing among men were risk factors.

It was only in the late 1980s that a test was developed to identify hepatitis C. While screening for hepatitis B and HIV has become routine at hospitals, drug centers, and blood banks, hepatitis C is sometimes overlooked. The Medical College study suggests it may be widespread among cocaine users, including those who smoke crack cocaine.

The Medical College study appeared in the June 2000 issue of *Community Mental Health Journal*. Co-authors of the study are John Pankiewicz, M.D.; Alan S. Bloom, Ph.D.; Charles Rainey, M.D.; Jung-Ki Cho, M.D.; Lori Sperry, Ph.D.; and Elliott A. Stein, Ph.D.

Section 31.4

Sex and HCV

Reprinted from "Sex and Hepatitis C Virus," VA National Hepatitis
C Program, Department of Veterans Affairs (VA), June 2004.

Many people with hepatitis C are worried about spreading the virus to their sex partners. This section talks about how likely it is to spread the hepatitis C virus through sex. If you have hepatitis C, it is not very likely that you will spread the virus through sex. But it is still possible. That is why it is very important to talk honestly and openly with your sex partner(s).

Can I give hepatitis C to my sex partner?

Yes, but it is not likely. Compared to hepatitis B virus and the human immunodeficiency virus (HIV), it is less likely that you will spread the hepatitis C virus to your sex partner.

If you have one long-term sex partner, you do not necessarily need to change your sex habits. But, if either you or your partner is worried about the small chance of spreading the hepatitis C virus, you can use latex condoms. This will make it almost impossible to spread the virus. Long-term partners of people with hepatitis C should get tested for the virus. If the test is negative, you will probably not need to repeat it.

If you have more than one sex partner, you are more likely to spread the virus. In this case, reduce the number of sex partners you have, practice safer sex, and always use latex condoms.

Can I get hepatitis C through other types of sexual contact, such as oral and anal sex?

We do not know if the virus can be spread by oral or anal sex. There is no proof that anyone has ever spread the virus through oral sex, although it may be possible. Anal sex may damage the lining of the rectum and make it easier to pass the virus through the blood. Using condoms will help prevent spreading the hepatitis C virus and will also protect you against other sexually transmitted diseases, such as HIV (human immunodeficiency virus) and hepatitis B.

You *cannot* spread the hepatitis C virus through other types of contact, such as hugging or kissing someone on the cheek.

I know the hepatitis C virus is in my blood, but is it in my saliva, semen, or vaginal secretions?

Some studies show that the virus may live in your saliva, semen, or vaginal secretions, but no one knows for sure. We also don't know exactly how much of the virus may live in these bodily fluids or if it can be passed on to a sex partner from these fluids.

If I have large amounts of virus in my blood, am I more likely to spread the disease to my sex partner(s)?

Some studies suggest that a lot of the virus in the blood might make it easier to spread the virus. But even with high levels of the virus, you are still not very likely to spread the virus through sex. You do not necessarily have to change your sex habits if you have higher levels of the hepatitis C virus.

What kind of birth control methods will prevent the spread of the hepatitis C virus?

If you are worried about the small risk of spreading the virus through sex, you should use latex condoms. Other types of birth control methods, like birth control pills, vasectomy, intrauterine devices (IUDs), or diaphragms do not decrease the risk of spreading the hepatitis C virus. Latex condoms will also help prevent the spread of hepatitis B, HIV, and other sexually transmitted diseases.

Can my partner get pregnant, and if so, what is the risk that the baby will get hepatitis C?

It is possible to get pregnant if you or your partner has hepatitis C. If you are a male with hepatitis C, and your female partner does not have hepatitis C (throughout the entire pregnancy), then there is no chance that the baby will contract the virus from the mother. If you are a pregnant female who already has hepatitis C (or gets hepatitis C at some point during the pregnancy), the chance of passing the virus to your baby is low, less than 5 percent. The risk becomes greater if the mother has both hepatitis C and HIV. With proper prenatal care, babies born to hepatitis C–positive mothers or fathers are usually quite healthy.

I am on combination treatment (ribavirin and interferon). Do I need to use birth control methods?

Yes! Ribavirin can cause severe birth defects, and you or your partner should *not* get pregnant while you are taking it. If you are taking ribavirin to treat your hepatitis C, you must use two effective forms of birth control, one for you and one for your partner. For example: the man uses a condom, and the woman uses a diaphragm or birth control pill. You must continue this type of birth control for six months after your last dose of combination treatment.

What makes me more likely to spread the hepatitis C virus to my sexual partner(s)?

You may be more likely to spread the virus if you:

- do not use latex condoms.
- have more than one sex partner.
- have had sexually transmitted diseases (STDs) before.
- also have another virus such as HIV.

How can I reduce the chances of spreading the hepatitis C virus through sexual contact?

To reduce this chance, use the following guidelines:

- Have sex with only one person, or not at all.
- Decrease the number of people with whom you have sex.
- Tell your sex partner(s) that you have hepatitis C and that it is unlikely, but still possible, to spread it to them.
- Use latex condoms correctly and every time, especially if
  - you have more than one sex partner;
  - you have "rough" sex, which might make one of you bleed;
  - you have sex during your menstrual period or your partner's menstrual period;
  - you have sex when you or your partner has an open sore or cut on either of your genitals.

The risk of spreading hepatitis C to your sex partner(s) is small. If you can talk openly about the disease, and are careful about your sex habits, you can have a safe, healthy sex life.

Section 31.5

Mother-to-Child Transmission of HCV

Hepatitis C virus (HCV) infection is common in the United States, estimated to affect some three million persons. Transmission of the virus is parenteral, that is, transmitted by blood. Statistically, the most common risk factor for HCV infection is current or remote drug use, but this mode of infection accounts for only half of known cases. It is clear that HCV can be transmitted via other exchanges of bodily fluids, including sexual contact and, the focus of this report, vertical (mother to infant) transmission.

Estimates of the prevalence of HCV infection in pregnant women vary widely among studies, ranging from 0.1 percent to 4.5 percent. Because the identified risk factors for HCV seropositivity in this group are identical to those of the general population, it is reasonable to conclude that the true seroprevalence in pregnant women is quite similar to that of the general public, or about 1.8 percent.

The rate of vertical transmission of HCV has also been estimated with widely varying results. The difficulty of obtaining accurate measurement of vertical transmission risk includes persistence of maternal antibodies in the newborn, failure to identify all infected mothers, and loss of infants born to HCV-positive mothers to follow-up. This being said, the best estimate of the prevalence of vertical transmission of HCV is in the range of 5 percent. Although HCV/HIV co-infection appears to increase the risk of vertical transmission, other risk factors have not been consistently identified. Even the identification of the timing of such transmission between intrauterine versus intrapartum exposure has not been satisfactorily delineated.

313

Previous Studies

Following is a summary of some of the largest studies of vertical transmission of HCV to date:

The Japanese Vertical Transmission of HCV Collaborative study, published in 1994, found a transmission rate of 5.6 percent in a small sample of 54 infants born to HCV-positive mothers. Transmission appears correlated with viral load.[1] The following year, the Lombardy Study on Vertical HCV Transmission reported the results from 116 infants born to HCV-positive mothers, 22 of whom were HCV/HIV co-infected. Vertical transmission was not seen in the HCV-only group, while a rate of 36 percent was seen in the co-infected group.[2] A Scandinavian study published in 1996 showed no transmission in 55 mothers, including two of whom were HCV/HIV co-infected.[3] A 1997 Italian study reported on a larger sample of 245 infants, with a vertical transmission rate of 3.7 percent, but higher figures in HCV/HIV co-infection (15 percent). This group also reported a higher risk in vaginal vs. cesarian delivery.[4] A 1998 Italian study of 75 HCV-infected pregnant women revealed a 4.4 percent vertical transmission rate in HCV-only infection and a more disconcerting 17 percent transmission rate in HCV/HIV co-infection.[5]

The largest study to date is a report published in the journal *Hepatology* in 2000 by Conte et al., in which 15,250 consecutive pregnant women were screened for HCV, 370 of whom had evidence of viral infection. Overall vertical transmission rate was 5.1 percent and was seen exclusively in mothers who had detectable viremia by PCR (polymerase chain reaction). Genotype, viral load, vaginal vs. cesarean delivery, breast-feeding or HIV co-infection were not associated with transmission.[6]

Recommendations

Based upon these and other studies, the following guidelines and recommendations can be made:

• HCV-positive mothers can transmit infection to their babies. The most accurate estimate of such an event is in the range of 5 percent. This risk is probably increased in the setting of HCV-HIV co-infection. It is not clear that high viral load increases the risk of transmission.

• The presence of HCV infection does not appear to result in a higher risk pregnancy or a higher incidence of poor obstetric outcome.

- Testing for the presence of HCV in infants born to HCV-positive mothers should not begin until at least one year following delivery. The natural history of HCV-infected infants is poorly understood at this time.

- Prophylactic caesarian section is not recommended in HCV-infected mothers. The role of cesarean delivery in HCV/HIV co-infected mothers remains controversial.

- Breast-feeding presents a low or negligible risk of transmission, and, given the well-documented benefits, should be routinely recommended.

References

1. Ohto H, Terazawa S, Sasaki N, Sasaki N, Hino K, Ishiwata C, Kako M, Ujiie N. Endo C. Matsui A. Transmission of hepatitis C virus from mothers to infants. *N Engl J Med.* 330(11): 744–50, 1994 Mar 17.

2. Zanetti AR, Tanzi E, Paccagnini S, Principi N, Pizzocolo G, Caccamo ML, D'Amico E, Cambie G, Vecchi L. Mother-to-infant transmission of hepatitis C virus. *Lancet.* 345(8945): 289–91, 1995 Feb 4.

3. Fischler B, Lindh G, Lindgren S, Forsgren M, Von Sydow M, Sangfelt P, Alaeus A, Harland L, Enockson E, Nemeth A. Vertical transmission of hepatitis C virus infection. *Scand J Infect Dis.* 28(4): 353–56, 1996.

4. Tovo PA, Palomba E, Ferraris G, Principi N, Ruga E, Dallacasa P, Maccabruni A. Increased risk of maternal-infant hepatitis C virus transmission for women co-infected with human immunodeficiency virus type 1. *Clin Infect Dis.* 25(5): 1121–24, 1997 Nov.

5. Mazza C, Ravaggi A, Rodella A, Padula D, Duse M, Lomini M, Puoti M, Rossini A, Cariani E. Prospective study of mother-to-infant transmission of hepatitis C virus (HCV) infection. Study Group for Vertical Transmission. *J Med Virol.* 54(1): 12–19, 1998 Jan.

6. Conte D, Fraquelli M, Prati D, Colucci A, Minola E. Prevalence and clinical course of chronic hepatitis C virus (HCV) infection and rate of HCV vertical transmission in a cohort of 15,250 pregnant women. *Hepatology.* 31(3): 751–55, 2000 Mar.

Chapter 32

Risks and Benefits of Screening for HCV

Background

Hepatitis C virus (HCV) is the most common blood-borne pathogen in the United States and is an important cause of patient morbidity and mortality, but it is unclear whether screening to identify asymptomatic infected persons is appropriate.

Introduction

Hepatitis C virus (HCV), the most common chronic blood-borne pathogen in the United States, is acquired primarily by large or repeated percutaneous exposures to blood. In the United States, approximately 2.3 percent of adults twenty years of age or older are positive for anti-HCV-antibody. Between 55 percent and 84 percent of these have chronic infection, but only 5 percent to 50 percent of infected adults are thought to know their status.

In the United States, HCV is associated with approximately 40 percent of cases of chronic liver disease and eight thousand to ten thousand deaths each year. Chronic HCV infection can also cause fatigue and decreased quality of life in the absence of cirrhosis or other complications.

Excerpted from "Screening for Hepatitis C Virus Infection: A Review of the Evidence for the U.S. Preventive Services Task Force," Agency for Healthcare Research and Quality, March 2004. The full text of this document, including references, can be found online at http://www.ahrq.gov/clinic/3rduspstf/hepcscr/hepcrev.htm.

The natural course of chronic HCV infection varies. Some patients never develop histologic evidence of liver disease even after decades of infection. In a meta-analysis of community-based cohort studies, 7 percent of patients with chronic HCV infection developed cirrhosis after twenty years. Factors that may be associated with a more progressive course include older age at acquisition; comorbid medical conditions, such as heavy alcohol use, HIV infection, and other chronic liver disease; male gender; and longer duration of infection. Mode of acquisition, viral load, aminotransferase levels, and viral genotype have not been consistently established as predictors of disease progression. The effects of ethnicity on the course of HCV infection have not been well studied in the United States.

In this systematic review, commissioned by the USPSTF [U.S. Preventive Services Task Force], we focus on whether it is useful to test for anti-HCV antibodies in asymptomatic adults who have no history of liver disease.

Methods

Briefly, relevant studies were identified from searches of MEDLINE® (1989 through February 2003) and the Cochrane Clinical Trials Registry (2002, Issue 2) and from the reference list of a recent evidence report commissioned by the National Institutes of Health. Reference lists of retrieved articles, periodic hand searches of relevant journals, and suggestions from experts supplemented the electronic searches.

We selected studies that provided direct evidence on the benefits of screening and studies on risk factors for HCV infection and the performance of third-generation HCV enzyme-linked immunoassay (ELISA) alone or followed by confirmatory recombinant immunoblot assay (RIBA). We focused on third-generation ELISAs because they are thought to be slightly more sensitive than second-generation tests, but included data on second-generation ELISAs from large, good-quality observational studies. We also selected studies evaluating noninvasive methods to evaluate active HCV infection and the harms associated with biopsy. For treatment, we focused on trials of pegylated interferon with ribavirin but included studies that examined the effect of other interferon-based treatment regimens on long-term clinical outcomes. We also reviewed studies evaluating effects of counseling on high-risk behaviors and benefits of immunizations.

We excluded studies of pregnant patients; children; and patients with occupational exposures, end-stage renal disease, or HIV infection, as well as studies focusing on patients who had already developed complications of chronic HCV infection.

Results

Studies of Screening

We identified no randomized trials or longitudinal cohort studies comparing outcomes between patients in the general adult population who were screened and not screened for HCV infection.

Risk Factor Assessment

The identification of risk factors for the presence of HCV infection could aid in the development of selective screening strategies. Independent risk factors for HCV infection found in the four large population-based studies include intravenous drug use and high-risk sexual behaviors (variably defined, but usually considered sex with multiple partners or sex with an HCV-infected person).

Since 1992, transfusions have not been an important mode of HCV transmission. There is insufficient evidence to determine the importance of tattoos, body piercings, shared razors, and acupuncture as risk factors. Nonpercutaneous risk factors such as gender, ethnicity, and socioeconomic status have inconsistent or weak associations with the prevalence of HCV infection.

Harms from HCV Antibody Testing

False-positive screening tests could result in harms that are difficult to measure (for example, labeling, anxiety, detrimental effects on close relationships). There are few data regarding harms in patients who have false-positive tests or HCV-positive patients who do not receive treatment, though one fair-quality observational study suggests worse quality of life in patients who are aware of their status. We found no studies investigating whether harms associated with learning HCV status could be reduced by effective patient education and counseling. However, data from one small trial of thirty-four patients found that a counseling program improved sense of well-being in women with HCV.

Proportion of Patients Qualifying for Treatment

In clinical practice, the number of referred patients who receive antiviral treatment depends on the degree of liver damage, the presence of serious co-morbid conditions, and patient preferences regarding treatment. Antiviral therapy is recommended for patients with chronic HCV infection who are at the greatest risk for progression to cirrhosis. These persons have HCV viremia, persistently elevated aminotransferase levels, or liver biopsy findings showing significant fibrosis or inflammation and necrosis. In patients with minimal or no biopsy abnormalities, the benefits of treatment are not clear, and decisions about therapy are individualized.

Harms from Work-Up for Active HCV Infection

In the work-up of patients with chronic HCV infection, percutaneous liver biopsy is associated with the highest risk for complications. The most common complication of liver biopsy is pain; approximately 30 percent of patients require strong analgesic medications. More serious but less common complications include bleeding (the most frequent major complication), biliary rupture, intestinal perforation, vasovagal hypotension, or infection.

Small studies suggest that ultrasound-guided biopsies may be associated with fewer complications than blind biopsies. Increased experience of the person performing the liver biopsy has also been associated with fewer complications.

Antiviral Treatment Efficacy for Clinical Outcomes

The long duration for important complications to develop and the relatively short time period that treatments have been available complicate our ability to assess the long-term benefits of antiviral treatment.

Efficacy of Counseling and Immunizations

Counseling asymptomatic patients found to have HCV infection might help prevent spread of disease or decrease the likelihood of progressive disease. Specifically, patients could be counseled to obtain immunizations for hepatitis A virus or hepatitis B virus, avoid excess alcohol, or avoid sharing needles or engaging in other risky practices.

Harms from Antiviral Treatment

Interferon-based treatments are commonly associated with self-limited adverse events. The most common adverse event is an influenza-like syndrome involving myalgias, fevers, and fatigue. A good-quality systematic review found that serious or life-threatening side effects occurred in 1 percent to 2 percent of patients receiving interferon monotherapy. Patients with significant comorbid conditions were generally excluded from randomized controlled trials. Because of the long duration (six months) of interferon regimens, adverse effects of treatment can have significant (although usually self-limited) effects on quality of life.

Relationship of Intermediate Outcomes to Clinical Outcomes

In five uncontrolled retrospective and prospective studies of patients who received antiviral treatment, complete responders (sustained virologic response and sustained biologic response) had a moderately decreased risk for hepatocellular cancer and cirrhosis compared with those who had relapses or those who did not respond. However, these studies did not consistently find a decreased risk for hepatocellular cancer in nonresponders compared with untreated controls. These studies were heterogeneous in design and had some methodologic limitations. Specifically, this body of literature does not exclude the possibility that favorable, unknown underlying prognostic factors led to a better response to treatment and better long-term outcomes.

Discussion

No direct evidence shows benefits of screening for HCV infection in the general adult population. There are inadequate data to accurately weigh the benefits and risks of screening for HCV in the otherwise healthy, asymptomatic adults. Although screening can accurately detect chronic HCV infection and antiviral treatment can successfully eradicate viremia, there are inadequate data to estimate benefits of treatment for long-term clinical outcomes such as death, cirrhosis, hepatocellular cancer, and quality of life. There are also no data to estimate benefits from vaccinations or counseling about alcohol use and high-risk behaviors.

Clinical trials of antiviral treatment have been performed in referred patients, who generally have more serious and progressive disease than patients followed in community-based cohorts. Even if treatment is equally effective for virology end points in patients identified by screening and those studied in clinical trials, the overall clinical benefit would be expected to be smaller since the underlying progression rate is lower. Although the proportion of screened patients found to have chronic HCV in selected high-risk populations, particularly intravenous drug users, would be substantially higher than in the general population, there are also no data to accurately weigh the risks and benefits of selective screening.

Important gaps remain in our understanding of the natural history of untreated patients with HCV infection who are likely to be identified by screening. If untreated chronic HCV infection causes important morbidity in the absence of cirrhosis, there may be other important goals to be obtained from treatment, but few studies have adequately assessed the impact of treatment on quality of life or symptoms. Additional studies are needed to define the progression from asymptomatic to symptomatic HCV infection and how long symptomatic patients remain unidentified without screening.

Many studies showing improvement in long-term clinical outcomes have been conducted in Japan. Chronic HCV infection appears to follow a substantially more aggressive course in Japan than in the United States. Although lead-time bias could explain some of the observed differences in disease progression rates, the case for screening would be greatly strengthened by data showing that treatment in earlier, asymptomatic stages of disease in western countries is associated with improved outcomes compared to treatment reserved for patients who have become symptomatic and could be identified without screening. Studies demonstrating important individual or public health benefits from counseling, immunizations, and behavioral changes after a diagnosis of HCV would also greatly strengthen the case for screening. Little is known about the benefits and risks of treatment in patients typically excluded from or under-represented in randomized trials, such as those with ongoing substance abuse, those with co-morbid conditions, elderly persons, and persons of non-white ethnicity).

No studies have adequately assessed the potential harmful effects of screening for HCV infection, such as anxiety, labeling, or damage to close relationships, and whether these factors can be minimized by appropriate counseling. Additional studies on the long-term effects of antiviral treatment in nonresponders are important because studies have not consistently found an improved outcome in this group compared with untreated controls.

Reasonable screening strategies might be to screen adults with established risk factors, adults in settings with a high prevalence of HCV, or all adults in the general population. Studies that adequately assess the usefulness of risk factor assessment to guide selective screening strategies and the harms and benefits of selective versus universal screening are needed. A potential barrier to screening patients on the basis of risk factors is the difficulty in obtaining accurate histories of intravenous drug use or high-risk sexual behaviors. Little is known about patient preferences for screening. There are no data to estimate risks and benefits of one-time screening versus other screening strategies.

Complications from chronic HCV present an enormous health burden that is expected to increase two- to fourfold over the next two to four decades. Further research to more accurately determine the benefits and harms of screening is of paramount importance.

Conclusions

Antiviral treatment can successfully eradicate HCV, but data on long-term outcomes in populations likely to be identified by screening are lacking. Although the yield from targeted screening, particularly in intravenous drug users, would be substantially higher than in the general population, data are inadequate to accurately weigh the overall benefits and risks of screening in otherwise healthy, asymptomatic adults.

Chapter 33

HCV Diagnosis and Testing

How Can I Get Tested?

There are several tests that your health care provider will do to diagnose hepatitis C, monitor the condition of your liver, and determine if you should consider treatment. Understanding the tests and what the results mean will help you become an active partner in managing your illness.

Antibody Tests

The first test usually done for hepatitis C is an antibody test such as an EIA. A reactive (positive) result means that, at some time in your life, you were exposed to hepatitis C and your body produced antibodies to fight off the virus. If the EIA test is reactive (positive), a second antibody test called the RIBA (which is more accurate) may be used to confirm the result. Most people who test reactive (positive) to both antibody tests are chronic carriers, meaning they carry the virus in their blood and can pass the virus on to others. However, some people (about 15 to 25 percent) who have a reactive (positive) result can clear the virus on their own without treatment. Further testing should be done to determine if you are chronically infected.

Reprinted from the Massachusetts Department of Public Health's Hepatitis C program website, http://www.mass.gov/dph/cdc/masshepc/.

PCR

A PCR (polymerase chain reaction) is a viral load test that detects the presence of hepatitis C in the blood. If the PCR is positive, you are infected with the hepatitis C virus, and are probably a chronic carrier. If you undergo treatment for hepatitis C, this test helps to monitor whether the medicines are working.

Liver Function Tests

Liver function tests (LFTs) help your health care provider determine whether your liver is working properly. These blood tests measure the levels of enzymes and other substances in your liver. When the liver is inflamed or damaged, certain enzymes will be released or the level of some substances will change. Some common LFTs include albumin, total protein, the enzymes ALT and AST, alkaline phosphatase, and bilirubin. Learn what your numbers mean and talk to your health care provider about how often the tests should be done.

Genotype

Genotype refers to the particular type of hepatitis C. There are at least six genotypes of hepatitis C. Most people (75 percent) in the United States have genotype 1. Genotypes 2 and 3 are the next most common. If you are infected with one genotype it is possible to become infected with another type. Therefore, it is important not to expose yourself to the blood of others. If you decide to be treated for your hepatitis C infection, knowing your genotype will help determine how you may respond to treatment, and how long your treatment will be. Your health care provider can find out your genotype by testing your blood.

Liver Biopsy

Your health care provider may want to do a liver biopsy. To do a biopsy, the provider takes a small piece of your liver to check for inflammation and scarring. It is a way for your health care provider to help you decide if and when you should begin treatment and what type of treatment you should receive. A biopsy is the only way to truly know the stage of liver disease. As with any medical procedure, there is a small risk associated with a biopsy, so be sure to ask your health care provider about the risks and what to expect before you decide to have a biopsy.

Questions to Ask Your Health Care Provider about Testing

The following questions relate to routine and one-time liver tests:

What is my hepatitis C viral load?

These questions pertain if you have already gotten a viral load test.

- What are the test results?
- How often should I have my viral load checked?
- May I have a copy of the test results for my records?

What is my hepatitis C genotype?

This is a one-time liver test.

- (If you have already gotten a genotype test) What are the test results?
- How does my genotype affect my illness and possible treatment?
- May I have a copy of the test results for my records?

What are my liver function test levels?

Liver function tests are ALT/AST (alanine transaminase/aspartate transaminase), ALP (alkaline phosphatase), and SGPT (serum glutamate pyruvate transaminase), bilirubin, albumin, and prothrombin time.

- (If you have already gotten liver function tests) What are the test results? How do they compare with normal levels?
- How often should I have liver function tests done?
- May I have a copy of the test results for my records?

Do you recommend I have a liver biopsy?

- If yes, why? If no, why not?
- What is involved in getting a biopsy?
- What are the risks?
- How is the procedure performed?

- How long does the procedure take?

- What experience do you have, or does the doctor performing the procedure have in doing liver biopsies? (The more experience they have, the better.)

- If a liver biopsy shows that I have fibrosis or cirrhosis (scarring), how does that affect my treatment options?

- (If you have already gotten a biopsy) What are the results of my liver biopsy and what does it mean? Will the result affect my treatment?

- May I have a copy of the biopsy report for my records?

Chapter 34

HCV Genotypes Explained

Introduction

Viruses are microscopic and no person could ever see them with the naked eye. Indeed, HCV is so small that around thirty billion would fit on a full stop.

Although it is much easier to talk of the hepatitis C virus as if it is a single organism, in fact it is a group of viruses, similar enough to be called hepatitis C virus, yet different enough to be classified into subgroups.

Genotypes

Several identifiable "families" of hepatitis C virus have been observed around the world, differing slightly from each other in their DNA sequencing (genetic makeup). The most commonly used classification system lists these "families" as HCV genotype 1, 2, 3, and so on.

Subtypes

Within each genotype, difference between viruses exists—too small to be seen as a different new genotype but significant enough and measurable, thus making the term *subtype* applicable. These lesser classifications are described as HCV subtype 1a or 1b, and so on.

329

Quasispecies

Among the viruses that make up a person's HCV infection, individual viruses will differ from each other very slightly. The differences are incredibly minute and not significant enough to form a distinct subtype. Instead they form what are known as quasispecies. It is believed that within an HCV subtype, several million quasispecies would exist.

Scientists predict that people who have hepatitis C have billions of actual viruses circulating within their body. Although there may be one or two predominant subtypes, the infection as a whole is not a single entity and is composed of many different quasispecies.

Global Patterns

It is believed that the hepatitis C virus has evolved over a period of several thousand years. This would explain the current general global patterns of genotypes and subtypes:

- 1a is mostly found in North and South America; also common in Australia
- 1b is common in North America, Europe, and Japan
- 2b is the most common genotype 2 in the United States and northern Europe
- 2c is the most common genotype 2 in western and southern Europe
- 3a is common in Australia and southern Asia
- 4a is highly prevalent in Egypt
- 4c is highly prevalent in Central Africa
- 6 is common in Asia

Genotype and Treatment

Current scientific belief is that factors such as duration of a person's HCV infection, their HCV viral load, age, grade of liver inflammation, or stage of fibrosis may play an important role in determining response to interferon treatment. Recent studies clearly show that a person's HCV subtype (or subtypes) influences his or her possible response to interferon, or to interferon-ribavirin combination treatment. For example, sustained response to interferon-ribavirin is 60 to 70 percent for people with genotypes 2 and 3, compared to 25 to 30 percent for people with genotype 1.

Source

Information taken from *Genotypes and Genetic Variation of Hepatitis C Virus* by G. Maerterns and L. Stuyver, reviewed by Dr. Greg Dore of the National Centre in HIV Epidemiology and Clinical Research.

Chapter 35

Patients with HCV:
Who Should Be Treated?

One may wonder why this question is being asked, as surely if one has hepatitis C, and a treatment is available, surely treatment would naturally be recommended? But unfortunately, although the success rates with antiviral therapy for chronic hepatitis C have improved markedly over the last ten years, a cure still cannot be achieved in everyone, the current therapies still carry with them many side effects, and there are still many infected individuals who have contraindications to their use. So some judgment has to be exercised regarding who will benefit most from therapy and who may suffer untoward consequences of therapy that could shift the risk-benefit ratio in the wrong direction.

Current Standard of Care for the Treatment of Hepatitis C

The most effective antiviral therapy regimen is a combination of long-acting pegylated interferon alpha and the oral nucleoside analogue ribavirin. A sustained virological response (SVR), which is defined as undetectability of HCV RNA in the blood both at the end of treatment and six months after cessation of therapy, occurs in 54 to 56 percent of individuals given this treatment. As with earlier forms of antiviral therapy, the response rate is very much dependent on the particular genotype of the hepatitis C infection.

Reprinted from "Patients with Hepatitis C: Who Should Be Treated?" by Jenny Heathcote, M.D., January 2003, with permission of the Hepatitis C Support Project, http://www.hcvadvocate.org, © 2003. All rights reserved.

Factors Influencing the Antiviral Response

As with all other antiviral therapies for hepatitis C, the particular genotype of the infecting virus has the greatest influence on the sustained virological response to therapy. In those individuals infected with genotype 1, the expected SVR ranges from 43 to 46 percent and in those with genotype 2 or 3 infections, from 76 to 82 percent. Other factors influencing this response include the height of the viral load (the higher the viral load, the lower the SVR), the severity of liver disease (individuals with cirrhosis have a somewhat lower overall response rate, 43 to 50 percent), and body habitus, the heavier the person, the lower the response rate.

Absolute Contraindications to Pegylated Interferon and Ribavirin Therapy

Interferon

Interferon is a natural cytokine produced whenever a viral infection is present, and when given by injection, typically causes flu-like symptoms. However interferon has some much more serious untoward effects which make it an unsuitable drug in certain individuals. It may impair bone marrow function. Red and white blood cells and platelets are all made in the bone marrow and so individuals who already have low values for any of these blood components may not be able to tolerate interferon therapy safely. A low white count or low platelet count is particularly common in individuals who have already developed cirrhosis of the liver. Other concomitant medications may lower the hemoglobin, for example, antiviral treatment for HIV, and it is for this and many other problems with drug interactions that treatment of hepatitis C in individuals co-infected with HIV is so problematic.

Interferon may affect the brain, which is why it is not given to individuals who have a seizure disorder that cannot be controlled with anti-epileptic therapy. Nor is IFN therapy thought wise in an individual who suffers from depression unless the latter is controlled with anti-depressant therapy. Interferon can also cause arrhythmias of the heart, and thus individuals that have had cardiac irregularities may be unsuitable for interferon therapy.

Interferon is a very potent immune stimulant, which is one of the reasons why it is so effective in viral hepatitis, but in individuals who already have some immune disorder, particularly those with auto-immune disease, for example, rheumatoid arthritis, systemic lupus

334

erythematosus, it is unwise to use interferon for fear of causing a flare-up of the autoimmune disease. Neither can one safely use IFN with an organ transplant in place for fear of precipitating rejection (except if it is a liver transplant).

Occasionally interferon, probably because of its immunological effect, may promote liver failure leading to sudden and rapid deterioration in liver function. Thus no patient who has even the mildest evidence of liver failure should receive interferon therapy.

Ribavirin

Ribavirin has two major side effects. It shortens the survival of red blood cells, which normally live 120 days. At least one-third of individuals given ribavirin have a markedly shortened red cell survival (called hemolysis). This may cause sudden onset of profound anemia, which leads to weakness and shortness of breath. Any individual who would become rapidly unwell with a sudden fall in hemoglobin, for example those who already have poor oxygen supply to their heart or to their brain from hardening of the arteries, should never be given ribavirin.

Unfortunately, ribavirin is also damaging to the unborn child (teratogenic), which means that neither a male or female may impregnate or conceive (as is appropriate for the gender) during treatment with ribavirin and for six months after stopping ribavirin (ribavirin remains in the blood for 120 days after the last dose).

Ribavirin is excreted via the kidneys. Hence if there is any impairment of renal function, ribavirin may be present in the blood perhaps even at high concentrations for a prolonged period of time, and this would enhance the likelihood of hemolysis; thus individuals with renal failure should not receive ribavirin therapy.

Would Antiviral Therapy be Helpful for Me?

As long as you have none of the contraindications to either interferon alpha or ribavirin then it is reasonable to consider therapy for your hepatitis C. But there are also a number of other factors that need to be taken into consideration before making the final decision.

Side Effects of Treatment

Treatment with pegylated interferon alpha and ribavirin is not easy. Side effects tend to be maximal in the first two weeks of therapy, but in most, some side effects continue throughout therapy. It is most important that treatment be started only during a relatively quiet and stable part of your life, that is not just prior to examinations, or just after taking on a new job. It is also unwise for couples living together who both require treatment to start treatment at the same time. Fortunately, the initial flu-like symptoms of fever, muscle aches, and headaches tend to diminish with time but most individuals undergoing therapy feel that they are under par for the entire treatment period, and some notice an effect on their mood such as becoming more irritable, occasionally developing overt depression. Whereas a past history of depression is no longer considered a contraindication to therapy, it may be wise in those who have such a history to consider going on antidepressant therapy prior to initiating treatment. Some individuals need to be started on an antidepressant during the course of their treatment. Other really irritating side effects include: dry itchy skin, cough, thinning of the hair, aphthous ulcerations of the mouth, diarrhea, and insomnia. Skin reactions at the injection site are particularly common with the pegylated interferon. Weakness and shortness of breath are generally associated with the anemia caused by the ribavirin. When ribavirin is added to interferon therapy, it really does worsen the overall fatigue and depressant effect of this treatment.

What Can Be Done to Combat Side Effects of Therapy?

The really best outcome with antiviral therapies occurs when patients receive excellent nursing care. Because we know that the successful outcome of treatment correlates well with the individual's ability to take a full course of treatment, it is most important that those persons undergoing antiviral therapy are given as much help as possible, are forewarned about potential side effects, and are taught how to prevent them and how to deal with side effects when they are present.

As previously mentioned, in those who have a tendency toward depression, pre-treatment with antidepressants is advisable. This of course, needs to be by prescription from your primary care physician or psychiatrist. Planning to start treatment at a suitable time in your life is appropriate. For the first two weeks individuals are advised to take an extra-strength Tylenol at the time of their injection and perhaps give the injection at bedtime. Because the pegylated interferon causes blood levels of interferon to remain high all week, the episodic occurrence of side effects seen commonly following standard interferon therapy given three times a week tend to be less. However, most patients find that the flu-like symptoms may last several days after the first few injections of pegylated interferon. If Tylenol helps, then this should be used for as long as is necessary, but no more than four extra-strength Tylenol should ever be taken within a twenty-four-hour period, and should never be taken with alcohol. As alcohol elevates the viral load, it is wise to abstain completely from alcohol while undergoing antiviral therapy for hepatitis C. It is most important to consume large amounts (at least three liters) of water daily during antiviral therapy. This markedly reduces the dry itchy skin, the skin rash, and sometimes even the nasal stuffiness. This quantity of water should be drunk on a daily basis from the first day of treatment. Most of the other side effects can be controlled by cutting back on the dose of either the interferon or the ribavirin. This may be either for the short-term or permanent.

New Stopping Rules

The good news is that if the viral load is measured just prior to starting therapy, and at twelve weeks into therapy, the physician can with a high degree of reliability predict whether or not treatment is likely to be successful. In those individuals whose viral load has not fallen by >2 logs, they are advised to stop their antiviral therapy and as a consequence all side effects will rapidly disappear. In those individuals whose HCV RNA has fallen by 2 logs or more, continued therapy at full dose is advised. If, however, because of adverse side effects the dose has to be reduced this does not seriously impair the overall response. Only stopping the drug completely after the first twelve weeks of therapy prior to completion reduces the chance of a successful antiviral response. Hence, if one passes the twelve-week mark with a >2 log fall in HCV RNA it is really important to continue treatment for the full term even if it has to be at a lower dose.

Should I Undergo a Liver Biopsy Prior to Deciding Whether or Not to Go for Antiviral Therapy?

Mainly because previous antiviral therapy was less than 50 percent effective was it recommended that a liver biopsy be done prior to deciding on treatment. This was because in those with very mild disease, it was considered quite safe to wait for better therapies coming along the pipeline, and for those who were found to have more severe disease, any treatment that could improve outcome was thought worthwhile. What was looked for on liver biopsy was either a high degree of inflammation that predicted later development of scar tissue or an already high degree of scarring (fibrosis). It is now thought that perhaps in those with genotype 2 and 3 infections a liver biopsy may be more appropriate in those who are shown not to respond to the complete course of pegylated interferon and ribavirin. However, in individuals with genotype 1 infections, the response rate is still less than 50 percent and so many patients opt for finding out whether or not they do in fact have evidence of progressive disease on liver biopsy before contemplating a full course of antiviral therapy. Unfortunately liver biopsy is the only way of diagnosing cirrhosis—it is very important to know if cirrhosis is present as this markedly affects both program and management.

Duration of Antiviral Therapy

It is likely that those who have genotype 2 and 3 need treatment only for a maximum of six months, and half dose, that is, 800 mg of ribavirin daily may be sufficient. The smaller dose of ribavirin is associated with far fewer side effects. For those with genotype 1 infections and probably those with genotype 4, full-dose ribavirin and interferon is required and for a full forty-eight weeks of treatment.

Summary

It should now be possible for you to determine whether or not you should opt for antiviral therapy for your hepatitis C infection. Unfortunately there remain individuals who often for various non-liver reasons cannot tolerate current treatments. There are others whose disease is so mild and who have infection with a genotype that is more likely not to respond than to respond, who may opt to not initiate antiviral therapy at the present time. Unfortunately there will be some whose liver disease is too advanced for antiviral therapy to be safe and for some, a liver transplant may be the better option.

Chapter 36

HCV Treatment: What You Need to Know

Before You Start Hepatitis C Treatment

What treatments can I get by prescription from my doctor?

There are three treatments that have been approved by the Food and Drug Administration (FDA) for hepatitis C virus infection:

- *Interferon alone* (called interferon monotherapy): Interferon is a protein that causes your body's immune system to attack infected liver cells and to protect healthy liver cells from new infection. There are several brands of interferon made by different drug companies.

- *Interferon combined with ribavirin* (called combination therapy): Overall, combination therapy is much more effective than interferon monotherapy. If you have already had monotherapy treatment and it didn't work, you may want to think about combination therapy or experimental treatments.

- *Long-acting interferon* (called pegylated interferon therapy): Most patients are treated with this type of interferon, usually in combination with ribavirin. This combination has shown the highest response rate of any treatment for hepatitis C.

Reprinted from "The Hepatitis C Treatment Series," VA National Hepatitis C Program, Department of Veterans Affairs (VA), June 2004.

How long does treatment take?

Treatment time varies. It depends on whether you get your medicine from your regular doctor or through a clinical trial. In general, standard combination therapy lasts between twenty-four and forty-eight weeks, with six months of follow-up after treatment has ended. Sometimes, if the treatment is not working or if you have too many side effects, your doctor may stop your treatment early.

If you are part of a clinical trial for new medicines, the treatment time will depend on the study design. Your doctor, nurse, or clinical trial coordinator will explain the schedule to you before your treatment begins.

How can treatment help me?

Hepatitis C treatments can remove (or *clear*) the hepatitis C virus from your blood, but this does not happen in all patients. If this does not happen, there are still some ways that treatment can help you. The treatment can:

- decrease the amount of liver damage.

- lower the amount of hepatitis C virus in your blood.

- improve your overall well-being and quality of your life.

- lower your alanine aminotransferase (ALT) liver enzyme level.

I've heard my doctor talk about different responses to treatment. What are they, and what do they mean?

There are three types of response to treatment that describe how treatment works for the patient, including the following:

- *Treatment naive:* This means that you have not yet taken medicine to treat hepatitis C.

- *Responders* (or sustained responders): This means that the treatment worked while you were taking the medicine and seemed to work even after you stopped taking it.

- *Nonresponders:* This means that the treatment did not work. Some of the different kinds of nonresponders include the following:

- *Relapsers* (or transient responders): The treatment only worked as long as you took it. When you stopped taking the medicine, the hepatitis C virus came back.

- *Breakthrough nonresponders:* The treatment worked in the beginning and then stopped working.

- *Complete nonresponders:* The treatment did not remove (or clear) the virus from your blood.

What will make the treatment more likely to work?

Not everyone will have the same results from hepatitis C treatment. There are some things that can affect the treatment and how well it works, including the following:

- *Viral genotype:* Not all hepatitis C viruses are exactly the same. We know of six different genotypes for hepatitis C. Some of them respond better to treatment than others.

- *Viral load:* This is the amount of virus in your blood. If you have lower levels of virus in your blood when you start treatment, you may have a better chance of getting rid of the virus. (Note: A high viral load does not necessarily mean you have worse liver damage.)

- *Iron:* If you have less iron in your blood or in your liver cells, your treatment may work better. Iron levels can be checked with a blood test or a liver biopsy.

- *Gender:* Hepatitis C treatment works slightly better for women than for men.

- *Age:* If you got the virus before the age of forty, the chance of treatment working for you may be better than if you became infected in older age.

- *Length of infection:* You may have a better chance of clearing the virus from your body if you haven't been infected with the hepatitis C virus for very long.

Do I have to get a liver biopsy to start treatment?

Sometimes your doctor may ask you to have a biopsy before you start treatment. This tells how much damage there is in your liver and can help you decide when to start treatment. Your doctor may also ask you to have a biopsy after treatment is finished.

When should I start treatment?

It is a good idea to talk about treatment with your doctor and family first. Only you can decide when to start. In general, doctors strongly suggest treatment if you

- have high liver enzymes, especially ALT levels;
- have a test that showed hepatitis C virus in your blood;
- have a liver biopsy that showed damage (or fibrosis) or inflammation;
- have *not* used alcohol or other drugs for at least six months.

If I want to start treatment, what should I do now?

If you want to start treatment for hepatitis C, speak with your doctor. It is a good idea to talk about any concerns you have before you start treatment. Your doctor and you will decide if treatment is right for you and which medicines might work.

While You Are on Hepatitis C Treatment

What should I know about treatment?

Following are some important things to know about treatment for hepatitis C:

- *You may have side effects:* Side effects will vary depending on what medicine you take for hepatitis C. Most patients on hepatitis C treatment have side effects, such as fatigue and flu-like symptoms. Some side effects go away and some of them last for the whole time you are treated.

- *Your treatment time may vary:* If you are on standard hepatitis C treatments, you will take them for twenty-four or forty-eight weeks. If you have too many side effects, or if the drugs don't seem to work for you, your doctor may suggest that you stop a little earlier than usual. After you finish taking the drugs, your doctor will usually follow your progress for six months. If you are in a clinical trial, you may take the medicine for only a month or for over a year. It depends on the kind of clinical trial and what type of medicine you are taking.

342

- *You will have several lab tests while you are on the medicine:* These lab tests are to make sure that the drugs are safe for you and also to find out if the treatment is working.

- *Your doctor will give you instructions:* Your doctor will give you instructions before you start treatment. It is important that you understand the risks and side effects of the drugs. For example, ribavirin can cause serious birth defects, and you or your partner should *not* get pregnant while taking it. If you start taking ribavirin to treat your hepatitis C, you must use two effective forms of birth control, one for you and one for your partner. An example is a condom for the man, and a diaphragm or birth control pill for the woman. You must keep using this type of birth control during the whole time you are on combination treatment and for six months after your last dose.

What lab tests will my doctor order to see if treatment is working?

Two blood tests that doctors use frequently to see if treatment is working:

- *ALT level* (Alanine aminotransferase): This test measures the amount (or level) of an enzyme called ALT that is made in liver cells. If liver cells are damaged or die, ALT leaks out into the bloodstream. One goal of treatment is to bring high levels of ALT back to normal. If the treatment is working, ALT levels should come down to normal. If the ALT level decreases quickly in the treatment process, you have a better chance of responding to treatment.

- *Viral load* (hepatitis C virus ribonucleic acid level or hepatitis C RNA level): This test measures the amount of hepatitis C virus in your blood. Treatment for hepatitis C tries to keep the viral load low or negative (undetectable). Undetectable means that no virus was found in your blood by the test used. Your doctor will check your viral load at different times during treatment.

How often will my doctor check my blood to see if treatment is working?

Doctors often take blood at certain time points to see if treatment is working. The most common tests look at your viral load and ALT levels. These checkpoints usually happen at the following times:

- *Week 1 or 2:* This is the first safety check to see how you are tolerating treatment.

- *Week 12:* If your viral load has decreased a lot, or become undetectable by Week 12, you have a better chance at sustained response. Sustained response means that treatment worked while you were taking the medicine and seemed to work even after you stopped taking it. The earlier you respond, the more likely it is that the treatment will fully work for you.

- *Week 24:* If your viral load is negative at Week 24, you will have a better chance of sustained response. If you still have detectable virus at this point, you have a very small chance of clearing it from your system. If the ALT is also still high, you and your doctor may want to consider stopping treatment. If your ALT level is normal, your doctor may keep you on treatment even if the virus is still present. Most studies have shown that if the treatment hasn't started to work by this checkpoint, it may not be right for you to continue.

- *Week 48:* If your viral load is negative, then you have a fairly good chance of showing a sustained response. If your virus is positive at the end of treatment, it is extremely rare to clear the virus once treatment has ended.

- *Week 72:* If your viral load is negative at Week 72 (or six months after the end of treatment), you are a sustained responder (there is a very small chance that the virus will reappear in your system). If the virus has come back, you are considered a relapser. This means that once the treatment stopped, the virus came back.

What other tests are important to know about while I'm on treatment?

Besides the ALT level and viral load, your doctor will also look at many other tests. Some of the most important tests look at your white blood cells, which may be affected by interferon treatment. If your white blood cells drop below a certain level, your doctor may change your interferon dose. Your doctor will also look at your red blood cells, which may be affected by ribavirin. If your red blood cells and hemoglobin levels drop below a certain point, your doctor may change your ribavirin dose.

Will I be able to work while I'm on treatment?

Some patients keep a normal work schedule while they are on treatment. Others may have to cut down their work hours or stop working altogether. The side effects are different for every patient, so it is hard to say how much hepatitis C treatment will affect your work schedule.

Will I have to take other medicines to help with my side effects?

You may not need any other medicines to help with your side effects. But if you have too many side effects, or they cause problems for you, your doctor may prescribe some extra drugs. These may include drugs to help you sleep better or to control skin itching caused by treatment. For more advice on how to manage side effects, speak with your doctor or nurse.

Will I need a liver biopsy during treatment?

Sometimes your doctor may ask you to have a liver biopsy before you start treatment or after treatment is finished. It is not likely that you will have a liver biopsy during the course of treatment.

Your liver may be healthier after treatment, showing less inflammation on a biopsy. So even if you haven't cleared the virus, a healthier liver is in itself a good benefit of treatment. Talk with your doctor and family to decide if you need a liver biopsy after treatment.

Common Questions about Finishing Hepatitis C Treatment

What should I know after I finish my hepatitis C treatment?

When you finish your treatment, your doctor will give you advice based on the type of drugs you took and whether they worked. This section of the chapter contains suggestions on what you should do after you have finished your treatment. Talk with your doctor if you have any questions about hepatitis C or the treatments you took.

What should I do if my treatment didn't clear the virus from my blood?

If you have finished your treatment and it did not clear the hepatitis C virus from your blood, you may want to take a break for a while or you may want to try another drug soon. Your decision will depend on several things, such as the results of your liver function tests and biopsy.

Some people with less severe liver damage decide to wait until better treatments are tested and become available. Other people decide to try new drugs right away. Keep in mind that even if the treatment didn't get rid of the virus, it may have improved the health of your liver.

What other kinds of treatment are being made?

Treatments for hepatitis C are changing, and new drugs are always being tested. But even after a new drug has been tested in clinical trials, it may take years before it gets the approval of the Food and Drug Administration (FDA).

There are also several new types of treatments that try to clear the virus or decrease the amount of liver damage. These new treatments work in different ways and may do the following things:

- Fight hepatitis C much like ribavirin does, but without causing anemia.
- Work with your body to naturally produce more interferon.
- Stop the virus from reproducing.
- Decrease the amount of liver injury.

If treatment didn't clear the virus from my blood, are there any herbal remedies that I can take?

Before you take herbs or any other medicine to treat your hepatitis C virus infection, talk to your doctor. Many herbs have not been carefully tested and may cause damage to your liver. In general, we don't know if certain herbs really work to help patients with hepatitis C.

If my viral test was negative six months at the end of treatment, will I stay negative?

Treatment for hepatitis C hasn't been available for very long, so doctors are just starting to understand the long-term effects. But studies show that if your viral load was negative six months after treatment, there is a good chance that it won't come back. Doctors don't yet call this a cure. They call it remission instead. A cure means that the virus will never come back. Remission means that the virus is not detectable now, and it is not known if it will come back in the future. The good news is that patients who cleared the virus on interferon treatment are still showing negative viral loads, up to ten years after the end of treatment.

Figure 36.1. Treatment for Hepatitis C.

If you tried any of these treatments:

- Interferon Monotherapy
- Combination Therapy (Ribavirin and Interferon)
- Pegylated Interferon Monotherapy
- Pegylated Interferon Combined with Ribavirin
- Other Type of Treatment

If the virus was cleared from your blood:

- Ask for liver function tests every six months or every year.

- Ask your doctor about a test for viral load if your liver test becomes abnormal.

- It is likely that you will stay virus free for at least three to five years.

- It is likely that the hepatitis C virus is no longer in your blood.

- Keep yourself healthy by
  - eating well
  - not drinking alcohol or using drugs
  - getting plenty of rest
  - staying active and exercising

- Keep your appointments with your doctor and get regular checkups.

If the virus is still in your blood:

- Talk with your doctor about other treatments.

- Ask for liver function tests every six months or every year.

- Think about having a liver biopsy every few years to check your liver's health.

- Ask about new clinical trials for hepatitis c treatments

- Talk with your doctor about tests for liver cancer if you have scarring of the liver (cirrhosis).

- Keep yourself healthy by
  - eating well;
  - not drinking alcohol or using drugs;
  - getting plenty of rest;
  - staying active and exercising.

- Keep your appointments with your doctor and get regular checkups.

Final Suggestions

Everyone has a slightly different experience with hepatitis C treatments. Side effects are different for everyone, and doctors can never predict how well a drug will work for a certain person. It always helps to know as much as you can and to keep yourself healthy by eating well, getting plenty of rest, and not using alcohol or drugs that can damage your liver.

At all stages—before, during, and after treatment—talk with your doctor or nurse to learn as much as possible about your disease and your treatment. Your doctor will give you advice after you finish treatment. You must understand that the risks and side effects of treatment may last even after you have finished treatment. For example, ribavirin can cause serious birth defects, so you or your partner should *not* get pregnant while on combination treatment and for six months after your last dose. You must practice two effective forms of birth control, one for you and one for your partner (an example is a condom, plus a diaphragm or birth control pill).

Try to find health care providers who know about hepatitis C and can give you up-to-date information and advice. With support from your family, friends, and a doctor that you trust, you can have a better treatment experience. If you have tried a treatment that didn't work, don't be discouraged. Every day new and better treatments are becoming available as we learn more about hepatitis C.

Chapter 37

Drugs Used to Treat HCV

Chapter Contents

349

Section 37.1

Ribavirin

Brand Names

In the U.S.:

- Copegus
- Rebetol
- Virazole

In Canada:

- Virazole

Another commonly used name is tribavirin.

Category

- Antiviral, systemic

Description

Ribavirin (rye-ba-VYE-rin) is used to treat severe virus pneumonia in infants and young children. It is given by oral inhalation (breathing in the medicine as a fine mist through the mouth), using a special nebulizer (sprayer) attached to an oxygen hood or tent or face mask.

Ribavirin taken by mouth (oral) treats a viral liver infection known as hepatitis C. It is used in combination with injectable interferon alfa-2b (in-ter-FEER-on AL-fa-2b) or with injectable peginterferon alfa-2b (peg-in-ter-FEER-on AL-fa-2b). Ribavirin is used to treat virus infections. Interferons are substances naturally produced by cells in the body to help fight infections and tumors. Interferon alfa-2b and peginterferon alfa-2b are synthetic (man-made) versions of these substances. Interferon alfa-2b and peginterferon alfa-2b are used to treat a variety of tumors and viruses including the hepatitis C virus.

Ribavirin is available in the following dosage forms:

- Inhalation
  - For inhalation solution (U.S. and Canada)
- Oral
  - Capsules (U.S.)
  - Oral solution (U.S.)
  - Tablets (U.S.)

Before Using This Medicine

In deciding to use a medicine, the risks of taking the medicine must be weighed against the good it will do. This is a decision you and your doctor will make. For ribavirin, the following should be considered:

Allergies

Tell your doctor if you or your child has ever had any unusual or allergic reaction to ribavirin. Also tell your health care professional if you or your child is allergic to any other substances, such as foods, preservatives, or dyes.

Pregnancy

Ribavirin for inhalation is not usually prescribed for teenagers or adults. However, women who are pregnant or may become pregnant may be exposed to ribavirin that is given off in the air if they spend time at the child's bedside while ribavirin is being given. Although studies have not been done in humans, ribavirin has been shown to cause birth defects and other problems in certain animal studies. Be sure you have discussed this with your doctor.

Ribavirin for oral use should not be used while you are pregnant, if you plan on becoming pregnant, or by men whose female partners are pregnant or are planning to become pregnant. It has been shown to cause serious birth defects and other problems in animals. Be sure you have discussed this with your doctor.

Breastfeeding

It is not known whether ribavirin passes into human breast milk. However, ribavirin passes into the breast milk of animals and has been shown to cause problems in nursing animals and their young. It may be necessary for you to take another medicine or to stop breastfeeding during treatment with ribavirin. Be sure you have discussed the risks and benefits of this with your doctor.

Children

Children may be sensitive to the effects of ribavirin. This may increase the chance of side effects or other problems during treatment. Be sure you have discussed the risks and benefits of this with your doctor.

Older Adults

Many medicines have not been studied specifically in older people. Therefore it may not be known if they work the same way that they do in younger adults or if they cause different side effects or problems in older people than they do in younger adults.

Other Medicines

Although certain medicines should not be used together at all, in other cases two different medicines may be used together even if an interaction might occur. In these cases, your doctor may want to change the dose, or other precautions may be necessary. When you are taking ribavirin it is especially important that your doctor and pharmacist know if you are taking any of the following:

- Didanosine (e.g., Videx): This medicine should not be used at the same time as ribavirin because serious side effects can occur.

- Stavudine (e.g., Zerit)

- Zidovudine (e.g., Retrovir): These medicines should not be used at the same time as ribavirin.

Tell your health care professional if you are taking any other prescription or nonprescription (over-the-counter [OTC]) medicine.

Other Medical Problems

The presence of other medical problems may affect the use of ribavirin. Make sure you tell your doctor if you have any other medical problems, especially:

- Anemia (blood disorder) or

- Autoimmune hepatitis (liver inflammation): Ribavirin could make these conditions worse and lead to very serious side effects.

- Heart disease: Patients with heart disease or a history of heart disease should not use ribavirin oral dosage forms because serious side effects can occur.

- Blood conditions such as

  - Sickle cell anemia (red blood cell disorder) or

  - Thalassemia major (genetic blood disorder): Ribavirin should not be used in patients with these conditions.

- Hepatic decompensation: Ribavirin medicine should not be used in patients with this condition.

- Mental depression: Ribavirin should be used carefully in patients with this condition, especially adolescents, as serious side effects can occur.

- Pancreatitis (inflammation of the pancreas): Ribavirin should be suspended in patients with symptoms of this condition and stopped in patients who have this condition.

Proper Use of This Medicine

To help clear up your infection completely, ribavirin must be given for the full time of treatment, even if you or your child begins to feel better after a few days. Also, ribavirin for inhalation works best when there is a constant amount in the lungs. To help keep the amount constant, ribavirin must be given on a regular or continuous schedule.

It is important that you read the patient information that comes with this medicine. Ask your doctor if you have any questions.

A negative pregnancy test is needed in women who are of childbearing age before starting treatment with oral ribavirin. Two forms of birth control must be used during oral ribavirin treatment and for six months after treatment ends.

Dosing

The dose of ribavirin will be different for different patients. Follow your doctor's orders or the directions on the label. The following information includes only the average doses of ribavirin. If your dose is different, do not change it unless your doctor tells you to do so.

353

For the Inhalation Dosage Form

- For treatment of respiratory syncytial virus (RSV) infection:
  - Adults and teenagers: Dose has not been determined since this medicine is not usually prescribed for teenagers or adults.
  - Infants and children: Dose must be determined by your doctor.

For the Oral Dosage Form

- For the treatment of Hepatitis C virus infection
- For oral dosage forms (capsules):
  - Adults and children: Dose must be determined by your doctor
- For oral dosage form (oral solution):
  - Adults and teenagers: Dose must be determined by your doctor. The oral solution form of this medicine is not usually prescribed for teenagers or adults.
  - Children: Dose must be determined by your doctor.
- For oral dosage form (tablets):
  - Adults: Dose must be determined by your doctor.
  - Children: Use and dose must be determined by your doctor. The tablet form of this medicine is not usually prescribed for children.

Precautions while Using This Medicine

It is very important that your doctor check your progress at regular visits. This will allow your doctor to see if the medicine is working properly.

This medicine may cause some people to become dizzy, drowsy, or less alert than they are normally. Make sure you know how you react to this medicine before you drive, operate machinery, or do anything else that could be dangerous if you are not alert.

It is very important that you stop this medicine and contact your doctor immediately if you think you might be pregnant.

Side Effects of this Medicine

Along with its needed effects, a medicine may cause some unwanted effects. Although not all of these side effects may occur, if they do occur they may need medical attention.

Check with your doctor as soon as possible if any of the following side effects occur:

- More common: Chest pain; difficult or labored breathing; pale skin; shortness of breath; tightness in chest; troubled breathing with exertion; unusual bleeding or bruising; unusual tiredness or weakness; wheezing.

Along with its needed effects, a medicine may cause some unwanted effects. The following side effects may go away during treatment as your body adjusts to the medicine. However, check with your doctor if any of the following side effects continue or are bothersome:

- More common: Acid or sour stomach; belching; discouragement; dizziness; feeling sad or empty; feeling unusually cold; heartburn; indigestion; irritability; itching skin; lack of appetite; loss of interest or pleasure; lack or loss of strength; shivering; stomach discomfort, upset, or pain; tiredness; trouble concentrating; trouble sleeping.

- Less common: Change in taste; cough; crying; depersonalization; difficulty in moving; dysphoria; euphoria; fatigue; fever; gastrointestinal effects; headache; insomnia; joint pain; mental depression; muscle aching or cramping; muscle pains or stiffness; nervousness; pain or tenderness around eyes and cheekbones; paranoia; quick to react or overreact emotionally; rapidly changing moods; rash; shortness of breath; stuffy or runny nose; swollen joints; vomiting.

- Rare: Itching, redness, or swelling of eyes; skin rash or irritation.

Other side effects not listed above may also occur in some patients. If you notice any other effects, check with your doctor.

Additional Information

Once a medicine has been approved for marketing for a certain use, experience may show that it is also useful for other medical problems. Although these uses are not included in product labeling, ribavirin is used in certain patients with the following medical conditions:

- Influenza A and B (given by aerosol inhalation)
- Lassa fever (either given orally or by injection)

For patients taking this medicine by mouth or injection for Lassa fever:

- Check with your doctor immediately if any of the following side effects occur:

  - More common: Unusual tiredness and weakness.

- Other side effects may occur that usually do not need medical attention. The following side effects may go away during treatment as your body adjusts to the medicine. However, check with your doctor if any of the following side effects continue or are bothersome:

  - Less common: Headache; loss of appetite; nausea; trouble in sleeping; unusual tiredness or weakness.

Other than the above information, there is no additional information relating to proper use, precautions, or side effects for these uses.

This medicine may also be used for other virus infections as determined by your doctor. However, it will not work for certain viruses, such as the common cold.

Section 37.2

Ribavirin and Interferon Alfa-2b, Recombinant

Reprinted with permission. Klasko RK (ed): USP DI® Vol II Advice for the Patient, Copyright 2005. USP DI® is a registered trademark used herein under license. Originally created and edited by the United States Pharmacopeia until January 1, 2004, and now entirely edited and maintained by Thomson Healthcare, Inc.

Brand Names

In the United States: In Canada:

- Rebetron   • Rebetron

Description

Ribavirin and interferon alfa-2b (rye-ba-VYE-rin and in-ter-FEER-on AL-fa) combination is used to treat a viral liver infection known as hepatitis C infection. Ribavirin is taken by mouth and interferon alfa-2b is administered beneath the skin (subcutaneously). Ribavirin is used to treat virus infections. Interferons are substances naturally produced by cells in the body to help fight infections and tumors. Interferon alfa-2b is a synthetic (man-made) version of these substances. Interferon alfa-2b is used to treat a variety of tumors and viruses including the hepatitis C virus.

Ribavirin is available for oral administration. Interferon alfa-2b is available only as an injectable form.

Before Using This Medicine

In deciding to use a medicine, the risks of taking the medicine must be weighed against the good it will do. This is a decision you and your doctor will make. For ribavirin and interferon alfa-2b combination, the following should be considered:

Allergies

Tell your doctor if you have ever had any unusual or allergic reaction to alpha interferons or ribavirin.

Pregnancy

Ribavirin should not be used while pregnant, if you plan on becoming pregnant, or by men whose female partners are pregnant.

Breastfeeding

It is not known whether ribavirin or interferon alfa-2b passes into breast milk. However, because these medicines may cause serious side effects, breastfeeding may not be recommended while you are receiving them. Discuss with your doctor whether or not you should breastfeed while you are receiving this combination medicine.

Children

Studies on this combination medicine have been done only in adult patients and there is no specific information comparing use of ribavirin and recombinant interferon alfa-2b combination in children younger than eighteen years of age with use in other age groups.

Older Adults

Many medicines have not been studied specifically in older people. Therefore, it may not be known whether they work exactly the same way they do in younger adults or if they cause different side effects or problems in older people. There is no specific information comparing use of ribavirin and interferon alfa-2b combination medicine in the elderly with use in other age group.

Other Medicines

Although certain medicines should not be used together at all, in other cases two different medicines may be used together even if an interaction might occur. In these cases, your doctor may want to change the dose, or other precautions may be necessary. Tell your health care professional if you are taking any other prescription or nonprescription (over-the-counter [OTC]) medicine.

Other Medical Problems

The presence of other medical problems may affect the use of ribavirin and interferon alfa-2b. Make sure you tell your doctor if you have any other medical problems, especially the following:

- Anemia, severe or

- Autoimmune hepatitis or

- Bleeding disorders: May worsen with ribavirin and/or recombinant interferon alfa-2b

- Diabetes (increased sugar in blood): May increase the risk of developing eye problems

- Heart disease: May worsen with ribavirin and/or recombinant interferon alfa-2b

- Hepatitis B or human immunodeficiency virus infection or

- Hepatitis C which has worsened or

- Hepatitis C which did not get better when treated with interferon alone: Safety and effectiveness in these conditions are unknown.

- High blood pressure: May increase the risk of developing eye problems

- Kidney problems: May worsen with ribavirin and/or recombinant interferon alfa-2b

- Liver or other organ transplant: Safety and effectiveness in these conditions are unknown.

- Lung problems: May worsen with ribavirin and/or recombinant interferon alfa-2b

- Mental problems (or history of): May result in depression, aggressive, violent, and suicidal behavior

- Problem with immune system or

- Psoriasis (inflammatory skin problem) or

- Thyroid problem: May worsen with ribavirin and/or recombinant interferon alfa-2b

- Virus infections, other: Use of ribavirin alone is not recommended

Proper Use of This Medicine

If you are injecting interferon alfa-2b yourself, use it exactly as directed by your doctor. Do not use more or less of it, and do not use it more often than your doctor ordered. The exact amount of medicine you need has been carefully worked out. Using too much will increase the risk of side effects, while using too little may not improve your condition.

Interferon alfa-2b often causes unusual tiredness. This effect is less likely to cause problems if you inject this medicine at bedtime. Also, your doctor may want you to drink extra fluids, especially during the early phase of treatment.

Dosing

The dose of ribavirin and interferon alfa-2b will be different for different patients. The dose that is used may depend on a number of things, including the patient's size and laboratory test. If you are receiving interferon alfa-2b at home, follow your doctor's orders or the directions on the label. If you have any questions about the proper dose of interferon alfa-2b, ask your doctor.

Missed Dose

If you miss a dose of ribavirin or interferon alfa-2b, do not inject the missed dose at all and do not double the next one. Check with your doctor for further instructions.

Storage

To store this medicine:

- Keep out of the reach of children.

- Store in the refrigerator.

- Keep the medicine from freezing.

- Do not keep outdated medicine or medicine no longer needed. Ask your health care professional how you should dispose of any medicine you do not use. Be sure that any discarded medicine is out of the reach of children.

Precautions while Using This Medicine

It is very important that your doctor check your progress at regular visits to make sure that this medicine is working properly and to check for unwanted effects.

This medicine may cause some people to become unusually tired or dizzy, or less alert than they are normally. Make sure you know how you react to this medicine before you drive, use machines, or do anything else that could be dangerous if you are dizzy or if you are not alert.

This medicine may make you feel very sad, depressed, or very angry. Call your doctor if you feel you cannot cope or you feel like you want to hurt yourself or someone else.

Interferon alfa-2b commonly causes a flu-like reaction, with aching muscles, fever and chills, and headache. To prevent problems from your temperature going too high, your doctor may ask you to take medicine for pain and fever such as acetaminophen (e.g., Anacin 3, Tylenol) before each dose of interferon alfa-2b. You may also need to take it after a dose to bring your temperature down. Follow your doctor's instructions carefully about taking your temperature, and how much and when to take the medicine such as acetaminophen.

Women of childbearing potential should use two reliable forms of effective contraception.

Alpha interferon can lower the number of white blood cells in your blood temporarily, increasing the chance of getting an infection. It can also lower the number of platelets, which are necessary for proper blood clotting. If this occurs, there are certain precautions you can take, especially when your blood count is low, to reduce the risk of infection or bleeding:

- If you can, avoid being close to people with infections. Check with your doctor immediately if you think you are getting an infection or if you get a fever or chills, cough or hoarseness, lower back or side pain, or have painful or difficult urination.

- Check with your doctor immediately if you notice any unusual bleeding or bruising; black, tarry stools; blood in urine or stools; or pinpoint red spots on your skin.

- Be careful when using a regular toothbrush, dental floss, or toothpick. Your medical doctor, dentist, or nurse may recommend other ways to clean your teeth and gums. Check with your medical doctor before having any dental work done.

- Do not touch your eyes or the inside of your nose unless you have just washed your hands and have not touched anything else in the meantime.

- Be careful not to cut yourself when you are using sharp objects such as a safety razor or fingernail or toenail cutters.

- Avoid contact sports or other situations where bruising or injury could occur.

Side Effects of This Medicine

Along with its needed effects, a medicine may cause some unwanted effects. Although not all of these side effects may occur, if they do occur they may need medical attention.

Check with your doctor as soon as possible if any of the following side effects occur:

More common:

- Chest pain; mood changes; trouble breathing; unusual tiredness or weakness

Rare:

- Thoughts of suicide, attempts at suicide, changes in behavior

Other side effects may occur that usually do not need medical attention. These side effects may go away during treatment as your body adjusts to the medicine. However, check with your doctor if any of the following side effects continue or are bothersome:

More common:

- Dizziness; fatigue; fever; headache; impaired concentration; impaired taste; influenza-like symptoms such as unusual tiredness or weakness; irritability; red itchy skin; large

361

swing in moods; loss of appetite; muscle or joint pain; nausea, vomiting, or upset stomach; nervousness; redness and warm feeling at the site of injection; shaking; temporary thinning of hair; stuffy nose; trouble sleeping

Other side effects not listed above may also occur in some patients. If you notice any other effects, check with your doctor.

Section 37.3

Pegylated Interferon Combination Therapy

What is pegylated interferon?

Interferon is a type of protein produced by the body's cells in response to viral hepatitis and other infections. Interferon stimulates the body's immune system to fight viral infections and affect the ability of viruses to divide in liver cells.

In pegylation, one or more chains of polyethylene glycol, or PEG (a gelatinous compound used to thicken food), are bonded to an interferon molecule. The PEG works to keep the interferon in the body longer, without reducing efficacy. Whereas three injections are normally required with regular interferon treatment, only one injection of pegylated interferon is required per week.

The U.S. Food and Drug Administration (FDA) has approved Schering-Plough's pegylated interferon product, PEG-INTRON (peginterferon alfa-2b), as well as Roche's product, Pegasys, for use alone or in combination with their antiviral drug, ribavirin.

For whom is pegylated interferon combination therapy prescribed?

The once-weekly pegylated injection and daily ribavirin pills are prescribed for the treatment of chronic hepatitis C in patients who are at least eighteen years of age, and have not previously been treated with alpha interferon.

Pegylated interferon is administered by injection once weekly for up to one year. When used in combination therapy, ribavirin is taken by mouth.

How effective is pegylated interferon combination therapy?

Overall, studies with pegylated combination therapy (peginterferon with ribavirin) have shown sustained response rates in about 55 percent of patients (42 percent in difficult-to-treat genotype 1 HCV; 82 percent in genotypes 2 and 3). Overall response rates for pegylated interferon alone are approximately 24 percent. It seems that both forms of pegylated interferon (PEG-INTRON and PEGASYS) are equally effective.

What are the side effects of treatment?

The safety profile of pegylated interferon combination therapy is similar to regular interferon treatment with no new adverse effects. Side effects can include "flu-like symptoms" such as fever, chills, headaches, muscle or joint aches, tiredness, and weakness. The ribavirin component of combination therapy can also cause a form of anemia. These side effects usually decrease in severity as treatment continues. Some patients may experience depression.

What's next in treatment of hepatitis C?

Future and ongoing clinical trials with pegylated interferon will study combination therapy with ribavirin dosages based on the patient's weight, HIV/HCV co-infected patients, dialysis patients, patients with normal ALT levels, patients with relapsing hepatitis, and patients who have previously not responded to regular interferon treatment.

Section 37.4

Attacking the HCV: Drugs in the Pipeline

A number of strategies for drug development have focused on the combination of antiviral therapy in the form of pegylated interferon with approaches to modulate or induce a cellular immune response.[4] These strategies have been based on the successful outcome of combination therapy of interferon or pegylated interferon with ribavirin, which has been the standard of care for treatment of hepatitis C in the United States and the European Union since 1998.[5–7] Challenges facing our current treatment of HCV include lack of efficacy in patients with difficult-to-treat disease, such as patients with cirrhosis or infected with HCV genotype 1 (who represent a majority of U.S. HCV infections), the toxicity of combination therapy, the expense and difficulty of therapy, and the poor reception of these treatments by many patients. The development of new hepatitis C antiviral agents is critical to our management of this disease. A number of approaches are under investigation, including long-acting interferons; immunomodulators such as Interleukin-12, IL-10 and IL-2, histamine, thymosin alpha-1, IMPDH (inosine-5'-monophosphate dehydrogenase) inhibitors, TNF antagonists, oral interferon-like molecules, ribavirin and ribavirin analogues, and hepatoprotectants; antifibrotics; specific HCV-derived enzyme inhibitors, drugs that either block HCV antigen production from RNA or prevent normal processing of HCV proteins; and other molecular approaches to treating HCV, such as ribozymes, short interfering RNAs, antisense oligonucleotides, immune blockers, and therapeutic vaccines.

New IFNs and IFN-Delivery Systems

A number of different technologies are being studied which might offer alternative strategies for sustained IFN (interferon) release into the circulation. These include the following:

- disposable infusion pumps which hold a three-day reservoir of drug
- controlled release injectables which would utilize a polymer matrix (e.g., a thermosensitive gel or a sucrose acetate isobutyrate-based system) delivered either im. or sc.
- a polyamino acid-based oral delivery system
- encapsulation in liposomes

Oral Interferon-Like Molecules

A number of compounds are known to induce interferon alpha and cytokines, including high molecular weight agents such as double-stranded RNA and oligonucleotides.[23] Because these compounds are not well absorbed with oral delivery or metabolized by the gastrointestinal tract, a more reasonable approach is to use low molecular weight molecules such as resiquimod. This compound is similar to imiquimod, which is currently approved as a topical agent for the treatment of external genitalia and perianal warts.[25]

The only data available regarding safety and efficacy of this oral interferon inducer is limited to that presented in 2003 in abstract form,[26] and in data submitted for publication which is derived primarily from two multicenter trials, one from the United States and one from the European Union (Patton H, Pockros PJ, et al., unpublished data). In the U.S. trial, resiquimod was tested at 0.01 mg/kg, both as a single dose and biweekly. At a higher dosage of 0.02 mg/kg used in the European trial the drug induced numerous cytokines including 2-5-AS, IL-12, IL-1-RA, IL-6, interferon alpha, TNF-alpha, and neopterin. A mean of approximately 1.5 log fall in HCV RNA was obtained by day 24 of biweekly therapy, with three of eleven patients obtaining a >2 log fall in HCV RNA, and two of eleven obtaining a >3 log fall in HCV RNA. Unfortunately, the typical interferon-like side effects were seen in all patients.

Immunomodulators and Anti-Fibrotics

Interleukin-12

Recombinant human interleukin-12 (IL-12) is a 70kD heterodimeric immunomodulatory cytokine which stimulates proliferation of activated virus-specific cytotoxic T lymphocytes and NK cells, as well as stimulating interferon alpha production.

Two hundred and twenty-five patients who were nonresponders to interferon alpha or combination interferon alpha plus ribavirin were randomized to receive 500 ng/kg IL-12 or placebo subcutaneously twice weekly for twelve weeks, and then unblinded. Only 1 percent of nonresponsive patients enrolled for treatment had a sustained virologic response to therapy (2 of 160), whereas 3 percent (7 of 225) developed severe adverse events probably related to treatment, which resulted in early termination of the trial.

Interleukin-10 and Interleukin-2

Interleukin (IL) 10 is a cytokine which down-regulates the pro-inflammatory response and therefore is thought to have a possible modulatory effect on hepatic fibrosis. In 2000, a pilot trial of twenty-four patients was performed by Nelson et al., suggesting that IL-10 treatment reduces fibrosis in patients with chronic hepatitis C.[16] Unfortunately, however, in the twelve-month follow-up study there was an increase in HCV RNA levels which led to titers >120 mEg/ml in some cases with significant ALT flares in two patients.

Gamma Interferon

Gamma interferon has activity both as an immunomodulator[34] and as an anti-fibrotic cytokine in both the murine and human hepatic stellate cells.[35] Data from a preliminary study of long-term treatment with gamma interferon 1b and low-dose prednisolone suggested this compound might be useful in patients with idiopathic pulmonary fibrosis.[36] Subsequent phase III trial data of interferon gamma 1b for idiopathic pulmonary fibrosis failed to reach significance. The results of a small pilot trial using gamma interferon as an anti-fibrotic failed to show significant benefit in data presented in 2003.[41] A large, phase 2b multicenter randomized, controlled trial using hepatic fibrosis as the primary endpoint in patients with advanced fibrosis or cirrhosis due to HCV has been completed and did not show any benefit of gamma interferon in reaching this endpoint.

Ribavirin-Like Molecules

IMPDH (Inosine-5'-monophosphate dehydrogenase) Inhibitors

Inhibition of the host inosine-5'-monophosphate dehydrogenase activity is a well-known effect of ribavirin induced by its monophosphate form.[27] Because of this, it would be sensible to study compounds which inhibit the IMPDH enzyme but do not have the adverse effect of hemolysis associated with ribavirin therapy. Two such compounds have been studied to date. One agent (VX-497, Vertex Pharm Inc., Cambridge, Mass.) has been shown to be safe in patients with hepatitis C. VX-497 is an orally bioavailable small molecule which is a potent IMPDH inhibitor. The results of a randomized, double-blind, placebo-controlled, multicenter trial of VX-497 plus interferon in treatment of naïve patients showed no significant additive reduction in HCV RNA and one patient with a significant rise in ALTs.[28] A second known IMPDH inhibitor is mycophenolate mofetil (CellCept, Hoffman-La Roche, Inc.). Mycophenolate Mofetil (MMF) is a well-known immunosuppressant compound currently used for management following organ transplantation. Because the compound has potent IMPDH inhibition, it has been studied as adjuvant therapy in patients treated with standard or PEG-interferon alpha-2a with or without ribavirin.[29,30] No data regarding sustained virologic response has been published to date. Because of the significant hemolytic effects related to bone marrow suppression, it is unlikely, in my opinion, that MMF will be suitable in combination with pegylated interferons, which by themselves have significant bone marrow suppression effects requiring dose reduction in many patients.

Ribavirin Analogues

In a search for analogues which would have the beneficial effects of ribavirin (RBV) without the adverse events, two key observations have been made which are critical to drug development: first, that RBV monotherapy is not effective at inducing a sustained virologic clearance, and second, that the hemolytic anemia caused by RBV has limited its dosing. The exact mechanism of action of RBV is unknown, although four proposed mechanisms have been described in detail.[27] The most important of these is the immune mediated activity which predisposes the Th2 to Th1 response. This in turn stimulates release of interferon gamma and TNF-alpha from the cytotoxic T lymphocyte, which stimulates immune clearance of HCV virus. As well, ribavirin also is rapidly taken up by the hepatocyte and phosphorylated. The monophosphorylated form of RBV acts as an inhibitor of IMPDH, which may be an important mechanism of its action, as noted above. The triphosphorylated form of RBV is a direct though mild inhibitor of HCV RNA dependent RNA polymerase, which may also be an important mechanism of action. As well, the triphosphorylated form of RBV acts as a RNA mutagen, creating defective HCV RNA particles that are unable to replicate. Both ribavirin and levovirin induce a Th1 cytokine bias favoring an antiviral response at similar concentrations. In chronic HCV infection, it is known that interferon-induced clearance is associated with increased cytotoxic T lymphocyte response and interferon-induced clearance is also associated with release of gamma interferon and diminished release of IL-10. Both of these immune responses have been mimicked in normal individuals receiving levovirin. Because the bioavailability of levovirin is less than that of RBV, the dose range for a phase II trial currently in progress is somewhat higher than that previously studied with RBV alone. No data are available regarding efficacy.

A second RBV analogue currently under study is viramidine, the amidine inversion of RBV. This prodrug is rapidly converted into RBV by the enzyme adenosine deaminase, as the liver is exposed to the first pass effect of oral dosing of the drug.[43] The strategy behind the use of this prodrug is simply to favor the concentration of ribavirin in hepatocytes over the rest of the body, including erythrocytes. In chimpanzees, this compound has been shown to concentrate in the liver, with a liver/RBC ratio three- to six-fold higher than that seen with RBV. In a phase I trial, viramidine showed similar adverse events as ribavirin, however, there was a diminished drop in hemoglobin over that seen with RBV (1.4 g/dl versus 2/5 g/dl) when it is used in a conventional weight-based dosing manner.[44,45] The advantage of viramidine over levovirin is that it will not be lacking any of the properties of RBV.

Molecular Therapies

Ribozymes

Stabilized ribozymes, small catalytic RNA molecules directed against a highly conserved region (5'UTR) of the HCV genome, are currently being tested as a novel therapeutic approach for HCV infection.[52] A ribozyme might effectively block the translation of viral gene products and subsequent replication in the host cell.[53] A pilot trial of an active ribozyme preparation (Heptazyme™) has been completed in humans and has demonstrated that the agent is safe and well tolerated. The results of the virological data of that study have not been released, although it is widely believed the compound was not very effective and was toxic in animals. The possible synergistic effects of the combined Heptazyme™ and Type 1 consensus IFN have been studied in a Phase 2 trial to compare three doses of Heptazyme™ with or without consensus IFN. No data are available regarding efficacy or safety at this time.

Antisense Oligonucleotides

Antisense drugs block the synthesis of disease-causing proteins by preventing translation of viral RNA. In the case of HCV, an antisense oligodeoxynucleotide directed against a specific HCV sequence effectively inhibits viral gene expression.[54] A number of HCV-infected patients have been infused with this antisense oligonucleotide in a Phase I/II trial at our center to demonstrate safety and tolerability (ISIS 14803).[55] The data from this trial indicate that treatment with ISIS 14803 results in significant reductions of HCV RNA (1 log or more) in some patients. A frequent and marked elevation of ALT occurred in association with a fall in HCV RNA in these cases, for currently unexplained reasons. The efficacy and safety of the compound is being further studied in a larger Phase II trial. No data are available for release at this time.

Protease Inhibitors

The NS2 and NS3 protease enzymes cleave the nonstructural proteins of the HCV polypeptide into functional proteins. Thus, inhibition of the NS2/3 proteases would block efficient viral replication. The x-ray crystallography structure of the proteases has been elucidated, allowing for the development of small molecule inhibitors. A serine protease inhibitor has been studied and reported in man in a phase I/II trial in HCV-infected patients. This compound (BILN 2061) caused a 2–3 log10 reduction of HCV RNA in all patients when given for a treatment duration of only forty-eight hours.[56] Many of the cases became HCV RNA undetectable in that brief period of treatment. Unfortunately, the compound has reportedly caused cardiotoxicity in this dose range and therefore must be studied at a lower concentration or must be replaced by alternative protease inhibitors. The key outcome of this pivotal trial is the proof-of-principle that a viral enzyme inhibitor has been extremely effective against HCV. It is very likely that viral resistance would occur after a relatively short period of use of any enzyme inhibitor given as monotherapy. Therefore, one can expect to see development programs of these compounds in combination with pegylated interferons with or without RBV.[57]

HCV Polymerase Inhibitors

Based on the fundamental knowledge of the action of HCV enzymes during viral replication, a number of viral enzyme inhibitors are being developed. The HCV RNA polymerase inhibitors are to be the first

369

enzyme inhibitors that were tested in patients. Phase I safety trials have been completed with a number of compounds. One of these (JTK-003, AkrosPharma, Inc.) has been studied in a randomized, double blind, placebo-controlled, ascending dose, multicenter trial of patients with HCV. Data from this trial have not been made publicly available at this time. Although a helicase inhibitor has been in development, it has not yet been placed in human trials.

Small Interfering RNA Compounds

Small interfering RNAs (siRNAs) are a new class of drug which inhibit gene expression by blocking specific mRNAs.[58] The 5'UTR is the most conserved region in the HCV genome across all genotypes and is therefore the ideal target for siRNA inhibition. An siRNA has been shown to specifically inhibit HCV RNA replication in a replicon model.[58] To date, no siRNA has been tested in man. It is possible that siRNA based gene therapy may be a promising approach to anti-viral therapy for HCV.

Summary

- The most important lessons learned regarding the use of immunomodulators can be drawn from our sizable knowledge base evaluating ribavirin.

- The most likely of these changes will be the use of a ribavirin analogue, at the earliest by 2007.

- Although a number of the other compounds discussed may ultimately show benefit, I believe this will take a longer period of time.

- New therapeutic approaches to HCV include antisense therapy, hammerhead ribozymes, oral IFNs, and specific enzyme inhibitors, such as protease, helicase, and polymerase.

- Ultimately, we need oral drugs that are easy to take, nontoxic, inexpensive, and efficacious.

References

1. Pockros P, Patel K, O'Brien CB: A multicenter study of recombinant human interleukin-12 for the treatment of chronic hepatitis C infection in patients with non-responsiveness to previous therapy. *Hepatology* 2003, 37:1368–74.

2. Thimme R, Bukh J, Spangenberg HC, Wieland S, Pemberton J, Steiger C, Govindarajan S, Purcell RH, Chisari FV: Viral and immunological determinants of hepatitis C virus clearance, persistence, and disease. *Proc. Natl. Acad. Sci. USA* 2002, 99:15661–68.

3. Erickson AL, Kimura Y, Igarashi S, Eichelberger J, Houghton M, Sidney J, McKinney D, Sette A, Hughes AL, Walker CM: The outcome of hepatitis C virus infection is predicted by escape mutations in epitopes targeted by cytotoxic T lymphocytes. *Immunity* 2001, 15:883–95.

4. Pockros PJ: Developments in the treatment of chronic hepatitis C. *Expert Opin. Investig. Drugs* 2002, 11:515–23.

5. McHutchison JG, Gordon SC, Schiff ER, et al: Interferon alfa-2b alone or in combination with ribavirin as initial treatment for chronic hepatitis C. *N. Engl. J. Med.* 1998, 339:1485–92.

6. Manns MP, McHutchison JG, Gordon SC, Rustgi AK, Shiffman M, Reindollar R, Goodman ZD, Koury K, Ling M, Albrecht JK: Peg-interferon alfa-2b plus ribavirin compared with interferon alfa-2b plus ribavirin for initial treatment of chronic hepatitis C: A randomised trial. *Lancet* 2001, 358:958–65.

7. Fried MW, Shiffman ML, Reddy KR, Smith C, Marinos G, Goncales FLJr, Haussinger D, Diago M, Carosi G, Dhumeaux D, Craxi A, Lin A, Hoffman J, Yu J: Peg-interferon alfa-2a plus ribavirin for chronic hepatitis C virus infection. *N. Engl. J. Med.* 2002, 347:975–82.

8. Kamal SM, Fehr J, Roesler B, Peters T, Rasenack JW: Peg-interferon alone or with ribavirin enhances HCV-specific CD4 T-helper 1 responses in patients with chronic hepatitis C. *Gastroenterology* 2002, 123:1070–83.

9. Schlaak JF, Pitz T, Lohr HF, Meyerzum Buschenfelde K.H., Gerken G: Interleukin 12 enhances deficient HCV-antigen-induced Th1-type immune response of peripheral blood mononuclear cells. *J. Med. Virol.* 1998, 56:112–17.

10. Fan XG, Tang FQ, Yi H, Liu WE, Houghton M, Hu GL: Effect of IL-12 on T-cell immune responses in patients with chronic HCV infection. *APMIS* 2000, 108:531–38.

11. Zeuzem S, Hopf U, Carreno V, Diago M, Shiffman M, Grune S, Dudley FJ, et al: A phase I/II study of recombinant human

interleukin-12 in patients with chronic hepatitis C. *Hepatology* 1999+, 29:1280–86.

12. Moscarella S, Buzelli G, Romanelli RG, Monti M, Giannini C, Careccia G, Marrocchi EM, et al: Interferon and thymosin combination therapy in naive patients with chronic hepatitis C: Preliminary results. *Liver* 1998, 18:366–69.

13. Pardo M, Castillo I, Oliva H, Fernandez-Flores A, Barcena R, de Peuter MA, Carreno V: A pilot study of recombinant inter-leukin-2 for treatment of chronic hepatitis C. *Hepatology* 1997, 26:1318–21.

14. Lurie Y, Pakula R, Malnick S: Efficacy and safety of the combi-nation of histamine dihydrochloride and interferon alpha-2b in a phase II trial in naive patients with chronic hepatitis C [abstract]. *Hepatology* 2001, 34:350A.

15. Rockey DC, Maher JJ, Jarnagin WR, Gabbiani G, Friedman SL: Inhibition of rat hepatic lipocyte activation in culture by interferon-gamma. *Hepatology* 1992, 16:776–84.

16. Nelson DR, Lauwers GY, Lau JY, Davis GL: Interleukin 10 treatment reduces fibrosis in patients with chronic hepatitis C: A pilot trial of interferon nonresponders. *Gastroenterology* 2000, 118:655–66.

17. Serrate SA, Schulof RS, Leondaridis L, Goldstein AL: Modula-tion of human natural killer cell cytotoxic activity, lymphokine production, and interleukin 2 receptor expression by thymic hormones. *J. Immunol.* 1987, 139:2338–43.

18. Moscarella S, Buzzelli G, Romanelli R, et al: Interferon and thymosin combination therapy in naive patients with chronic hepatitis C. *Liver* 1998, 18:366–69.

19. Rasi G, Divigilio D, Mutchnick MG, et al: Combination thy-mosin alpha 1 and lymphoblastoid interferon treatment in chronic hepatitis C. *Gut* 1996, 39:679–83.

20. Sherman K, Sjogren M, Creager R, et al: Combination ther-apy with thymosin alpha1 and interferon for the treatment of chronic hepatitis C infection: A randomized, placebo-controlled double-blind trial. *Hepatology* 1998, 27:1135.

21. Pockros PJ, Reindollar R, McHutchison JG, Reddy R, Wright T, Boyd DG, Willett WC: The safety and tolerability of daily

infergen plus ribavirin in the treatment of naive chronic hepatitis C patients. *J. Viral Hepatitis* 2003, 10:55–60.

22. Su AI, Pezaki JP, Wodicka L, Brideau AD, Supekova L, Thimme R, Weiland S, Bukh J, Purcell RH, Schultz PG, Chisari FV: Genomic analysis of the host response to hepatitis C virus infection. *Proc. Natl. Acad. Sci. USA* 2002, 99:15669–74.

23. Guidotti LG, Chisari FV: Non-cytolytic control of viral infections by the innate and adaptive immune response. *Ann. Rev. Immunol.* 2001, 19:65–91.

24. Tompkins WA: Immunomodulation and therapeutic effects of the oral use of interferon-alpha: Mechanism of action. *J. Interferon Cytokine Res.* 1999, 19:817–28.

25. Goldstein D, Hertzog P, Tomkinson E, Couldwell D, McCarvile S, Parrish S, Cunningham P, Newell M, Owens M, Cooper DA: Administration of imiquimod, an interferon inducer, in asymptomatic human immunodeficiency virus-infected persons to determine safety and biologic response modification. *J. Infect. Dis.* 1998, 178:858–61.

26. Pockros PJ, Tong M, Wright T, et al: A phase IIa placebo-controlled, double-blind trial to determine the safety, tolerability, PK/PD of an oral interferon inducer, Resiquimod, in chronic HCV. *Gastroenterology* 2003, 124 (Suppl 1):A-766.

27. Lau JYN, Tam RC, Liang TJ, Hong Z: Mechanism of action of ribavirin in the combination treatment of chronic HCV infection. *Hepatology* 2002, 35:1002–9.

28. McHutchison JG, Cheung R, Shiffman ML, et al: A 4-week trial of VX 497 (an IMPDH inhibitor) combined with interferon in previously untreated patients with chronic hepatitis C. *Hepatology* 2001, 34 (Suppl): 329A.

29. Afdhal N, Flamm S, Imperial JC, et al: Analyses of 40 KDA peginterferon alfa-2a in combination with ribavirin, mycophenolate mofetil, amantadine or amantadine plus ribavirin in patients that relapsed or did not respond to Rebetron therapy: A report of two randomized, multicenter, efficacy and safety studies. *Hepatology* 2001, 34 (Suppl):243A.

30. Cornberg M, Hinrichsen H, Teuber G, Berg T, Naumann U, Falkenberg C, Zeuzem S, Manns MP: Mycophenolate mofetil

in combination with recombinant interferon alfa-2a in interferon-nonresponder patients with chronic hepatitis C. *J. Hepatol.* 2002, 37:843–47.

31. Fabris C, Del Forno M, Falleti E, Toniutto P, Pirisi M: Kinetics of serum soluble tumour necrosis factor receptor (TNF-R) type-I and type-II after a single interferon-alpha (IFN-alpha) injection in chronic hepatitis C. *Clin. Exp. Immunol.* 1999, 117:556–60.

32. Tilg H, Vogel W, Dinarello CA: Interferon-alpha induces circulating tumor necrosis factor receptor p55 in humans. *Blood* 1995, 85:433–35.

33. Zein NN, ETANERCEPT Study Group: A phase II randomized, double-blind, placebo-controlled study of tumor necrosis factor antagonist (Etanercept, Enbrel as an adjuvant to interferon and ribavirin in naive patients with chronic hepatitis C. *Hepatology* 2002, 36:304A.

34. Shi Z, Wakil AE, Rockey DC: Strain-specific differences in mouse hepatic wound healing are mediated by divergent T helper cytokine responses. *Proc. Natl. Acad. Sci. USA* 1990, 94:10663–68.

35. Rockey DC: Hepatic fibrogenesis and hepatitis C. *Semin. Gastrointest. Dis.* 2000, 11:69–83.

36. Ziesche R, et al: A preliminary study of long-term treatment with interferon gamma-1b and low-dose prednisolone in patients with idiopathic pulmonary fibrosis. *N. Engl. J. Med.* 1999, 341:1264–69.

37. Saez-Royuela F, et al: High doses of recombinant alpha-interferon or gamma-interferon for chronic hepatitis C: A randomized, controlled trial. *Hepatology* 1991, 13:327–31.

38. Di Biscegli AM, Rustgi AK, Kassianides C, et al: Therapy of chronic hepatitis B with recombinant human alpha and gamma interferon. *Hepatology* 1990, 11:266–70.

39. Kakumu S, et al: Treatment with human gamma interferon of chronic hepatitis B: Comparative study with alpha interferon. *J. Med. Virol.* 1991, 35:32–37.

40. Frese M, Schwarzle V, Barth K, Krieger N, Lohmann V, Mihm S, Haller O, Bartenschlager R: Interferon-gamma inhibits

replication of subgenomic and genomic hepatitis C virus RNAs. *Hepatology* 2002, 35:694–703.

41. Muir AJ, Sylvestre PB, Rockey DC: Interferon gamma-1 for the treatment of chronic hepatitis C infection. *Gastroenterology* 2003, 124 (Suppl 1):A-718.

42. Davis GL, Wong JB, McHutchison JG, Manns MP, Harvey J, Albrecht J: Early virologic response to treatment with peginterferon alfa-2b plus ribavirin in patients with chronic hepatitis C. *Hepatology* 2003, 38:645–52.

43. Arora S, Lau D, Gish R, et al: Phase I clinical studies of viramidine—A liver-targeting prodrug of ribavirin. *Hepatology* 2002, 36:356A.

44. Arora S, Lau D, Gish R, Rossi S, Lin C-C, Lau JYN, Fang JWS: Phase I clinical studies of viramidine—A liver targeting prodrug of ribavirin [abstract]. *Hepatology* 2002, 36:356A.

45. Watson J: Prospects for hepatitis C virus therapeutics: Levovirin and viramidine as improved derivatives of ribavirin. *Curr. Opin. Investig. Drugs* 2002, 3:680–83.

46. Lemon SM, Chisari FV, Lai MMC, Nishioka K, Mishiro S, Johnson L: The Nineteenth United States-Japan Joint Hepatitis Panel Meeting. *Hepatology* 1998, 28:881–87.

47. Arase Y, Ikeda K, Murashima N, Chayama K, Tsubota A, Koida I, et al: The long term efficacy of glycyrrhizin in chronic hepatitis C patients. *Cancer* 1997, 1997:1494.

48. Valentino K, Gutierrez M, Sanchez R, Pockros P, Winship MS: First clinical trial of IDN-6556: First anti-apoptotic caspase inhibitor improves liver function. *Gastroenterology* 2002, 122:A-622.

49. Poupon RE, Bonnand AM, Queneau PE, Trepo C, Zarski JPi, Vetter D, et al. Randomized trial of interferon-alpha plus ursodeoxycholic acid versus interferon plus placebo in patients with chronic hepatitis C resistant to interferon. *Scand J Gastroenterol.* 2000 Jun; 35(6):642–49.

50. Nelson DR, Tu Z, Soldevila-Pico C, Abdelmalek M, Zhu H, et al: Long-term interleukin 10 therapy in chronic hepatitis C patients has a proven proviral and anti-inflammatory effect. *Hepatology* 2003, 38:859–68.

51. Lesburg CA, Radfar R, Weber PC: Recent advances in the analysis of HCV NS5B RNA-dependent RNA polymerase. *Curr. Opin. Investig. Drugs* 2000, 1:289–96.

52. Lyons AJ, Lytle JR, Gomez J, Robertson HD: Hepatitis C virus internal ribosome entry site RNA contains a tertiary structural element in a functional domain of stem-loop II. *Nucleic Acids Res.* 2001, 29:2535–41.

53. Macejak DG, Jensen KL, Jamison SF et al: Inhibition of hepatitis C virus (HCV)-RNA-dependent translation and replication of a chimeric HCV poliovirus in synthetic stabilized ribozymes. *Hepatology* 2000, 31:769–76.

54. Zhang H, Hanekak R, Browndriver V et al: Antisense oligonucleotide inhibition of hepatitis C virus (HCV) gene expression in livers of mice infected with an HCV-vaccinia virus recombinant. *Antimicrob. Agents Chemother.* 1999, 43:347–53.

55. McHutchison JG, Pockros PJ, Nyberg LM: A dose-escalation study of ISIS 14803, an antisense inhibitor of HCV, in chronic hepatitis C patients. *Hepatology* 2001, 34:350A.

56. Lamarre D, Anderson PC, Bailey M, et al: An NS3 protease inhibitor with antiviral effects in humans infected with hepatitis C virus. *Nature* 2003, 426:186–89.

57. Casbarra A, Piaz FD, Ingallinella P, et al: The effect of prime-site occupancy on the hepatitis C virus NS3 protease structure. *Protein Sci* 2002, 11:2102–12.

58. Kapadia SB, Brideau-Anderson A, Chisari FV: Interference of hepatitis C virus RNA replication by short interfering RNAs. *Proc Natl Acad Sci USA* 2003, 100:1024–28.

59. Tong MJ, Reddy KR, Lee WM, Pockros PJ, et al. Treatment of chronic hepatitis C with consensus interferon: a multicenter, randomized, controlled trial. *Hepatology* 1997, 26:747–54.

60. Pepinsky RB, LePage DJ, Gill A, Chakraborty A, Vaidyanathan S, Green M, Baker DP, Whalley E, Hochman PS, Martin P. Glycol-modified form of interferon-beta 1a with preserved in vitro bioactivity. *J Pharmacol Exp Ther* 2001, 297:1059–66.

Chapter 38

HCV and Complementary and Alternative Medicine

Introduction

Hepatitis C is a disease of the liver that is caused by the hepatitis C virus. The disease occurs in acute and chronic forms; symptoms can range from mild (or even no symptoms) to severe. There are conventional medical treatments available for hepatitis C, but some patients also try complementary and alternative medicine (CAM). This chapter answers some frequently asked questions on hepatitis C and CAM, reviews findings from scientific research on some dietary supplements that have been used as CAM treatments for hepatitis C (milk thistle, licorice root, ginseng, thymus extract, schisandra, and colloidal silver), and suggests sources for further information.

Note: Conventional medicine is medicine as practiced by holders of M.D. (medical doctor) or D.O. (doctor of osteopathy) degrees and their allied health professionals, such as physical therapists, psychologists, and registered nurses. Other terms for conventional medicine include allopathy; Western, mainstream, orthodox, and regular medicine; and biomedicine. Some conventional medical practitioners are also practitioners of CAM. CAM, as defined by the National Center for Complementary and Alternative Medicine (NCCAM), is a group of diverse medical and health care systems, practices, and products that are not presently considered to be part of conventional medicine.

Reprinted from "Hepatitis C and Complementary and Alternative Medicine: 2003 Update," National Center for Complementary and Alternative Medicine, National Institutes of Health, NCCAM Publication No. D004, May 2004.

Key Points

- Conventional medical treatment (consisting of a combination drug regimen) for hepatitis C has shown sustained benefit in approximately 55 percent of patients.

- Some of the reasons hepatitis C patients try CAM are that they find conventional drug treatment difficult to tolerate or they do not experience a sustained response to treatment.

- No CAM treatment has yet been proven safe and effective for treating hepatitis C.

- There are many CAM treatments for which benefits for health are claimed. However, it is important to find out what scientific studies have been done on the safety and effectiveness of the CAM treatment in which you are interested. Clinical trials are needed of CAM therapies that may show some potential for benefit for hepatitis C, such as milk thistle. The National Center for Complementary and Alternative Medicine (NCCAM) is sponsoring a clinical trial of milk thistle.

- It is important to inform all of your health care providers about any therapy that you are currently using or considering, including any dietary supplements. This is to help ensure a safe and coordinated course of care.

Frequently Asked Questions about Hepatitis C and Complementary and Alternative Medicine

What is hepatitis C?

Hepatitis C is a communicable (contagious) disease of the liver caused by the hepatitis C virus (HCV). The liver, the largest organ in the body, is found behind the ribs on the right side of the abdomen. It has many important functions, including removing harmful material from the blood and converting food into substances needed for life and growth. The term "hepatitis" means inflammation of the liver. There are other viruses in the hepatitis family (such as hepatitis A and hepatitis B), but HCV is not related to them.

Quick Facts about Hepatitis C

- Hepatitis C is the most common blood-borne infection in the United States. About thirty-five thousand new cases are diagnosed in the United States each year.

378

- Hepatitis C is transmitted primarily when an infected person's blood comes into contact with the blood of a noninfected person.

- People who are at the highest risk for HCV infection are those who have used or experimented with injection drugs; received a blood transfusion, blood product, or organ transplant before July 1992; worked in health care and had a needlestick accident involving HCV-infected blood; or had multiple sex partners.

- A risk exists but is low (1 to 5 percent) for babies born to a mother with hepatitis C and for people who are in a monogamous sexual relationship with someone with hepatitis C; who have had other sexually transmitted diseases; who have had tattooing or body piercing done with unsterilized tools; or who have used cocaine intranasally (i.e., "snorted" it).

- Hepatitis C is not spread through sneezing, coughing, kissing, hugging, food or water, or casual contact.

- People who are newly infected have what is called acute hepatitis C. For about 15 to 40 percent of this group, the infection is short-term, goes away, and does not return. Others develop chronic (or long-lasting) hepatitis C, in which the virus stays in the liver, replicates itself, and injures the liver over time.

- Among people with chronic hepatitis C, most show no symptoms for up to twenty to thirty years; some have mild symptoms; and some have more serious symptoms.

- Chronic hepatitis C can cause liver disease, cirrhosis (scarring of the liver), liver cancer, and liver failure. However, persons who have been diagnosed with hepatitis C need to know that serious illness or death from the disease is by no means inevitable—especially if they take proper care of themselves and get the health care they need.

What does conventional treatment for chronic hepatitis C consist of?

People who have a mild case of hepatitis C may need only to manage it by visiting their doctor regularly and following their doctor's recommendations—such as eating a nutritious diet, avoiding alcohol (because of its impact on the liver), and getting regular exercise.

For people with more severe hepatitis C, however, drug therapy may be needed. A drug called interferon is the mainstay of conventional treatment. Interferon is often combined with an antiviral (virus-fighting) drug called ribavirin. Such combination therapies are usually taken for six months to one year. Approximately 55 percent of patients treated with the combination of interferon and ribavirin for one year will achieve a sustained response (that is, a sustained benefit from treatment).[1] If a patient does not achieve a sustained response, his or her doctor may decide whether another course of treatment (re-treatment) is appropriate.

Combination regimens benefit many patients. However, their side effects can be difficult for some patients to tolerate. These side effects can include flu-like symptoms (such as body aches, fever, chills, and fatigue); nausea and other gastrointestinal problems; hair loss; emotional changes; skin reactions; and, in more severe cases, depression, organ damage, blood conditions, and other problems.

Why do people use CAM for hepatitis C?

There are various reasons why people use CAM for hepatitis C, including:

- They have not had a response to initial treatment or to re-treatment with drugs.

- They are not willing to have drug treatment or continue it—for example, because of the side effects or length of treatment.

- They would like to support their body's fight against damage by hepatitis C, and they hear of benefits claimed for some CAM treatments—such as "strengthens the immune system" or "cleanses or rejuvenates the liver" (or other organs).

- They are experiencing problems from other diseases and conditions that can be caused by or worsened by hepatitis C.

- They are not satisfied with their conventional medical treatment.

How commonly do people with hepatitis C use CAM therapies, and what do they use?

While there have been no surveys yet on the use of CAM by persons with hepatitis C specifically, there is some data from a survey published in 2002 on the use of CAM by persons who have chronic liver diseases (such as hepatitis, liver cancer, alcoholic liver disease, or cirrhosis).[2] This survey of 989 patients being treated for various liver diseases at six clinics in the United States found that 39 percent

380

used some form of "alternative therapy." The therapy they used the most (21 percent) was herbals or botanicals. (Herbs are plants or plant parts valued for their flavor, scent, or therapeutic properties. "Herbals" and "botanicals" are synonyms and mean herbal and botanical products.) However, the herbals and botanicals were used for reasons besides liver disease, such as depression. Thirteen percent of all survey participants used herbals or botanicals specifically for their liver disease, and they used only milk thistle (12 percent) or licorice root (1 percent). The other most commonly used CAM therapies were self-prayer (18 percent), and (from 6 to 9 percent each) relaxation, megavitamins, massage, chiropractic, and spiritual healing.

What CAM therapies are discussed in this chapter?

There is a range of medical concerns associated with hepatitis C, and the number of CAM therapies that are tried is large. Therefore, it is beyond the scope of this chapter to discuss all possible CAM therapies used for hepatitis C. The chapter focuses on a number of dietary supplements that are used: milk thistle, licorice root, ginseng, thymus extract, schisandra, and colloidal silver.

About Dietary Supplements

Dietary supplements were defined in a law passed by Congress in 1994. A dietary supplement must meet all of the following conditions:

- It is a product (other than tobacco) intended to supplement the diet, which contains one or more of the following: vitamins, minerals, herbs or other botanicals, amino acids, or any combination of the above ingredients.

- It is intended to be taken in tablet, capsule, powder, softgel, gelcap, or liquid form.

- It is not represented for use as a conventional food or as a sole item of a meal or the diet.

- It is labeled as being a dietary supplement.

Sources for this chapter consist of the peer-reviewed medical and scientific journals indexed in the National Library of Medicine's MEDLINE/PubMed database, in English, from January 1999 through May 2003. Sources that you can use to research additional science-based information are in the "Sources" sections.

What is known from the scientific evidence about CAM modalities for hepatitis C?

- No CAM treatment has been scientifically proven to success-fully treat hepatitis C.

- Authors who have done recent analyses of the scientific work have found some results that are intriguing and even promis-ing, but they have noted that more research—especially in the form of controlled clinical trials—is needed before firm conclu-sions can be drawn.

  - The authors of a 2003 systematic review of medicinal herbs for hepatitis C concluded that there is not enough evidence to support using herbs to treat the disease. This team identi-fied thirteen clinical trials that were of sufficient quality for them to analyze. Compared to placebo, they found that none of the herbs tested showed effects on liver enzymes or reduced the amount of HCV in the bloodstream, except for milk thistle, which did show a significant reduction of liver enzymes in one trial.[3]

  - Two general reviews from 2000 that covered a variety of CAM modalities for hepatitis C concluded that conventional therapies are the only scientifically proven treatments for the disease.[4,5]

  - NIH released a Consensus Statement in 2002 on the man-agement of hepatitis C. This assessment by a panel of medical and scientific experts found that "alternative and nontradi-tional medicines" should be studied.

What should I do to take care of myself if I have hepatitis C?

- Make sure you have received an accurate diagnosis. Hepatitis C can be diagnosed reliably only through sophisticated blood tests used in conventional medicine.

- See your health care provider regularly.

- Discuss treatment options with your provider. Ask any questions you have to make sure you understand any treatment and pos-sible side effects. Follow his or her recommendations for any changes to your diet or lifestyle.

- Tell your provider about any herbal supplements, other di-etary supplements, or medications (whether prescription or over-the-counter) that you are using or considering. This is important for your safety. Even if your provider does not know about the actions or interactions of an herbal supplement or other CAM treatment, he or she can access the most current medical guidance.

- Get vaccinated against hepatitis A and B. Infection with hepatitis C does not prevent a person from becoming infected with other types of hepatitis; if this happens, it can be serious, even life-threatening.

- Be an informed consumer. Seek high-quality, science-based information on any CAM modality that you are using or considering. There is free information available from NCCAM, the National Library of Medicine, and other federal sources to help you distinguish science-based information from other types, including word-of-mouth and manufacturers' claims.

- If you decide to try herbal supplements, do so with care.

Scientific Research Findings: Selected CAM Treatments for Hepatitis C

This section describes six CAM therapies that people have used to treat hepatitis C. More-detailed discussions of individual studies are available in the Table 38.1. Reviews are discussed where available.

Note: There are different types of review articles: In a general review, a broad picture of the scientific studies and evidence available on a particular topic is presented. In a systematic review, data from a set of studies on a particular question or topic are collected, analyzed, and critically reviewed. A meta-analysis uses statistical techniques to analyze results from a collection of individual studies.

Milk Thistle

Milk thistle (scientific name *Silybum marianum*) is a plant from the aster family. The active extract of milk thistle believed to be responsible for the herb's medicinal qualities is silymarin, found in the fruit.[6] Milk thistle has been used in Europe as a treatment for liver disease and jaundice since the sixteenth century.[7]

Summary of the Research Findings

- The results of scientific studies to date do not definitively find that milk thistle is beneficial in treating hepatitis C in humans.

- Studies in laboratory animals suggest that silymarin may have various benefits to the liver, such as promoting the growth of certain types of liver cells, having a protective effect upon liver cells, fighting a chemical process called oxidation that can damage cells, and inhibiting inflammation.[7-14] However, in some cases, a consistent pattern of benefit was not seen, and these studies did not specifically examine the effects of silymarin on hepatitis C.

- There have been some studies on silymarin or milk thistle in humans. These studies have generally been small and on liver diseases rather than on hepatitis C infection specifically, and the results have been contradictory (with some positive and some negative).[15-17] A review and a meta-analysis published in 2001 on silymarin in the treatment of liver diseases found it to be generally safe, but contained no firm conclusions with regard to its use to treat viral hepatitis.[18,19] A 2002 systematic review on milk thistle for liver disease found "no reduction in mortality (frequency of death as an outcome), in improvements in histology (tissue studies) observed through liver biopsy, or in biochemical markers of liver function" and that the data was too limited to support recommending milk thistle for treatment of liver disease.[20]

To obtain more extensive and reliable data, NCCAM is sponsoring a clinical trial on the use of milk thistle for hepatitis C.

Side Effects and Other Risks

Milk thistle is generally well tolerated and has shown few side effects in clinical trials. It can cause a laxative effect; less common effects include nausea, diarrhea, abdominal bloating, fullness, and pain. Milk thistle can produce allergic reactions, which tend to be more common among people who are allergic to plants in the same family (e.g., ragweed, chrysanthemum, marigold, and daisy).

Licorice Root

Licorice root is the peeled or unpeeled dried root of the licorice plant (*Glycyrrhiza glabra*). The primary active component of licorice root is a substance called glycyrrhizin. Licorice root has been in use in China since the second and third century B.C. and in the West since Egyptian, Greek, and Roman times.[21]

Summary of the Research Findings

- Laboratory studies of glycyrrhizin in cell cultures suggest that it may have antiviral properties.[21]

- In a review of several randomized controlled trials, researchers reported that glycyrrhizin has potential for reducing long-term complications in chronic hepatitis C in those patients who may not respond to interferon.[22] Several of the trials reviewed indicated improvements in liver tissue damaged by hepatitis. Some also showed improvements in how well the liver did its job after treatment.

- A 1997 study and a 2002 review suggest that long-term administration of glycyrrhizin might prevent liver cancer in patients with chronic hepatitis C.[23,24]

- The use of glycyrrhizin as a complementary therapy (i.e., used in addition to conventional interferon therapy) has been studied, but no significant benefit has been found.[25,26]

- Recent clinical trials have shown that taking glycyrrhizin lowers the levels of liver enzymes (increased levels of certain liver enzymes indicate liver damage or inflammation). However, taking the herb did not reduce the amount of HCV in patients' blood, a critical indicator of the long-term progress of the infection.[27–29]

Side Effects and Possible Risks

Taking licorice over a prolonged period of time can lead to potentially serious side effects, including high blood pressure, salt and water retention, swelling, depletion of potassium, headache, or sluggishness.[30] Glycyrrhizin can worsen ascites, the accumulation of fluid in the abdominal cavity, a condition that can be caused by cirrhosis.[31] The herb also can interact with certain drugs, such as diuretics, digitalis, antiarrhythmic agents, and corticosteroids.

Ginseng

The herb ginseng comes in two types: American ginseng (*Panax quinquefolius*) and Asian ginseng (*Panax ginseng*). Among the Asian forms of ginseng are Chinese, Japanese, and Korean ginseng. (So-called Siberian ginseng is not a true ginseng.) Ginseng has been used for thousands of years in Asia. It is usually used with the belief that it will boost the immune system and increase stamina; such properties are thought to be more useful for the elderly and those recovering from illness.[32]

385

Summary of the Research Findings

- The research on ginseng that has been done to date has been primarily in animal models and human tissue in the laboratory. Some beneficial effects of ginseng on the liver were seen in these studies. Researchers concluded that ginseng may also help strengthen glandular systems and the ability to resist disease.[33–36]

- One study found that ginseng may be helpful for elderly people with liver conditions similar to hepatitis.[37]

- No conclusions can be drawn about the possible usefulness and safety of ginseng as a treatment in people who have hepatitis C, because it has not yet been studied formally in people.

Side Effects and Possible Risks

General adverse (negative) effects of ginseng can include insomnia, headache, nosebleed, nervousness, and vomiting. Prolonged use of caffeine and a high dose of ginseng may be associated with hypertension, which is of particular concern for people with cardiovascular disease or diabetes. In addition, people with diabetes who use insulin should be aware that ginseng has demonstrated hypoglycemic effects (lowering of the blood sugar). Ginseng has been shown in laboratory studies to inhibit grouping of platelets in the blood, increasing bleeding risk. Because of this, using ginseng along with NSAIDs (non-steroidal anti-inflammatory drugs), such as aspirin or ibuprofen, should be discussed with your health care provider.[32]

Thymus Extract

The thymus is a gland that is involved in the regulation of the body's immune response. Thymus extract products consist of peptides taken from the thymus glands of cows or calves and are sold as dietary supplements. Often, these products carry claims of boosting immune system functioning to combat diseases, such as hepatitis C. These over-the-counter supplements should not be confused with the prescription drug thymosin alpha-1.

Summary of the Research Findings

There has been little testing of bovine thymus extract for treatment of hepatitis C. A small clinical trial of a product called Complete Thymic Formula, which contains bovine thymus extracts along with

vitamins, herbs, minerals, and enzymes, did not find the product beneficial for hepatitis C patients who had not responded previously to
interferon therapy.[38] However, this small study does not provide sufficient evidence to draw firm conclusions about either Complete Thymic Formula or thymus extracts in general.

Side Effects and Possible Risks

In the study of Complete Thymic Formula, one adverse event was
reported: a patient developed thrombocytopenia, a drop in the number of platelet cells in the blood; the patient recovered after treatment
was stopped.[38] In general, no adverse effects from thymus extracts
have been reported. However, since thymus extracts are derived from
animals, there can be concern related to possible contamination from
diseased animal parts. Accordingly, people on immunosuppressive
drugs or who have suppressed immune systems, such as transplant
recipients or persons with HIV/AIDS, should use caution about thymus extracts and consult with their health care provider.

Schisandra

Schisandra is a plant that has been used (through extracts from
its fruit) in traditional Chinese medicine and in Kampo, traditional
Japanese medicine. There are several species, including *Schisandra
chinensis*, native to northeastern China and Korea, and *Schisandra
sphenanthera*, native to China.

Summary of the Research Findings

- Research has primarily focused on the various lignans (a class
  of plant nutrients) and essential oils in the dried fruit of schisandra.[39] Major constituents include the lignans gomisin A, schi-
  zandrins and schizandrol, vitamins C and E, and others.

- Studies of the effects of schisandra in the liver have mostly
  been in animal models. These studies have suggested that extracts of the fruit have a liver-protective effect, a helpful effect
  on some liver enzymes, and an antioxidant effect (antioxidants
  are substances [such as vitamin E] that help prevent oxygen
  from reacting with other chemicals in cells [oxidation], a process that can have negative effects).[39,40]

- Schisandra is also used in herbal formulas. For example, an herbal medicine called TJ-108 (Ninjin-yomei-to is one of its Japanese

Table 38.1. Research Findings on Selected CAM Treatments for Hepatitis C

Citation: Liu et al., 2003[3]q
Description: Systematic review
Findings: The researchers conducted searches in several databases to identify thirteen randomized trials of medicinal herbs for hepatitis C (trial quality was rated adequate in only four trials). The selected trials, involving a total of 818 patients with mainly HCV, evaluated fourteen different medicinal herbs versus various control interventions such as placebo. Compared to placebo, they found that none of the herbs tested showed effects on liver enzymes or in reducing the amount of HCV, except for milk thistle, which did show a significant reduction of liver enzymes in one trial. The authors concluded, "There is no firm evidence supporting medicinal herbs for HCV infection, and further randomized trials are justified."

Milk Thistle (Silymarin)
Citation: Letteron et al., 1990[11]
Description: Animal study
Findings: Researchers tested the liver-protective effects of silymarin against the damaging effects of carbon tetrachloride by administering 800 mg/kg of silymarin to mice before administering carbon tetrachloride. The researchers concluded that giving silymarin to mice prior to exposure to carbon tetrachloride prevented in part both lipid peroxidation (damage to the membrane) and liver cell death.

Citation: Davila et al., 1989[12]
Description: Animal study
Findings: Using cultures of liver cells from newborn rats, researchers studied the protective effects of an active component of silymarin. Pretreatment of the liver cells with silybin before exposure to liver cell toxins led to less damage and reduction of leakage of liver enzymes. The researchers concluded that the silymarin component "may act by stabilizing the plasma membrane against toxic insult."

Citation: Fuchs et al., 1997[13]
Description: Animal study
Findings: Using a specific type of liver cell (hepatic stellate cells) whose proliferation and transformation are associated with progression to fibrosis in liver disease, researchers studied the effects of an active component of silymarin. The component reduced the proliferation of rat hepatic stellate cells by about 75 percent and reduced the transformation of the cells to myofibroblasts.

Citation: Boigk et al., 1997[14]
Description: Animal study
Findings: Using an animal model of liver fibrosis, researchers studied the effects of silymarin on collagen accumulation, which occurs during the progression of liver fibrosis. After the six-week experiment, the researchers found that rats with induced liver fibrosis who were given silymarin had from 30 percent to 35 percent reduction in the amount of collagen accumulated. This suggests that silymarin may have antifibrotic activity.

Table 38.1. Research Findings on Selected CAM Treatments for Hepatitis C (*continued*)

Milk Thistle (Silymarin) (*continued*)

Citation: Ferenci et al., 1989[15]
Description: Randomized, controlled trial
Findings: Eighty-seven patients with cirrhosis of the liver from various causes, including alcohol abuse, were given 140 mg of silymarin three times a day for two years, and 83 patients received placebo. A total of 146 patients completed the two-year study. The researchers noted that the four-year survival rate of patients in the treatment group was approximately 58 percent and the four-year survival rate in the placebo group was approximately 39 percent. The beneficial effects of silymarin were especially seen in patients with cirrhosis as a result of alcohol. According to the researchers, results suggest "mortality of patients with cirrhosis was reduced by treatment with silymarin."

Citation: Pares et al., 1998[16]
Description: Randomized, double-blind, controlled trial
Findings: Researchers studied 200 patients with cirrhosis of the liver caused by alcohol. In the two-year trial, 103 patients received 150 mg of silymarin 3 times a day, and 97 patients received a placebo. A total of 125 patients finished the trial. The researchers measured time to death and worsening of the disease to test effectiveness of silymarin. They found that survival of patients was similar in the treatment and placebo groups, and silymarin did not seem to improve the course of the disease in the treatment group.

Citation: Buzzelli et al., 1993[17]
Description: Randomized, controlled, pilot study
Findings: This small trial of hepatitis patients suggests that a component of silymarin may be beneficial in managing chronic hepatitis. Ten patients with chronic hepatitis were assigned to receive 240 mg of the silymarin component two times a day for one week, and ten other patients received placebo. The results of tests that show how well the liver is functioning showed significant improvement in the treatment group.

Citation: Wellington and Jarvis, 2001[18]
Description: Review
Findings: The authors reviewed the properties of silymarin and its uses in treating liver diseases and concluded that the "antioxidant properties of silymarin . . . have been demonstrated in vitro and in animal and human studies. However, studies evaluating relevant health outcomes associated with these properties are lacking." Furthermore, they stated "silymarin was largely ineffective in the treatment of patients with viral hepatitis."

Citation: Saller et al., 2001[19]
Description: Meta-analysis
Findings: Thirty-six studies were analyzed. Regarding viral hepatitis, the authors concluded, "Several small trials involving silymarin . . . have been published. Most of them are methodologically outdated." Furthermore, they stated, "In spite of some

Table 38.1. Research Findings on Selected CAM Treatments for Hepatitis C (*continued*)

positive results in patients with acute viral hepatitis, no formally valid conclusion can be drawn regarding the value of silymarin in the treatment of these infections."

Citation: Jacobs et al., 2002[20]
Description: Systematic review, meta-analysis
Findings: Fourteen randomized, placebo-controlled trials in patients with chronic liver disease met inclusion criteria. Authors found "no reduction in mortality, in improvements in histology and liver biopsy, or in biochemical markers of liver function." They found the data to be too limited to support recommending milk thistle for treatment of liver disease.

Licorice Root (Glycyrrhizin)

Citation: van Rossum et al., 1998[22]
Description: Review
Findings: In this review the authors found treatment with glycyrrhizin to be effective in easing liver disease in some people. Some trials reviewed indicated improvements in liver tissue that had been damaged by hepatitis. Others showed improvements in liver function. The authors concluded "glycyrrhizin is a potential drug in reducing long-term complications in chronic viral hepatitis C in patients who do not respond with viral clearance to interferon therapy."

Citation: Arase et al., 1997[23]
Description: Retrospective study
Findings: This retrospective study examined the long-term preventive effect of glycyrrhizin on the development of liver cancer (hepatocellular carcinoma). Of 453 patients with chronic hepatitis C identified, 84 had been treated with glycyrrhizin. A control group of 109 patients not treated long-term with either glycyrrhizin or interferon was identified. At ten years out from diagnosis, the researchers found 7 percent of those treated with glycyrrhizin had developed liver cancer compared to 12 percent in the control group. At fifteen years, the rates were 12 percent and 25 percent, respectively. They concluded that glycyrrhizin may help prevent the development of liver cancer.

Citation: Kumada, 2002[24]
Description: Nonrandomized clinical trial
Findings: The author assessed clinical data from nonrandomized chronic hepatitis C patients who received glycyrrhizin in the form of a Japanese pharmaceutical product called Stronger Neo-Minophagen C (SNMC). He concluded, "SNMC can suppress necro-inflammation in chronic hepatitis C. Long-term treatment with SNMC, therefore, would be able to prevent liver cirrhosis and the development of HCC [liver cancer]."

Citation: van Rossum et al., 1999[27]
Description: Double-blind, randomized, placebo-controlled phase I/II trial
Findings: Fifty-seven chronic hepatitis C patients were randomized to receive 240, 160, or 80 mg of glycyrrhizin or placebo for four weeks with four weeks of

Table 38.1. Research Findings on Selected CAM Treatments for Hepatitis C (*continued*)

follow-up. Glycyrrhizin lowered liver enzymes during treatment, but did not decrease the level of HCV. The authors concluded that glycyrrhizin was safe and that further investigation is needed.

Citation: Tsubota et al., 1999[28]
Description: Randomized, controlled clinical trial
Findings: One hundred sixty-seven patients completed this twenty-four-week study. Eighty-four patients received glycyrrhizin alone, and 83 took glycyrrhizin plus ursodeoxycholic acid. Liver enzyme levels were significantly decreased by both treatments. However, levels of HCV did not change in either group.

Citation: van Rossum et al., 2001[29]
Description: Part I: randomized, double-blind, placebo controlled trial; Part II: open trial
Findings: Part I: Sixty-nine patients with chronic hepatitis C received glycyrrhizin as SNMC three times per week for four weeks with a four-week follow-up. Part II: Fifteen of the original patient group then participated in an open trial where they received 200 mg of glycyrrhizin six times per week for four weeks. Researchers' overall conclusion is that glycyrrhizin induces significant decreases in liver enzyme (ALT) levels in patients with chronic hepatitis C. Administering glycyrrhizin six times per week appeared more effective than three times per week.

Ginseng

Citation: Nguyen et al., 2000[35]
Description: Animal study
Findings: This study showed that treating mice with either crude ginseng extract or total saponins (ginseng's active ingredients) before receiving the liver-damaging chemical carbon tetrachloride decreased carbon tetrachloride-induced increase of certain liver enzyme levels by 50 percent and 49 percent, respectively. According to the researchers, the data suggest that Panax vietnamensis could be used as a hepatoprotectant.

Citation: Tran et al., 2002[36]
Description: Animal study
Findings: A mouse model of liver failure, which is applicable to a broad range of liver diseases, was used to test the liver protective effect of Vietnamese ginseng. Mice were pretreated with a ginseng extract, Majonoside R2, at twelve hours and one hour before being given a liver cell death and failure inducing combination of D-galactosamine and lipopolysaccharide. The ginseng extract was seen to significantly inhibit liver cell death.

Thymus Extract

Citation: Raymond et al., 1998[38]
Description: Randomized, double-blind, placebo-controlled trial
Findings: Thirty-eight patients who had not responded or did not tolerate interferon received Complete Thymic Formula (CTF) for three or six months or placebo

Table 38.1. Research Findings on Selected CAM Treatments for Hepatitis C (*continued*)

for three months. No differences were noted at three months between the placebo group and the treatment group. Nineteen patients who completed six months of treatment with CTF still had levels of HCV similar to those they had when treatment began. The researchers concluded that CTF did not benefit patients who had previously received interferon therapy.

Schisandra

Citation: Cyong et al., 2000[41]
Description: Two clinical studies, not controlled or randomized. Additional studies done *in vitro* and in animal models.
Findings: In a short-term study thirty-four hepatitis C patients were treated with one of three Kampo medicines for six months (TJ-108, TJ-48, or TJ-8). Eight patients had a decrease in virus levels; six of these were treated with TJ-108.

In a long-term study thirty-seven patients were treated with Kampo medicines, mainly TJ-108, for one year. The researchers determined that after one year of Kampo medicine, eight patients (about 21 percent) tested negative for the virus and symptoms were improved in all patients.

The researchers then tested the ability of TJ-108 to inhibit virus infection *in vitro* by adding TJ-108 to MOLT-4 cells (human lymphoblastoma cells) followed by HCV. They found that TJ-108 inhibited virus infection in a dose-dependent manner.

Researchers identified the active ingredient in TJ-108 as schisandra fruit. The researchers then identified gomisin A as the active ingredient in the fruit. They then tested it in a mouse model of induced acute hepatic failure and concluded it increased survival.

Colloidal Silver

Citation: Fung and Bowen, 1996[42]
Description: Review
Findings: Authors review the history of silver products in conventional medicine and the marketing of oral colloidal silver protein supplements for the prevention and treatment of numerous diseases. Also address its chemistry, pharmacology, toxicology, and case reports of adverse events. Authors emphasize "the lack of established effectiveness and potential toxicity of these products."

Citation: Gulbranson et al., 2000[43]
Description: Review and case report
Findings: Authors review the historical use of silver for medicinal purposes and discuss the case of a man who developed argyria after taking colloidal silver supplements for his allergies and colds.

Citation: White et al., 2003[44]
Description: Case report
Findings: History of a man who developed argyria after taking colloidal silver to prevent and treat various diseases, including cancer.

names) used in Kampo has schisandra fruit among its herbal components. In one very small study, TJ-108 was compared with two other Kampo herbal formulas for effects in thirty-seven patients who had chronic hepatitis C and had been treated before with interferon.[41] The findings were that TJ-108 may have antiviral properties, which the authors attributed to schisandra fruit and its lignan gomisin A.[7,41] These findings need to be interpreted with caution because of the study's small size and because use of an herbal formula, not schisandra alone, was evaluated; herbal formulas contain many ingredients that could cause a variety of effects.

There are no reports on the safety and effectiveness of using schisandra alone for treatment of hepatitis C in humans in the sources reviewed for this chapter.

Side Effects and Other Risks

Schisandra is considered generally safe. In some people, however, it may cause heartburn, acid indigestion, decreased appetite, stomach pain, or allergic skin rashes.

Colloidal Silver

Silver is a metallic element that is mined as a precious metal. People are exposed to silver, usually in tiny amounts, through their environment, drinking water, food, and possibly work or hobbies. Colloidal silver supplements consist of tiny silver particles suspended in a liquid base. They are often marketed with a variety of unproven health claims, including for immunity, diabetes, cancer, and AIDS.

Summary of the Research Findings

Silver has had some medicinal uses going back for centuries. However, more modern and less toxic drugs have eliminated the vast majority of these uses. Reviews in the scientific literature on colloidal silver have concluded that:[42,43]

- Silver has no known function in the body.

- Silver is not an essential mineral supplement or a cure-all and should not be promoted as such.

- Claims that there can be a "deficiency" of silver in the body and that such a deficiency can lead to disease are unfounded.

- Claims made about the effectiveness of colloidal silver products for numerous diseases are unsupported scientifically.

- Colloidal silver products can have serious side effects (discussed in the following).

- Laboratory analysis has shown that the amounts of silver in these supplements vary greatly, which can pose risks to the consumer.

Side Effects and Other Risks

Animal studies have shown that silver builds up in the tissues of the body. In humans, this accumulation can have a serious side effect called argyria, a bluish-gray discoloration of the body, especially of the skin, other organs, deep tissues, nails, and gums. How this happens is not fully known, but silver-protein complexes are thought to deposit in the skin and then be processed by sunlight (similar to traditional photography).[44,45] Argyria is not treatable or reversible. Other possible problems include neurologic problems (such as seizures), kidney damage, stomach distress, headaches, fatigue, and skin irritation. Colloidal silver may interfere with the body's absorption of the following drugs: penicillamine, quinolones, tetracyclines, and thyroxine.

Sources

General

1. National Institutes of Health. National Institutes of Health Consensus Development Conference Statement. Management of Hepatitis C: 2002. National Institutes of Health Web site. Accessed at odp.od.nih.gov/consensus/cons/116/116cdc_intro .htm on July 15, 2003.

2. National Institute of Diabetes and Digestive and Kidney Diseases. Viral Hepatitis: A Through E and Beyond. National Digestive Diseases Information Clearinghouse Web site. Accessed at digestive.niddk.nih.gov/ddiseases/pubs/viralhepatitis/index. htm on July 15, 2003. NIH publication no. 03-4762, 2003.

3. National Institute of Diabetes and Digestive and Kidney Diseases. What I Need To Know About Hepatitis C. National Digestive Diseases Information Clearinghouse Web site. Accessed at digestive.niddk.nih.gov/ddiseases/pubs/hepc_ez/index.htm on July 15, 2003. NIH publication no. 02-4229, 2002.

4. National Institute of Allergy and Infectious Diseases. What You Should Know About Hepatitis C. National Institute of Allergy and Infectious Diseases Web site. Accessed at www.niaid .nih.gov/dmid/hepatitis/hepcfacts.htm on July 15, 2003.

5. Gruenwald J, Brendler T, Jaenicke C, eds. *PDR for Herbal Medicines*. 2nd ed. Montvale, N.J.: Medical Economics Company, Inc.; 2000.

6. Natural Medicines Comprehensive Database. Accessed at www.naturaldatabase.com on May 15, 2003.

7. Herrine SK. Approach to the patient with chronic hepatitis C virus infection. *Annals of Internal Medicine*. 2002; 136(10): 747–57.

8. Bren L. Hepatitis C: an update. *FDA Consumer*. July–August 2001. Accessed at www.fda.gov/fdac/features/2001/401_hepc .html on July 15, 2003.

References

1. National Institute of Diabetes and Digestive and Kidney Diseases. Chronic Hepatitis C: Disease Management. National Institute of Diabetes and Digestive and Kidney Diseases Web site. Accessed at digestive.niddk.nih.gov/ddiseases/pubs/ viralhepatitis/index.htm on September 3, 2003.

2. Strader DB, Bacon BR, Lindsay KL, et al. Use of complementary and alternative medicine in patients with liver disease. *American Journal of Gastroenterology*. 2002; 97(9):2391–97.

3. Liu J, Manheimer E, Tsutani K, et al. Medicinal herbs for hepatitis C virus infection: a Cochrane hepatobiliary systematic review of randomized trials. *American Journal of Gastroenterology*. 2003; 98(3):538–44.

4. Kasahara A. Treatment strategies for chronic hepatitis C virus infection. *Journal of Gastroenterology*. 2000; 35(6):411–23.

5. Sarin SK. Management of hepatitis C: what should we advise about adjunctive therapies, including herbal medicines, for hepatitis C? *Journal of Gastroenterology and Hepatology*. 2000; 15(suppl):E164–E171.

6. Bean P. The use of alternative medicine in the treatment of hepatitis C. *American Clinical Laboratory*. 2002; 21(4):19–21.

7. Seeff LB, Lindsay KL, Bacon BR, et al. Complementary and alternative medicine in chronic liver disease. *Hepatology.* 2001; 34(3):595–603.

8. Flora K, Hahn M, Rosen H, et al. Milk thistle (*Silybum marianum*) for the therapy of liver disease. *American Journal of Gastroenterology.* 1998; 93(2):139–43.

9. O'Hara M, Kiefer D, Farrell K, et al. A review of 12 commonly used medicinal herbs. *Archives of Family Medicine.* 1998; 7(6):523–36.

10. Muriel P, Garciapina T, Perez-Alvarez V, et al. Silymarin protects against paracetamol-induced lipid peroxidation and liver damage. *Journal of Applied Toxicology.* 1992; 12(6):439–42.

11. Letteron P, Labbe G, Degott C, et al. Mechanism for the protective effects of silymarin against carbon tetrachloride-induced lipid peroxidation and hepatotoxicity in mice: evidence that silymarin acts both as an inhibitor of metabolic activation and as a chain-breaking antioxidant. *Biochemical Pharmacology.* 1990; 39(12):2027–34.

12. Davila JC, Lenherr A, Acosta D. Protective effect of flavonoids on drug-induced hepatotoxicity in vitro. *Toxicology.* 1989; 57(3): 267–86.

13. Fuchs EC, Weyhenmeyer R, Weiner OH. Effects of silibinin and of a synthetic analogue on isolated rat hepatic stellate cells and myofibroblasts. *Arzneimittel-Forschung.* 1997; 47(12):1383–87.

14. Boigk G, Stroedter L, Herbst H, et al. Silymarin retards collagen accumulation in early and advanced biliary fibrosis secondary to complete bile duct obliteration in rats. *Hepatology.* 1997; 26(3):643–49.

15. Ferenci P, Dragosics B, Dittrich H, et al. Randomized controlled trial of silymarin treatment in patients with cirrhosis of the liver. *Journal of Hepatology.* 1989; 9(1):105–13.

16. Pares A, Planas R, Torres M, et al. Effects of silymarin in alcoholic patients with cirrhosis of the liver: results of a controlled, double-blind, randomized and multicenter trial. I. 1998; 28(4): 61521.

17. Buzzelli G, Moscarella S, Giusti A, et al. A pilot study on the liver protective effect of silybin-phosphatidylcholine complex

(IdB1016) in chronic active hepatitis. *International Journal of Clinical Pharmacology, Therapy and Toxicology.* 1993; 31(9): 456–60.

18. Wellington K, Jarvis B. Silymarin: a review of its clinical properties in the management of hepatic disorders. *BioDrugs: Clinical Immunotherapeutics, Biopharmaceuticals and Gene Therapy.* 2001; 15(7):465–89.

19. Saller R, Meier R, Brignoli R. The use of silymarin in the treatment of liver diseases. *Drugs.* 2001; 61(14):2035–63.

20. Jacobs BP, Dennehy C, Ramirez G, et al. Milk thistle for the treatment of liver disease: a systematic review and meta-analysis. *American Journal of Medicine.* 2002; 113(6):506–15.

21. Shibata S. A drug over the millennia: pharmacognosy, chemistry, and pharmacology of licorice. *Yakugaku Zasshi (Journal of the Pharmaceutical Society of Japan).* 2000; 120(10):849–62.

22. van Rossum TG, Vulto AG, de Man RA, et al. Review article: glycyrrhizin as a potential treatment for chronic hepatitis C. *Alimentary Pharmacology & Therapeutics.* 1998; 12(3):199–205.

23. Arase Y, Ikeda K, Murashima N, et al. The long-term efficacy of glycyrrhizin in chronic hepatitis C patients. *Cancer.* 1997; 79(8):1494–1500.

24. Kumada H. Long-term treatment of chronic hepatitis C with glycyrrhizin [stronger Neo-Minophagen C (SNMC)] for preventing liver cirrhosis and hepatocellular carcinoma. *Oncology.* 2002; 62(suppl 1):94–100.

25. Abe Y, Ueda T, Kato T, et al. Effectiveness of interferon, glycyrrhizin combination therapy in patients with chronic hepatitis C. *Nippon Rinsho (Japanese Journal of Clinical Medicine).* 1994; 52(7):1817–22.

26. Okuno T, Arai K, Shindo M. Efficacy of interferon combined glycyrrhizin therapy in patients with chronic hepatitis C resistant to interferon therapy. *Nippon Rinsho (Japanese Journal of Clinical Medicine).* 1994; 52(7):1823–27.

27. van Rossum TG, Vulto AG, Hop WC, et al. Intravenous glycyrrhizin for the treatment of chronic hepatitis C: a double-blind, randomized, placebo-controlled phase I/II trial. *Journal of Gastroenterology and Hepatology.* 1999; 14(11):1093–99.

28. Tsubota A, Kumada H, Arase Y, et al. Combined ursodeoxycholic acid and glycyrrhizin therapy for chronic hepatitis C virus infection: a randomized controlled trial in 170 patients. *European Journal of Gastroenterology & Hepatology.* 1999; 11(10):1077–83.

29. van Rossum TG, Vulto AG, Hop WC, et al. Glycyrrhizin-induced reduction of ALT in European patients with chronic hepatitis C. *American Journal of Gastroenterology.* 2001; 96(8):2432–37.

30. Radix glycyrrhizae. In: *WHO Monographs on Selected Medicinal Plants.* Vol. 1. Geneva, Switzerland: World Health Organization; 1999:183–94.

31. Lewis JH. Licorice for hepatitis C: yum-yum or just ho-hum? *American Journal of Gastroenterology.* 2001; 96(8):2291–92.

32. Abebe W. Herbal medication: potential for adverse interactions with analgesic drugs. *Journal of Clinical Pharmacy and Therapeutics.* 2002; 27(6):391–401.

33. Jeong TC, Kim HJ, Park JI, et al. Protective effects of red ginseng saponins against carbon tetrachloride-induced hepatotoxicity in Sprague Dawley rats. *Planta Medica.* 1997; 63(2): 136–40.

34. Matsuda H, Samukawa K, Kubo M. Anti-hepatitic activity of ginsenoside Ro. *Planta Medica.* 1991; 57(6):523–26.

35. Nguyen TD, Villard PH, Barlatier A, et al. Panax vietnamensis protects mice against carbon tetrachloride-induced hepatotoxicity without any modification of CYP2E1 gene expression. *Planta Medica.* 2000; 66(8):714–19.

36. Tran QL, Adnyana IK, Tezuka Y, et al. Hepatoprotective effect of majonoside R2, the major saponin from Vietnamese ginseng (Panax vietnamensis). *Planta Medica.* 2002; 68(5):402–6.

37. Zuin M, Battezzati PM, Camisasca M, et al. Effects of a preparation containing a standardized ginseng extract combined with trace elements and multivitamins against hepatotoxin-induced chronic liver disease in the elderly. *Journal of International Medical Research.* 1987; 15(5):276–81.

38. Raymond RS, Fallon MB, Abrams GA. Oral thymic extract for chronic hepatitis C in patients previously treated with

interferon: a randomized, double-blind, placebo-controlled trial. *Annals of Internal Medicine*. 1998; 129(10):797–800.

39. Sinclair S. Chinese herbs: a clinical review of Astragalus, Ligusticum, and Schizandrae. *Alternative Medicine Review: A Journal of Clinical Therapeutics*. 1998; 3(5):338–44.

40. Liu GT. Pharmacological actions and clinical use of fructus schizandrae. *Chinese Medical Journal*. 1989; 102(10):740–49.

41. Cyong JC, Kim SM, Iijima K, et al. Clinical and pharmacological studies on liver diseases treated with Kampo herbal medicine. *American Journal of Chinese Medicine*. 2000; 28(3–4): 35160.

42. Fung MC, Bowen DL. Silver products for medical indications: risk-benefit assessment. *Journal of Toxicology. Clinical Toxicology*. 1996; 34(1):119–26.

43. Gulbranson SH, Hud JA, Hansen RC. Argyria following the use of dietary supplements containing colloidal silver protein. *Cutis*. 2000; 66(5):373–74.

44. White JM, Powell AM, Brady K, et al. Severe generalized argyria secondary to ingestion of colloidal silver protein. *Clinical and Experimental Dermatology*. 2003; 28(3):254–56.

45. Hori K, Martin TG, Rainey P, et al. Believe it or not—silver still poisons! *Veterinary and Human Toxicology*. 2002; 44(5): 291–92.

Chapter 39

HCV Treatment Challenges for People in Drug and Alcohol Recovery

This chapter addresses some specific challenges that people in recovery might face during treatment for hepatitis C infection.

Why is treatment for hepatitis C infection challenging?

Currently, combination therapy is the most effective treatment for hepatitis C. Combination therapy is when you take more than one medicine. Patients who are on combination therapy for hepatitis C take both ribavirin and interferon.

- Ribavirin comes in a pill that you swallow.
- Interferon is given as an injection (or shot).

Both interferon and ribavirin can cause side effects. In addition, since interferon is given as an injection, it may be uncomfortable for some people, especially people who are in recovery for injection drug use.

What are some of the side effects of hepatitis C treatment?

Some of the side effects may include the following:

- Feeling tired

Reprinted from "Treatment Challenges for People in Drug and Alcohol Recovery," VA National Hepatitis C Program, Department of Veterans Affairs (VA), June 2004.

- Having a fever and chills
- Feeling sick to your stomach or vomiting
- Not feeling hungry or eating less than usual
- Feeling anxious, irritable, or depressed
- Having headaches and muscle aches
- Losing your hair
- Not being able to sleep (insomnia)
- Having dry, itchy, or irritated skin, or rash
- Having problems with thyroid disease or diabetes
- Having shortness of breath
- Having chest pain

How can I manage the side effects of my treatment?

Many people have a difficult time with the side effects of hepatitis C treatment. If you experience any of these side effects, talk to your doctor. Your doctor will be able to give you suggestions on how to deal with the side effects. Your doctor may also suggest prescription drugs to lessen your side effects and make you feel better.

If you feel that taking medicine for the side effects of anxiety, irritability, or depression contradicts your recovery program, speak with your doctor and support people. Some recovering addicts practice total abstinence from drugs that may alter mood or feelings. This may include medicines that your doctor might prescribe for interferon side effects, such as depression, anxiety, or irritability. Taking medicine for these side effects may not be right for you.

Learning how to deal with the side effects of your hepatitis C treatments can take time. Talk to your friends or support people about the side effects you are experiencing. You may find that people in your own recovery program are coping with hepatitis C and may also be on treatment.

Important Note: If you were prescribed medicines for a mental or emotional disorder prior to starting hepatitis C treatment, you should not skip or change the doses of your medicines without speaking with your doctor first.

What do others in recovery say about hepatitis C treatment?

The following people talk about how they deal with their recovery and the side effects of hepatitis C treatment:

- The side effects from the interferon injections are similar to those of heroin withdrawal...the fever, the hot/itchy skin, and aching muscles and joints. For me, an attitude of gratitude has helped me immensely. I remind myself that I am taking treatment so I can have a normal life. I go to meetings.

  —Ted, hepatitis C-positive person in recovery

- I was really having a hard time with the treatment. I was having a really bad depression. I couldn't even get out of bed in the morning. I talked to my doctor and he prescribed a medication for my depression. It has made it easier for me to deal with my treatment and focus on my recovery.

  —Mark, hepatitis C-positive person in recovery

- I experience some depression on my therapy, but I feel that taking antidepressants contradicts my program. I take my commitment to NA's [Narcotics Anonymous] philosophy of total abstinence very seriously. Taking the side effects of hepatitis C therapy day-by-day helps me through some of the dark periods.

  —Matt, hepatitis C-positive person in recovery

- I know a lot of people who are in my program with hepatitis C infection. I have talked to many members of my fellowship for support and advice on this disease.

  —Pat, hepatitis C-positive person in recovery

What are some other ways of dealing with the side effects?

Here are some other suggestions for dealing with the side effects of hepatitis C treatment:

- Talk with your doctor or nurse about whether you would benefit from talking with a social worker, psychologist, or other mental health professional to help you cope with the side effects of your hepatitis C treatment and your recovery.

- Talk openly about your feelings with your sponsor, fellowship, a family member, friend, or someone else you trust.

- Tell people close to you that you are taking medicine to treat hepatitis C that may affect your moods.

- Join a support group for people with liver disease.

- Avoid people, places, or things (called triggers) that can make you feel stressed.

- Try to avoid too much caffeine, sugar, and tobacco.

- Learn ways to relax. Meditate or breathe quietly. Go for a walk or do some other light exercise.

- Take care of your body. Eat healthy meals, get lots of sleep, and drink plenty of water.

- Talk with your doctor about other ways to deal with the side effects that may be appropriate for you.

Will the act of injecting interferon bring up old memories?

Sometimes, the act of injecting interferon can bring up memories and feelings of your "using" days. It might be difficult for you. Here are some tips to make taking interferon easier on you:

- Remind yourself that interferon is working to heal your liver from the damage caused by hepatitis C.

- Try not to isolate yourself while injecting interferon. It may be helpful to inject interferon around people you trust, such as family members.

- Talk openly about your feelings of injecting interferon with your sponsor, fellowship, and other people you trust.

- Remind yourself that being clean and sober is the best thing you can do to keep yourself healthy when you have hepatitis C.

- Get help managing side effects. Remember to talk with your doctor if you are experiencing any side effects from your hepatitis C treatment.

- Don't skip or change doses of interferon. Try to make the injections part of your schedule and routine.

Chapter 40

Future of Western
Treatment for HCV

Introduction

Despite current advances in treatment options, more effective and
safer antiviral agents for hepatitis C are clearly still needed. About
40 percent of people who are infected with the hepatitis C virus (HCV)
worldwide will not respond (viral clearance) long-term to our best
current Western therapy in spite of compliance with full dosing and
duration of therapy. Clearly, new therapies are needed to obliterate
this global disease. A discussion of some of the treatments currently
under investigation for hepatitis C is presented below.

Therapies that Modulate the Immune Response

Interferon

Recently, polyethylene glycol molecules of different sizes have been
attached to interferon at different sites forming "pegylated" interferon.
This has allowed the development of biologically active interferon
molecules. These molecules are not cleared by the kidneys as quickly
and remain active in the body longer than standard alpha-2a and 2b
interferon. The response rates of PEG IFN with ribavirin are in the
54 to 56 percent range according to the recent licensing trials. Amgen,

---

in coordination with Intermune Pharmaceuticals, may bring PEG IFN alfa con-1 to market as well. An albumin-interferon combination is being developed by Human Genome Sciences.

Vaccines

The development of a vaccine remains a challenge for several practical and scientific reasons. The hepatitis C virus can mutate to avoid detection by the body's immune system and the body's neutralizing antibodies (specific CD4 and CD8 T-cells) are not efficiently produced. The virus is found only in humans and chimpanzees and the virus replicates poorly in cell cultures in the laboratory. It is also important to note that the viral envelope proteins (E1/E2) are highly susceptible to mutation, making it difficult for antibodies to provide long-term protective immunity. This current scientific information highlights why vaccine development will be difficult. Chiron Corporation has published phase one trial data about an HCV vaccine in high-risk patients, demonstrating safety. Recent advances in recombinant protein technology, novel adjuvants, and DNA-based vaccines will play a major role in providing new techniques for the development of vaccines. HCV antibody preparations are in clinical testing at this time to prevent recurrent disease after liver transplantation.

Products Derived from Thymus Extracts

Two thymus gland derivatives, thymosin fraction 5 and thymosin a-1, are cytokines that produce specific reactions in the cells of the body, including within the thymus gland itself. These thymus-derived proteins appear to be able to change a person's response to an HCV infection. A series of clinical trials using Thymosin a-1 have led to the approval of this medication in more than twenty countries for the treatment of patients with viral hepatitis C infection. Combination therapy with interferon is currently being studied in the United States in a large clinical trial.

Targeting Specific Sites in the HCV Genome

The HCV genome has been studied extensively over the last nine years. From these studies, we have been able to identify various HCV protein products involved in viral replication, translation, and packaging. One enzyme, the HCV RNA-dependent RNA polymerase, is responsible for the replication of the entire HCV genome. It may be possible to develop drugs that target this enzyme and prevent the replication of the hepatitis C virus including a medication by AKROS Pharmaceutical. Other areas within the HCV genome are also likely targets for drug development. These are the helicase enzyme, protease inhibitors, the internal ribosomal entry site (IRES), and the interferon sensitivity-determining region (ISDR). Despite the promise of these proteinase, helicase, and RNA-dependent RNA polymerase inhibitors, development of these agents is slowed by the lack of suitable cell culture or animal models, although recent advances in this will markedly speed up drug development. This means that it is difficult for drug developers to test the many thousands of possible compounds that must be developed before one is found that is effective and safe.

Alpha glucosidase inhibitors (DNJ and related compounds) are candidates to treat and suppress HCV replications due to their apparent ability to inhibit viral packaging although their mechanism of action may be through blocking viral envelope stabilization. This approach may greatly reduce the ability of HCV to infect other cells and also to decrease the development of resistance. New ribavirin-like products such as vx497 may also have a role in expanding combination therapy for HCV. Mycophenolate mofetil is a new immunosuppressant that also blocks inosine monophosphate dehydrogenase (IMPDH), but appears to a have a very weak effect on HCV replication. HCV attaches to liver cells and other cells through the CD81 receptor.

The development of molecules that block the attachment of the virus to the human cell would block viral entry. This product could work alone or in combination with other medications to aid in viral suppression or clearance. Analogues to ribavirin, levovirin and a prodrug of ribavirin, targeting the infected liver cells are being developed by ICN Pharmaceuticals to advance HCV therapy

Although there are many variations of the hepatitis C virus (HCV), one part is the same in all variations. This part is called the 5' untranslated region, or UTR. Scientists have learned how to add molecules, called "antisense" molecules, to this and other regions of the virus and are being developed by ISIS Pharmaceuticals in cooperation with Elan Pharmaceuticals. Another approach uses a normal cell enzyme called a ribozyme. Ribozymes are RNA molecules that can be modified to attach to and break a specific RNA sequence such as the one the hepatitis C virus must make to reproduce (replicate) itself in order to cause disease. Recently, synthetic ribozymes have been developed to specifically target and break up the 5'UTR portion of the HCV RNA. These synthetic anti-HCV ribozymes have been tested in cell cultures and in animal by RPI Pharmaceuticals. These additions cut existing viral copies of HCV and prevent the virus from replicating. Early clinical trials have recently been started to evaluate the safety of this new approach in humans. There have been no serious side effects in the animals tested. Ribozymes are currently in phase I human studies for HCV.

Chapter 41

Side Effects of HCV Treatments

What are side effects?

Medicines can cause different changes or effects in the body. Some effects, like making you feel better, are the ones that you want and expect to happen. Other effects are ones that you don't want or don't expect. The effects that you don't want or expect are called side effects.

Almost all medicines have side effects. Some people take aspirin for a headache, but it gives them an upset stomach. The upset stomach is a side effect of the aspirin. Not all side effects are unpleasant, though. Even the side effects that make you feel sick aren't always bad. Some side effects mean that your medicine has started to work.

Will I have side effects from treatment for hepatitis C (HCV)?

Most people who get treated for hepatitis C have side effects. These side effects can be mild or they can be severe. The same treatment can cause different side effects in different people. There is no way of knowing which side effects you might have. If you have side effects from your hepatitis C treatment, you should tell your doctor. If you think you might forget them, write them down. Your doctor needs to know as much as possible about your side effects to help your treatment work better.

Reprinted from "Side Effects of Hepatitis C Treatments," VA National Hepatitis C Program, Department of Veterans Affairs (VA), June 2004.

409

What are some of the side effects of hepatitis C treatment?

Side effects of hepatitis C treatment may include any of the following:

- Feeling tired
- Having a fever and chills
- Feeling sick to your stomach, nausea, or vomiting
- Not feeling hungry or not eating as much as usual
- Feeling anxious, irritable, depressed, or moody
- Having headaches and muscle aches
- Losing your hair
- Not being able to sleep (insomnia)
- Having dry, itchy, or irritated skin or a rash
- Having problems with thyroid disease or diabetes
- Having shortness of breath
- Having chest pain

If you have any of these side effects, tell your doctor.

How can I reduce the side effects of my hepatitis treatment?

Your doctor might give you special advice or medicines to help you reduce (or manage) the side effects from your treatment. Other side effects might go away by themselves or become less unpleasant with time. In the meantime, here are some ways to handle unpleasant side effects:

- Drink plenty of clear liquids. Try to drink between eight and ten glasses of water or another clear liquid every day. Drink even more if you are vomiting.
- Do not drink beverages that have alcohol, caffeine (coffee, cola, and strong tea), or a lot of sugar (most soft drinks).
- Try to get plenty of sleep at night. Take short naps during the day.
- Eat small, healthy meals. Crackers, dry toast, or ginger ale can help settle your stomach. Greasy, high-fat foods (including most

"fast food") can make you feel worse. Try to eat healthy meals even if you are not very hungry.

- Exercise regularly but lightly. Walking and lifting light weights are good choices.

- Take any pain relievers that your doctor suggests. Try taking your medicine before you go to bed, so that you can sleep through the side effects. Taking a pain reliever about a half-hour before your interferon injection can help make the side effects less severe. Don't take any pain relievers until you check with your doctor.

- Stay away from things that make you feel worse (called triggers). These may include loud noises, bright lights, strong smells, or skipped meals.

- Don't color or perm your hair until your treatment is finished.

- Don't use strong detergents or soaps that might irritate your skin. If you need suggestions for mild products, ask your doctor.

- Try to use simple, unscented lotions to help dry and itchy skin.

What can I do if I feel irritable, anxious, depressed, or moody from my treatment?

Your hepatitis C treatment might make you feel irritable, angry, anxious, depressed, or confused. You may also have mood swings. Try to remember that these are only the side effects of your treatment. They should go away, but if you need help dealing with them, please tell your doctor or nurse. He or she can refer you to someone who can help.

Here are more suggestions on how to deal with these feelings:

- Talk with your health care provider about these and other side effects.

- Talk about your feelings with a family member, friend, or someone else you trust.

- Tell people close to you when you are taking your treatment. Tell them that it can affect your moods.

- Join a support group to learn from others who have been through this.

- Avoid things that can make you feel stressed, like too much caffeine, sugar, or nicotine.

- Learn ways to relax. Meditate or breathe quietly. Go for a walk or do some other light exercise.

- Take care of your body. Eat healthy meals, get lots of sleep, and drink plenty of water.

- If you are taking medicine because you are depressed, be sure not to skip a dose.

- Keep all of your appointments with your psychiatrist or therapist.

If your mood swings or depression get very severe, or if you ever think about suicide, call your doctor right away. There are other ways your doctor can help you.

If I have side effects, can I just reduce the amount of medicine I am taking?

No. If you take less medicine or stop taking it, then your treatment might not work as well. You must talk with your doctor about your side effects. He or she will work with you to find the best way to deal with them.

Chapter 42

Clinical Trials and HCV Treatment

You may wonder how you can get treatment for your hepatitis C virus infection. One thing you can do is to enroll in a clinical trial. This chapter answers some questions about clinical trials and may help you decide if joining one is a good idea for you.

What is a clinical trial?

A clinical trial is a research program that tests a new medicine to see if it is safe and works well. When a new medicine (or drug) is first discovered, you cannot get it by prescription. Researchers must first test it in a laboratory with animals. Then, they must do a clinical trial in a hospital or clinic to test it in people. They test it to see if it is safe and to see how much of the medicine (or what dose) is enough to work.

The Food and Drug Administration (FDA) is a government agency that decides if a new drug is safe enough to give to patients by prescription. It looks at the results of the clinical trials to make this decision. Testing drugs for hepatitis C is very important, and clinical trials are a way to find new and better medicines. All medicines that you can now get for hepatitis C were first tested in clinical trials.

Reprinted from "Clinical Trials and Hepatitis C Treatment," VA National Hepatitis C Program, Department of Veterans Affairs (VA), June 2004.

How do clinical trials work?

Clinical trials follow a set of rules called a protocol. The protocol says who can participate, how long the study is, and which tests need to be done.

Clinical trials are managed by doctors and are usually run by nurses or other health care professionals. The clinical trial staff will follow your progress closely and can help tell your regular doctor what is happening with your treatment.

Trials are also checked by an institutional review board (IRB). This is a group of people who reviews the clinical trial regularly to protect your rights, safety, and well-being.

When you are in a clinical trial, you may need to see the doctor more often and sometimes stay overnight in the hospital. This is because they want to check the effects of the medicine carefully. Because clinical trials are research, they will often test the real drug against a placebo (or sugar pill). Usually you will not know if you are taking the medicine or the placebo until the clinical trial is over.

How do I begin a clinical trial?

Before you start a clinical trial, you will go through a screening process. This is to make sure that it is safe for you to start taking the medicine. The staff will ask you about your health history, and you may have a blood test, urine test, or others (such as a physical exam or a heart test).

What is informed consent?

You will also go through a process called informed consent. The doctors and nurses will explain exactly what will happen during the clinical trial. They will answer your questions and tell you about the risks and benefits of the clinical trial. They will ask you to sign a document called a consent form. When you sign this form, you are saying that you understand what is going to happen and that you agree to participate. Even after you have started a clinical trial, you are free to quit at any time for any reason. Quitting early will not affect your medical care in the future.

Does it cost anything to participate in a clinical trial?

No. It will not cost you anything because you are helping the researchers to test a new medicine. Sometimes you may even get extra money to pay for your time or travel.

How long do clinical trials last?

Clinical trials can last from a few weeks to several months. After the treatment is over, they will usually ask you to come back for some follow-up visits. The follow-up period may be as short as a few weeks or as long as six months and helps to make sure that you are safe.

What are the different types of clinical trials?

There are four different types of clinical trials: Phase I, Phase II, Phase III, and Phase IV.

Phase I

- is the first time they have tried the drug in people
- tests for the drug's safety and helps find the right dose
- may ask for frequent tests or a stay in the hospital to check for safety and effectiveness
- lasts a fairly short time
- has a small number of patient volunteers

Phase II

- happens when early studies show that the drug may work well to fight hepatitis C
- tests for safety and effective dose level
- lasts longer than Phase I trials
- tries to find out what kind of side effects you get with this medicine
- has several hundred patients

Phase III

- happens if the drug worked well in Phase I and II
- compares standard treatments (medicines that you can already get by prescription) or sugar pills (placebos) with the new medicine
- may last longer than Phases I and II
- looks for ways to reduce the side effects and improve the quality of your life while you are taking the medicine

- is the last phase of study before a drug is sent to the FDA
- has many patients (sometimes thousands)

Phase IV

- happens when the drug is already available by prescription
- happens less often than other phases
- checks other safety issues and long-term side effects
- may be used to check higher or lower amounts (or doses) of the medicine

How long does it take for a medication to be approved by the FDA?

It usually takes about ten years for a drug to be developed and approved for prescription. Many people would like to take the newest medicine as soon as it is proven to work. However, even after a drug has been successful in a Phase III trial, it still may take six to twelve months before that drug is approved for prescription.

Who pays for clinical trials?

Trials are paid for by government agencies, pharmaceutical (or drug) companies, individual doctors and hospitals, or clinics. Most hepatitis C clinical trials are paid for by the companies that make the drugs. The doctors and nurses will tell you who is paying for the study before you begin a trial.

If I want to be in a clinical trial, will I definitely be able to participate?

Not necessarily. Most clinical trials have eligibility criteria. These are rules about who can participate, based on health, age, and maybe other things. They are designed to keep you safe and to help you get the best results. If you do not meet these criteria, you will probably not be able to participate. If you do qualify for a trial and decide to participate, you should be willing to follow the guidelines of the study.

What are the benefits and risks of being in a clinical trial?

Before you start a clinical trial, you should think about the positive and negative things that may happen.

Benefits

- You may get frequent free checkups from hepatitis C specialists.
- You can get free medicine.
- You can get new medicine that is not yet available from your regular doctor and may work better than the old medicine.
- You may learn a lot about your hepatitis C disease and how to take care of yourself.
- You may help medical researchers to find better treatments for all patients with hepatitis C.

Risks

- You may have side effects from the medicine that you did not expect.
- You may have to have frequent office visits, blood tests, and other medical exams.
- You may not get better from the treatment.

How can I find out about participating in a hepatitis C clinical trial?

Many trials are being conducted at medical centers across the country. There are trials in all phases, studying many different drugs. Ask your doctor about what trials may be appropriate for you.

The decision to participate in a clinical trial is an important personal choice. It is a good idea to know as much as possible about the trial before beginning. You may want to have a list of questions for the health care providers and study coordinators when you meet with them. You may also want to talk with your regular doctor, friends, and family to help you make your decision.

Chapter 43

Management of Chronic HCV: Diagnosis and Testing

Overview

Hepatitis C, a viral disease, is the most common blood-borne infection in the United States, affecting more than four million Americans. Approximately thirty-six thousand cases of acute hepatitis C infection occur each year in the United States and 85 percent of those with acute hepatitis C develop a chronic infection. Chronic hepatitis C is often asymptomatic but may lead to cirrhosis of the liver as well as hepatocellular carcinoma (HCC). The natural history is variable, and progression to cirrhosis is estimated to occur in approximately 20 percent of patients. Prognosis of those with hepatitis C-related cirrhosis often depends on the development of hepatic decompensation or HCC. The ten-year survival of those with chronic hepatitis C is approximately 50 percent for those with uncomplicated cirrhosis, and the median survival for HCC is approximately six to twenty months. Chronic hepatitis C is the leading cause of liver transplants and HCC in the United States and accounts for between eight thousand and ten thousand deaths per year. Without advances in treatment, the number of deaths could triple in the next ten to twenty years.

The National Institutes of Health (NIH) conducted a Consensus Development Conference in 1997 on the management of hepatitis C. Missing from the conclusions and recommendations of the 1997 conference was discussion of the utility of liver biopsy in determining the

Excerpted from "Management of Chronic Hepatitis C," Agency for Healthcare Research and Quality, AHRQ Publication No. 02-E030, June 2002.

appropriateness of treatment or the best protocols for screening for hepatocellular carcinoma. In addition, medical research has made significant progress in the past five years regarding treatment modalities for chronic hepatitis C, with pegylated (peg) interferon and ribavirin showing promising results. Recent research has shown that certain subgroups of patients may be more or less likely to benefit from treatment based on clinical factors such as ethnicity, hepatitis C virus (HCV) genotype, or initial response to therapy. In addition, a substantial number of patients treated with initial therapies either relapsed after treatment or never responded. The NIH is convening another Consensus Development Conference on the management of hepatitis C to update the recommendations on prevention, diagnosis, and treatment of hepatitis C. The purpose of this chapter is to review and synthesize the recent literature on several key questions on the management of chronic hepatitis C that will be addressed at the Consensus Development Conference.

Reporting the Evidence

This chapter addresses the following key questions in the management of chronic hepatitis C:

Role of Initial Liver Biopsy

Question 1b: *How well do the results of initial liver biopsy predict outcomes of treatment in patients with chronic hepatitis C, taking into consideration patient characteristics such as viral genotype?*

Initial biopsy means the biopsy that occurs at initial evaluation before treatment decisions are made. The main outcomes of interest were virologic and histologic measures of disease activity and progression.

Question 1e: *How well do biochemical blood tests and serologic measures of fibrosis predict the findings of liver biopsy in patients with chronic hepatitis C?*

The focus was on biochemical and serologic tests that clinicians could use to estimate the likelihood of fibrosis in patients with chronic hepatitis C.

Treatment Options

Question 2a: *What is the efficacy and safety of current treatment options for chronic hepatitis C in treatment-naive patients, including:*

peginterferon plus ribavirin, peginterferon alone, standard interferon plus ribavirin, and standard interferon plus amantadine?

Efficacy was assessed in terms of virologic and histologic response to treatment as well as other clinical outcomes including the incidence of cirrhosis, hepatic decompensation, HCC, death, and adverse effects of treatment.

Question 2c: *What is the efficacy and safety of current interferon-based treatment options (including interferon alone) for chronic hepatitis C in selected subgroups of patients, especially those defined by the following characteristics: age less than or equal to eighteen years, race or ethnicity, HCV genotype, presence or absence of cirrhosis, minimal versus decompensated liver disease, concurrent hepatitis B or HIV infection, nonresponse to initial interferon-based therapy, and relapse after initial interferon-based therapy?*

Efficacy was assessed in terms of virologic and histologic response to treatment as well as other clinical outcomes.

Question 2d: *What are the long-term clinical outcomes (greater than or equal to five years) of current treatment options for chronic hepatitis C?*

The main outcomes of interest were the incidence of cirrhosis, hepatic decompensation, HCC, and death. This question included studies of the natural history of chronic hepatitis C because observation is an option.

Screening for Hepatocellular Carcinoma

Question 3a: *What is the efficacy of using screening tests for hepatocellular carcinoma to improve clinical outcomes in patients with chronic hepatitis C?*

The review on this question focused on alpha-fetoprotein, other serological markers, ultrasonography, computerized tomography, and other imaging studies. The outcomes of interest were mortality and the rate of resectable versus nonresectable HCC.

Question 3b: *What are the sensitivity, specificity, and predictive values of tests that could be used to screen for hepatocellular carcinoma (especially resectable carcinoma) in patients with chronic hepatitis C?*

The review on this question focused on the same screening tests listed previously.

Findings

Question 1b: *How well do the results of initial liver biopsy predict outcomes of treatment in patients with chronic hepatitis C, taking into consideration patient characteristics such as viral genotype?*

- A moderate number of randomized controlled trials addressed this question.

- These studies varied widely in how they reported the relation of initial histological findings to the outcomes of treatment.

- The analyses for this question had important limitations including frequent lack of reporting of parameter estimates and confidence intervals.

- The studies that used multivariate analysis were relatively but not entirely consistent in suggesting that the presence of advanced fibrosis or cirrhosis on initial liver biopsy may predict a modest decrease in the likelihood of having a sustained virological response to treatment. The studies suggested that there is no interaction between pretreatment liver histology and the effect of different treatment regimens on the rate of sustained virological response.

Question 1e: *How well do biochemical blood tests and serologic measures of fibrosis predict the findings of liver biopsy in patients with chronic hepatitis C?*

- Numerous studies evaluated the value of biochemical tests and serologic measures of fibrosis in predicting fibrosis on liver biopsy in chronic hepatitis C.

- The studies had some important limitations and varied widely in published evidence: they covered numerous tests and used a variety of methods for reporting results.

- The studies were relatively consistent in showing that:
  - Serum liver enzymes have only modest value in predicting fibrosis on liver biopsy.
  - The extracellular matrix tests hyaluronic acid and laminin have modest value in predicting fibrosis on liver biopsy.
  - Cytokines have less value than the extracellular matrix tests in predicting fibrosis on liver biopsy.

- Panels of tests may have the greatest value in predicting the absence of more than minimal fibrosis on liver biopsy and in predicting the presence versus absence of cirrhosis on biopsy.

Question 2a: *What is the efficacy and safety of current treatment options for chronic hepatitis C in treatment-naive patients, including peginterferon plus ribavirin, peginterferon alone, standard interferon plus ribavirin, and standard interferon plus amantadine?*

Peginterferon Plus Ribavirin

- Two published trials evaluated the efficacy of peginterferon plus ribavirin for the treatment of hepatitis C. The results of an additional large trial have not yet been published.

- The largest of these two trials had a relatively high score in all five categories of study quality, but generalizability was limited by the exclusion of patients with HIV infection, previous interferon treatment, mental illness, or other significant co-morbidity (among other exclusions).

- The studies were consistent in showing a significant increase in efficacy with peginterferon plus ribavirin compared with standard interferon plus ribavirin or peginterferon alone.

Peginterferon Alone

- A few randomized controlled trials evaluated the efficacy of standard peginterferon alone for the treatment of chronic hepatitis C.

- The studies had relatively high study quality scores, but differed significantly in the distribution of patients by race or ethnicity, HCV genotype, and presence of cirrhosis.

- The studies were somewhat consistent in showing a large relative increase in virological sustained response and a modest increase in histological response with peginterferon compared with standard interferon.

Standard Interferon Plus Ribavirin

- A large number of trials evaluated the efficacy of standard interferon and ribavirin therapy for the treatment of hepatitis C.

- A previous systematic review demonstrated an increased efficacy of standard interferon plus ribavirin compared with standard interferon alone in treatment-naive patients.

- The additional studies reviewed were somewhat consistent in showing at least a modest increase in virological sustained response with standard interferon plus ribavirin compared with standard interferon alone.

- The magnitude of the relative treatment effect may depend on the dose and duration of treatment as each study used a different treatment regimen.

Standard Interferon Plus Amantadine

- A moderate number of trials evaluated the efficacy of standard interferon plus amantadine therapy for the treatment of chronic hepatitis C.

- Evidence on the efficacy of standard interferon and amantadine was fairly homogeneous with relatively high study quality scores and some variation in treatment protocols.

- The studies were relatively consistent in showing that standard interferon plus amantadine is not more effective than standard interferon monotherapy and is not more effective than standard interferon plus ribavirin in treatment-naive patients.

Question 2c: *What is the efficacy and safety of current interferon-based treatment options (including interferon alone) for chronic hepatitis C in selected subgroups of patients, especially those defined by the following characteristics: age less than or equal to eighteen years, HCV genotype, presence or absence of cirrhosis, minimal versus decompensated liver disease, concurrent hepatitis B or HIV infection, nonresponse to initial interferon-based therapy, and relapse after initial interferon-based therapy?*

Standard Interferon Plus Ribavirin: Relapsers and Nonresponders

- A moderate number of trials evaluated the efficacy of standard interferon plus ribavirin for the treatment of chronic hepatitis C in patients who previously failed to respond to interferon or who relapsed after interferon treatment.

- Evidence of the efficacy of standard interferon plus ribavirin in nonresponders is heterogeneous and has methodologic limitations including differences in HCV genotype, gender, and treatment protocols among the studies.

- Efficacy data was stronger for sustained virological response than for clinical outcomes like cirrhosis and hepatitis C specific mortality.

- Previous systematic reviews suggested a small but significant increase in sustained virological response in nonresponders receiving combination therapy with standard interferon plus ribavirin.

- The additional studies reviewed were consistent in showing combination therapy has greater efficacy than standard interferon monotherapy in improving end-of-treatment response in nonresponders; however, this response was not consistently sustained through follow-up.

- Evidence of the efficacy of standard interferon plus ribavirin in relapsers and nonresponders combined was heterogeneous and had methodologic limitations.

- A previous systematic review reported that this type of combination therapy had a greater efficacy than standard interferon monotherapy for relapsers and nonresponders combined.

- The additional studies reviewed were relatively consistent in demonstrating that longer duration of interferon and ribavirin therapy has a greater efficacy than shorter duration in both interferon relapsers and nonresponders. Furthermore, the evidence was consistent in showing that interferon relapsers have a better response to therapy than previous nonresponders.

Standard Interferon Plus Amantadine

- Two studies evaluated the efficacy of standard interferon plus amantadine for treatment of chronic hepatitis C in patients who did not respond to previous interferon treatment. These studies were small but one had a high study quality score.

- The studies suggested that amantadine plus standard interferon is not more effective than standard interferon alone.

- Only one small study evaluated the efficacy of standard interferon in combination with ribavirin and amantadine compared to interferon and ribavirin in nonresponders.

Interferon Monotherapy

- A moderate number of studies evaluated the efficacy of standard interferon therapy for the treatment of chronic hepatitis C in selected subgroups of clinical interest.

- The evidence of the efficacy of standard interferon in specific clinical subgroups is heterogeneous and had important limitations.

- Few randomized controlled trials of standard interferon therapy focused on HIV-infected patients, renal patients, hemophiliacs, or intravenous drug users.

- The studies that have been done were consistent in showing that standard interferon monotherapy is relatively ineffective in the retreatment of nonresponders and relapsers.

Question 2d: *What are the long-term clinical outcomes (greater than or equal to five years) of current treatment options for chronic hepatitis C?*

Interferon-Treated Patients

- The evidence of the effect of interferon-based therapy on long-term outcomes in hepatitis C is heterogeneous and has important methodologic limitations, including variable lengths of follow-up within and among studies, variable numbers of patients with cirrhosis, different doses and durations of therapy (and this information is frequently missing), varying amounts of alcohol consumption, and little description of the population that was not treated.

- These studies were nonetheless somewhat consistent in suggesting that treatment with interferon-based therapy decreases the risk of HCC and cirrhosis in complete responders.

- The evidence also suggested that biochemical responders may also have a decreased risk of HCC and decreased progression of liver disease.

- The data were inconsistent regarding the impact of interferon therapy in nonresponders and relapsers compared with each other and with untreated controls. One long-term randomized trial suggested that all patients treated with interferon, regardless of response, derive long-term benefits; other studies suggested that relapsers but not nonresponders or controls derive long-term benefit from interferon therapy.

Natural History

- The evidence on the natural history of hepatitis C is very heterogeneous and has important methodologic limitations. The studies, however, were consistent in suggesting that older age, cirrhosis, hepatitis B coinfection, HIV infection, alcoholism, male sex, and initial fibrosis all predict worse long-term outcomes in hepatitis C.

- The studies were somewhat consistent in showing that HCV genotype does not increase the rate of fibrosis progression in patients with chronic hepatitis C.

- Studies were somewhat consistent in showing that HBV coinfection hastens the progression of liver disease in patients with chronic hepatitis C.

- Studies were consistent in showing that patients with chronic hepatitis C who have a normal ALT have a lower incidence of HCC at five years.

Question 3a: *What is the efficacy of using screening tests for hepatocellular carcinoma to improve clinical outcomes in patients with chronic hepatitis C?*

- Only one prospective cohort study and no randomized controlled trials evaluated the efficacy of screening for HCC in patients with chronic hepatitis C.

- The prospective cohort study had important limitations, especially the fact that it included patients with chronic liver disease—primarily due to hepatitis B or C, but also due to other causes—and thus may not be representative of the development of HCC in patients with hepatitis C.

- This study suggested that HCC was detected earlier and was more often resectable in patients who underwent routine screening with AFP and hepatic ultrasound than in those who had usual care.

Question 3b: *What are the sensitivity, specificity, and predictive values of tests that could be used to screen for hepatocellular carcinoma (especially resectable carcinoma) in patients with chronic hepatitis C?*

- Numerous trials evaluated the performance characteristics of serum AFP in screening for HCC in patients with chronic hepatitis C.

427

- These studies had important methodologic weaknesses and varied widely in study design and patient eligibility criteria.

- The studies were relatively consistent in suggesting that a serum AFP level of greater than 10 ng/mL has a moderate sensitivity of 75 to 80 percent and a specificity of approximately 95 percent in screening for HCC, and that a serum AFP level of greater than 400 ng/mL has a low sensitivity with a specificity of nearly 100 percent.

- Several other serologic and urinary screening tests have been evaluated, but none of these has been evaluated in more than two studies.

- Few of these studies had a large enough population of patients with chronic hepatitis C to provide reliable estimates of the performance characteristics of the tests.

- The studies on use of soluble interleukin-2 receptor level and protein induced in vitamin K absence (PIVKA-II) suggested that these tests could be useful in screening for HCC if combined with serum AFP or ultrasonography.

- A few studies evaluated the performance characteristics of ultrasonography in screening patients with hepatitis C.

- These studies had some limitations in that they varied by screening frequency, experience of the ultrasonographer, and extent of liver disease in the screened patients.

- The studies using ultrasonography were relatively consistent in demonstrating high specificity but variable sensitivity depending on the population screened.

- Combination screening with AFP and ultrasonography demonstrated an increase in sensitivity in at least one trial of patients with hepatitis B or C.

- Two studies reported on the performance characteristics of computerized tomography and magnetic resonance imaging.

- These studies were limited in that they were not designed to assess the efficacy of screening, but to evaluate the incidence of HCC.

- The studies were consistent, however, in demonstrating both a high sensitivity and specificity in patients with hepatitis C.

Future Research

Relation of Initial Liver Biopsy Findings to Outcomes of Treatment

Future treatment studies need to be designed to appropriately answer this question using initial liver biopsy findings in analysis of factors associated with a virologic or histologic response to therapy. These studies should use standard techniques for obtaining adequate liver biopsy samples and standardized reporting of liver biopsy results. The studies also should report the details of both univariate and multivariate analyses of the relation of initial biopsy findings to outcomes, including adjusted and unadjusted parameter estimates of the relation of each histological variable to the outcome variable, and whether the analysis considered potential interaction effects. Such studies would help to provide better estimates of the independent value of liver biopsy in predicting outcomes of treatment options.

Tests to Predict Fibrosis on Liver Biopsy

Future studies will need to be designed to more directly address this question. Such studies should give attention to the methodologic limitations we encountered in trying to extract meaningful information from the studies performed to date. In particular, the studies should provide enough details about the liver biopsy methods to convince readers of the adequacy of the reference standard. Future studies also should give more attention to the potential value of a panel of tests for predicting fibrosis on liver biopsy.

Treatment of Chronic Hepatitis C

Future studies will need to further address the questions of the optimal doses and duration of therapies. In addition, randomized controlled trials should include traditionally understudied populations with high rates of hepatitis C, such as blacks, injection drug users, alcoholics, and those with renal disease or HIV. In particular, randomized controlled trials of treatments for chronic hepatitis C should include subgroup analysis by gender and race or ethnicity, as some studies have suggested different response rates between women and men, and between different racial or ethnic groups. Such studies should give attention to the methodologic limitations we encountered in trying to extract meaningful information from the studies performed to date.

429

Long-Term Outcomes of Chronic Hepatitis C

Future studies will need to assess the long-term outcomes of current treatment options, particularly studies with standard interferon plus ribavirin, as well as new studies with peginterferon. Although some data has suggested that longer treatment is better for improving virologic outcomes, little is known regarding the long-term outcomes of different treatment durations. Finally, although natural history studies may no longer be practical in the current treatment era, following certain subgroups at high risk for complications, such as patients co-infected with HIV or HBV, injection drug users, and alcoholics, will be useful in making clinical recommendations regarding follow-up for these patients.

Efficacy of Screening for HCC

Randomized controlled trials of screening of patients with hepatitis C will be most useful in helping to determine screening recommendations for these patients; however, it is difficult to conduct large, randomized controlled trials of screening strategies. Therefore, conducting trials on the patients at greatest risk may yield the most significant results. At the present time, serum AFP and ultrasonography appear to hold the most promise.

Performance Characteristics of Screening Tests

Future studies should include randomized controlled trials of screening for HCC in patients with chronic hepatitis C. Although it may be difficult to conduct randomized controlled trials in all patients with hepatitis C, including patients at highest risk for HCC in screening trials makes it more likely that future research will determine definitively the benefits of screening. Future studies should consider the use of a combination of screening tests and should consider examining the relative cost-effectiveness of alternative strategies.

Future studies also should consider examining promising new tests such as soluble Interleukin-2 receptor compared to and possibly combined with the currently most sensitive screening options, including serum AFP and ultrasonography.

Overall Areas of Future Research

Most studies reviewed provided limited information on the type and degree of involvement of the funding source. Consistent with new reporting guidelines accepted by many major journals, this information should become part of the standard data report in future trials.

In addition, to improve the quality of publications on these study questions, standardized methods should be developed and disseminated to investigators. Journals should encourage standardized approaches to presenting data on these questions. For published articles, full copies of protocols should be made available, perhaps on the Web. This is important because the pressure to shorten manuscripts often results in reduced descriptions of study methods.

Chapter 44

Complications of Chronic HCV Infection

Although most patients with chronic hepatitis C are asymptomatic, an appreciable number will experience symptoms that are due to the liver disease or extrahepatic manifestations of HCV infection. Recognition of these symptoms will lead to early diagnosis and treatment of hepatitis C. Fatigue is the most common symptom of chronic hepatitis C and is most often mild. Intermittent right upper quadrant pain, anorexia, and nausea occur less commonly.

Chronic hepatitis C (CHC) infection predisposes patients to the development of diseases involving other organ systems including the kidneys, the skin, eyes, joints, immune system, and the nervous system. There are many extrahepatic manifestations of hepatitis C: some are relatively common (e.g., cryoglobulinemia), whereas others are infrequent and their association with hepatitis C has not been clearly defined. Only the common extrahepatic manifestations with clear association with hepatitis C will be discussed in this review.

Cryoglobulinemia

Cryoglobulins are antibody complexes that precipitate as serum is cooled and that dissolve on rewarming.[1] These complexes contain hepatitis C virus (HCV) particles and can precipitate in the walls of

Reprinted from "Extrahepatic Manifestations of Chronic Hepatitis C" by Roderick Remoroza, M.D., and Herbert Bonkovsky, M.D., August 2003, with permission of the Hepatitis C Support Project, http://www.hcvadvocate.org, © 2003. All rights reserved.

small- and medium-sized vessels. There are three types (I, II, III) of cryoglobulinemia. Type II or "mixed" cryoglobulinemia (MC) is the one most commonly associated with chronic hepatitis C infection. This type is called "mixed" because the antibodies that are found are of two kinds. One antibody is a polyclonal (i.e., from more than one group of cells) antibody (IgG), and the other antibody is a monoclonal (IgM) directed against the IgG. The frequency with which cryoglobulins are detectable in serum of patients with CHC depends on how carefully samples are handled and upon the methods used for detection of cryoglobulins. Because these proteins precipitate from serum as it is cooled, the blood must be kept at body temperature after it has been obtained until it has clotted and the serum has been drawn off. Then the serum is tested for the abnormal proteins. If this precaution is not observed, the test may be spuriously negative.

The skin, kidney, nerves, and joints can be affected by cryoglobulins. Cutaneous leukocytoclastic vasculitis is a skin lesion that appears as palpable purpura (hemorrhages in the skin that result in the appearance of purplish spots or patches) that usually affects the lower extremities over the shins. These lesions are caused by plugging of the dermal capillaries (very small blood vessels in the skin). Successful treatment of the hepatitis C infection with interferon (plus ribavirin) usually results in resolution of the skin lesions.

Cryoglobulins also affect the nervous system in some HCV-infected patients. The most frequent symptoms and signs are those of chronic sensory polyneuropathy, although acute or subacute encephalopathy has been reported as well.[2,3] "Restless leg syndrome" and Guillain-Barré syndrome have also been reported.[4] The mechanism of nerve involvement is thought to be MC-well-established related vasculitis of the small blood vessels that supply the nerves. There is no well-established treatment. Treatment with interferon, corticosteroids, or cyclophosphamide (cytoxan) has not shown any consistent results although some patients appear to respond to one or a combination of these drugs.[5]

Kidney Manifestations

The kidneys are also affected in some patients with hepatitis C. The most common kidney disease related to hepatitis C infection is membranoproliferative glomerulonephritis (MPGN).[6] The prevalence of MPGN varies with geographical location. It is more common in Japan and is less frequently seen in France. Patients with MPGN usually complain of weakness, edema and have systemic arterial hypertension. Urine of such patients contains a lot of protein (>3.5 g/day), a condition called nephritic syndrome. Other abnormalities include low serum albumin (due to losses in the urine), decreased complement levels, and the presence of rheumatoid factor and cryoglobulins. MPGN may sometimes occur in the absence of cryoglobulinemia. Another kidney disease called membranous nephropathy (MN) is less common in HCV-infected patients and is not associated with cryoglobulinemia or rheumatoid factor but is associated with heavy proteinuria.[7] The mechanism of the disease is still unclear, but some studies suggest that it is caused by circulating complexes of antibodies and HCV particles directly causing damage to the kidneys as they are deposited in the glomerulus and tubules of the kidneys. Some authors recommend treatment of patients with HCV-related kidney disease even in the absence of active liver disease. The current treatment of choice for HCV infection is interferon and ribavirin. However, in patients with severe renal failure, only interferon monotherapy is recommended because ribavirin cannot be removed by dialysis. Thus, it accumulates and causes severe breakdown of red blood cells (hemolysis) and anemia.

Skin Lesions

Porphyria cutanea tarda (PCT) is the most common form of the porphyrias, a group of diseases characterized by defects in one or more of the enzymes involved in the production of heme. This results in the overproduction of porphyrins or its precursors. Patients with PCT often present with blisters and vesicles on the dorsal aspects of the hands, forearms, back of the neck, and face. These lesions develop in areas that are exposed to the sun and that sustain minor trauma. Increased facial hair and pigmentation changes are also noted. In some patients, as the injury becomes chronic, scarring, alopecia, and thickening of the skin may occur. The skin lesions may be further complicated by deposition of calcium and formation of nonhealing ulcers. Patients with PCT who are of northern European origin were also found to have increased prevalence of *HFE* gene mutation, the gene found to be responsible in most cases of hereditary hemochromatosis. In addition to iron, heavy alcohol use and use of estrogens are also major risk factors for the development of PCT. The treatment of PCT involves dietary restriction of foods rich in iron, and avoidance of alcohol and estrogen use. Phlebotomy to remove iron is the first treatment for most patients with PCT. In patients with PCT, we recommend iron depletion by phlebotomy before initiating antiviral therapy with interferon and ribavirin. Antimalarial drugs like chloroquine have been used in the treatment of PCT as well.[8]

In a large case-control study of 34,204 veterans, lichen planus, vitiligo, and PCT are the skin disorders that have been found to have significant association with HCV infection.[9] Lichen planus is a disease of the skin and mucous membranes that appears as violaceous, scaling papules usually located on the limbs and white reticular lesions on the mucous membranes. It is suggested that this is an autoimmune response to an antigen shared by HCV particles and the basal cell layer of the skin. Vitiligo is an acquired loss of pigmentation of the skin. The loss of pigmentation is usually found around body orifices like the mouth, eyes, and nose and on the extensor surfaces of the elbows and knees as well as the wrists. Interferon has not been found to be uniformly effective in the treatment of lichen planus.

Rheumatologic and Autoimmune Manifestations

Myalgia (muscle pains), fatigue, and arthralgias (joint pains) are common manifestations of HCV infection. HCV-related arthritis commonly presents as symmetrical inflammatory arthritis involving small joints. The joints involved in HCV-related arthritis are similar to rheumatoid arthritis (RA). This sometimes makes it difficult to differentiate true RA from HCV patients with positive rheumatoid factor but without RA. HCV-related arthritis is usually nondeforming and there are no bony erosions in the joints. A marker called anti-keratin antibodies has been studied to differentiate true RA from HCV-related arthritis. In a recent study, seventy-one patients who were rheumatoid factor positive were tested for anti-keratin antibodies. Anti-keratin antibodies were detected in twenty of thirty-three (60.6 percent) patients with true RA and only two of twenty-five (8 percent) patients with HCV-related arthritis.[10] Patients with HCV-related arthritis seldom respond to anti-inflammatory medications, and although there are no controlled trials to address this issue, it has been recommended to treat these patients with combination antiviral therapy of interferon and ribavirin.[11]

Sjögren syndrome (SS), an autoimmune disease characterized by dry eyes and dry mouth, has been found in some studies to be more common in HCV-infected patients. They differ from primary SS in that they do not have lung and kidney involvement. Thus it is recommended to test for HCV infection in patients with SS or primary SS. A study by El-Serag of thirty-four thousand veterans failed to show a significant association between HCV infection and diabetes, SS, or autoimmune thyroid disease.[9]

Interferon therapy of HCV infection may also trigger the development of autoimmune diseases, the most frequent of which is autoimmune thyroiditis (Hashimoto thyroiditis). This may lead transiently to hyperthyroidism, but eventually to hypothyroidism (underactive thyroid) and to the need for lifelong thyroid replacement therapy (Bonkovsky & Mehta).

Lymphoma

B-cell non-Hodgkin's lymphoma (NHL) has been linked to HCV infection. This is probably due to the long-standing stimulation of B cells caused by chronic HCV infection, although other factors must be important because most patients with CHC do not develop such lymphomas. A high prevalence of HCV was found in patients with immunocytomas, a low-grade type of lymphoma, which was associated with cryoglobulinemia. Another study linked HCV infection and splenic B-cell lymphomas. Seven of nine patients with splenic lymphoma were treated with interferon monotherapy. Two patients who had detectable HCV RNA after treatment received combination therapy of interferon and ribavirin. All nine patients had sustained virological responses and had remission of their lymphoma, as well. On the other hand, six control patients with splenic lymphoma without HCV infection did not respond to interferon treatment at all.[12] It is therefore reasonable to screen for HCV infection in patients with splenic lymphoma as well as other low-grade NHL.

Eye Manifestations

HCV infection has been associated with several eye disorders. Keratoconjunctivitis sicca (dry eyes) is part of SS. Mooren ulcer is a rapidly progressive, painful ulceration of the cornea. The diagnosis is made by exclusion of other causes of corneal ulcer. A few cases of Mooren ulcer and HCV infection have been reported. In at least two of these patients, the ulcers did not respond to steroid and cyclosporine drops but did respond to interferon alfa-2b.[13] Damage to the retina of the eye (retinopathy, which includes cotton-wool spot formation, hemorrhages, and arteriolar occlusion) is a frequent complication of interferon therapy. Fortunately, the retinopathy is usually reversible once treatment is stopped and sometimes even improves despite continuation of therapy. However, patients receiving interferon who experience visual symptoms should hold treatment and undergo careful eye examinations by eye specialists.

Summary

In summary, extrahepatic manifestations of chronic hepatitis C are varied and involve a number of organ systems. Physicians and patients should be aware of these signs and symptoms, and testing for HCV should be done in patients who manifest these. This may lead to early diagnosis and successful treatment of chronic hepatitis C infection.

References

1. Ferri C, Zignego AL, Pileri SA. Cryoglobulins. *J Clin Pathol.* 2002; 55:4–13.

2. Authier FJ, Pawlotsky JM, Viard JP, Guillevin L, Degos JD, Gherardi RK. High incidence of hepatitis C virus infection in patients with cryoglobulinemic neuropathy. *Ann Neurol* 1993; 34:749–50. (Abstract)

3. McKee DH, Young AC, Alonso-Dominguez A, Tembl JI, Ferrer JM, Sevilla MT, Lago A, Vilchez JJ, and Mayodomo F. Neurologic complications associated with hepatitis C virus infection *Neurology* 2000; 55: 459.

4. Lacaille F, Zylberberg H, Hagege H, et al,. Hepatitis C associated with Guillain-Barré syndrome. *Liver* 1998; 18:49. (Abstract)

5. Levey JM, Bjornsson B, Banner B, Kuhns M, Malhotra R, Whitman N, Romain PL, Cropley TG, and Bonkovsky HL. Cryoglobulinemia in chronic hepatitis C infection: A clinicopathological analysis of 10 cases and review of recent literature. *Medicine* (Baltimore) 1994; 73:53–67.

6. Johnson RJ, Gretch DR, Yamabe H, et al. Membranoproliferative glomerulonephritis associated with hepatitis C virus infection. *N Engl J Med* 1993; 328:465–70.

7. Stehman-Breen C, Alpers CE, Couser WG, Willson R, Johnson RJ. Hepatitis C virus associated membranous glomerulonephritis. *Clin Nephrol* 1995; 44:141–47.

8. Bonkovsky HL and Mehta S. Hepatitis C: a review and update. *Journal of the American Academy of Dermatology* 2001; 44:159–79.

9. El-Serag HB, Hampel H, Yeh C, Rabeneck L. Extrahepatic manifestations of hepatitis C among United States male veterans. *Hepatology* 2002; 36:1439–45.

10. Kessel A, Rosner I, Zuckerman E, et al., Use of antikeratin antibodies to distinguish between rheumatoid arthritis and polyarthritis associated with hepatitis C infection. *J Rheumatol* 2000; 27:610–12.

11. Zuckerman E, Yeshurun D, Rosner I. Management of hepatitis C virus-related arthritis. *BioDrugs* 2001; 15:573–84.

12. Hermine O, Lefrere F, Bronowicki JP, et al. Regression of splenic lymphoma with villous lymphocytes after treatment of hepatitis C virus infection. *N Engl J Med* 2002; 347:89–94.

13. Wilson SE, Lee WM, Murakami C, et al. Mooren type hepatitis C virus associated corneal ulceration. *Ophthalmology* 1994; 101:736–45. (Abstract)

Chapter 45

Cirrhosis in Chronic HCV Infection

Diagnosing Cirrhosis

Cirrhosis is the presence of large amounts of scar tissue in the liver as a result of many years of liver inflammation and injury. Cirrhosis is usually diagnosed by doing a liver biopsy. The normal liver has no evidence of scar tissue. When bands of scar tissue develop and surround groups of liver cells (also known as regenerative nodules), the diagnosis of cirrhosis is established. The liver biopsy may miss the diagnosis of cirrhosis if the sample obtained is too small or it is fragmented.

In some cases, a liver biopsy is not performed and the presence of cirrhosis is presumed based on laboratory test results and physical exam findings that suggest advanced liver disease. In cases of advanced cirrhosis, a liver biopsy may be contraindicated as the likelihood of complications is increased.

There are many causes of cirrhosis. Virtually any liver disease that persists for years may eventually lead to the formation of cirrhosis. Chronic hepatitis C is a common cause of cirrhosis.

Cirrhosis in Hepatitis C Infection

Only the minority of patients with hepatitis C infection progress to cirrhosis. Studies have shown that 20 percent to 25 percent of people

Reprinted from "Cirrhosis in Chronic Hepatitis C Infection" by Jorge L. Herrera, M.D., April 2003, with permission of the Hepatitis C Support Project, http://www.hcvadvocate.org, © 2003. All rights reserved.

with hepatitis C will develop cirrhosis.[1] There are some individuals that are more likely to progress to cirrhosis than others.[2] The current or past use of significant amounts of alcohol is the single most important factor in accelerating progression to cirrhosis.[3] For this reason, we recommend that all patients with chronic hepatitis C abstain totally from alcohol.

Other factors that may increase the likelihood of progression to cirrhosis include co-infection with HIV (human immunodeficiency virus) or hepatitis B virus. Recent research suggests that excessive iron in the liver may also accelerate progression to cirrhosis.[4] In some patients, progression to cirrhosis occurs despite none of these factors being present. Virus-specific factors or the type of immune response to the infection may be responsible for the progression to cirrhosis in these individuals.

More recently it has been observed that progression to fibrosis (scar tissue) and cirrhosis appears to accelerate after age forty-five. The reasons for this are not clear, but it is suspected that changes in the immune response to the hepatitis C infection may cause increased fibrosis after age forty-five.[5] This is another reason why we are becoming more aggressive in treating hepatitis C in young people, even if fibrosis has not yet developed.

Factors that are associated with a lower likelihood of progression to cirrhosis include young age at time of infection, female gender, no history of alcohol use, and past treatment with interferon. It should be noted that the genotype of the virus and the viral load have no relationship whatsoever to the development of cirrhosis.

What Are the Symptoms of Cirrhosis?

In early cases of cirrhosis, there are no specific symptoms that would make the physician suspect cirrhosis. At an early stage, even laboratory tests may not show evidence of cirrhosis. Currently we do not have an accurate way of diagnosing cirrhosis by doing a blood test. Even though there is a commercially available blood test for detecting advanced fibrosis in the liver, the accuracy of this test in patients with hepatitis C is still unknown, and currently it is unable to differentiate cirrhosis from less-advanced stages of fibrosis.

As the cirrhosis becomes more advanced, symptoms from the complications of cirrhosis may develop. By this time, laboratory test abnormalities suggestive of decreased liver function (abnormal levels of bilirubin and albumin and abnormal coagulation parameters) also develop. Complications from cirrhosis include ascites, variceal bleeding, encephalopathy, and liver cancer.

The severity of the cirrhosis is determined based on laboratory test results and findings on physical exam. The liver biopsy plays no role in determining the severity of the cirrhosis. Factors that are taken into account to determine the severity of cirrhosis include the serum albumin (albumin is a protein produced by the liver), the PT or INR (measures the ability of the blood to clot), and the level of serum bilirubin (bilirubin is a substance excreted by the liver, which, when it accumulates, causes jaundice). In addition, the presence or absence of ascites (fluid accumulation in the abdomen) and encephalopathy (confusion caused by toxins not filtered by the liver) are also used to grade the severity of cirrhosis.

A point system known as the Child-Pugh-Turcotte score (CPT score) has been devised to determine the severity of the cirrhosis. Depending on the total score, a patient is classified as Class A (early cirrhosis) through Class C (advanced cirrhosis).

Table 45.1. Child-Pugh-Turcotte Criteria

	1 Point	2 Points	3 Points
Albumin (g/dl)	>3.5	2.8–3.5	<2.8
Bilirubin (mg/dL)	<2	2–3	>3
Ascites	None	Minimal	Moderate
Encephalopathy	None	Grade 1–2	Grade 3–4
PT (sec prolonged)	<4	4–6	>6
INR	<1.7	<1.7–2.3	>2.3

Note: Class A: 5–6 points; Class B: 7–9 points; Class C: 10–15 points

Prognosis of Cirrhosis

Patients with early cirrhosis (CPT Class A) from hepatitis C infection who have no complications from cirrhosis have an excellent prognosis. Even without treating the hepatitis C infection, ten years after diagnosing cirrhosis the majority (more than 75 percent) continue to do well with no liver-related complications.[6] It is believed that treatment of the hepatitis C with interferon will provide an even better prognosis.

The diagnosis of early cirrhosis should not be considered a fatal diagnosis. Most patients will continue to do well for decades. There is no reason to refer a person with cirrhosis to a liver transplant center unless the cirrhosis is advanced (CPT class C) or complications from cirrhosis have developed.

Medical Care of the Patient with Cirrhosis from Hepatitis C

The medical care of the hepatitis C patient with well compensated (CPT class A and B) is designed to keep them healthy as long as possible and to monitor for possible complications of cirrhosis and intervene early when they develop. The treatment of the hepatitis C infection should also be addressed. Patient education, preventive medicine, and routine monitoring every six months by a gastroenterologist or hepatologist are the main components of the care of these patients.

Patient Education

Alcohol Use

All patients with cirrhosis should totally abstain from alcohol use. It is not known if there is a safe level of alcohol intake for patients with liver disease. Alcohol is a well-known toxin to the liver, and total abstinence for patients with liver disease is mandatory.

Acetaminophen Use

Contrary to popular belief, acetaminophen (the active ingredient in Tylenol®) is perfectly safe for patients with cirrhosis as long as it is used cautiously. Any person who drinks alcohol regularly should not consume any acetaminophen. For patients with early cirrhosis (CPT class A or B), the use of acetaminophen is safe as long as the recommended dose is not exceeded (1,000 mg per dose, repeated no more often than every six hours). Patients with more advanced cirrhosis should take only half of the recommended dose. In fact, for patients with cirrhosis, acetaminophen, when used as described, is the preferred medication for the treatment of pain.

Vibrio Vulnificus *Infection*

Vibrio vulnificus is an organism that lives in saltwater, particularly in the Southeast Atlantic and the waters of the Gulf of Mexico. However, infections have been reported from all coastal areas in the

United States. This infection can be acquired by eating raw or poorly cooked seafood (raw oysters, sushi) or by going in seawater with open skin sores. In patients with cirrhosis this infection can be lethal. Patients with cirrhosis should not eat raw seafood and should abstain from going in the ocean if open sores are present.

Multivitamin Use

Many patients with cirrhosis take multivitamins in an attempt to feel better. While there is no evidence that multivitamins make people with cirrhosis feel any better, taking too many vitamins may worsen the liver disease. Vitamin A is toxic to the liver, and patients with cirrhosis should not take more than 5,000 Units per day. Vitamin A as beta-carotene is not toxic to the liver and can be taken in any amount. Vitamin E, if taken in doses over 1,200 IU per day, could cause bleeding. Iron promotes the formation of scar tissue in the liver. Persons with cirrhosis who are not iron deficient should not take multivitamins with iron.

Preventive Care

Keeping patients with cirrhosis healthy is important and can often be achieved if we take measures to prevent other diseases that can affect the liver or threaten the health of patients with cirrhosis. Often, the medical care of these patients is centered on the liver disease and doctors may forget to screen for preventable diseases that affect other organs.

Immunizations

Patients with hepatitis C infection should be immunized against hepatitis A and hepatitis B infections unless blood tests show that they are already immune. Influenza vaccine (flu shot) should be administered once a year. Pneumococcal vaccination (prevents the most common type of bacterial pneumonia) should be given once every five years. It has been shown that patients with cirrhosis who develop influenza or pneumococcal pneumonia are much more likely to die than otherwise healthy people who develop these diseases.

Dental Examination

Gingivitis or infection of the gums can seed bacteria into the bloodstream. In healthy individuals this is of minor consequence, but in cirrhotics, it can cause severe infections. Moreover, if a patient with cirrhosis needs a liver transplant, the presence of gingivitis will prevent him or her from receiving a liver. We recommend our patients with cirrhosis visit a dentist once a year. As the liver disease becomes more advanced (CPT Class B or C) we recommend dental exams every six months.

Prevention of Bleeding

As the cirrhosis progresses, blood is unable to pass through the liver on its way to the heart. As a result, the blood finds other ways of getting to the heart. One of these paths could be through veins in the esophagus and stomach. As a result these veins become engorged and may rupture, leading to severe internal bleeding, a complication that can cause death. These large vessels are called varices. People with early cirrhosis have a 5 percent to 45 percent chance of having varices; the risk increases to over 60 percent in people with advanced cirrhosis. Varices can be detected by doing upper endoscopy, a test that examines the inside of the esophagus and stomach. If varices are found, medications or endoscopic treatment can reduce the chances of bleeding.[7]

Detection of Liver Cancer

Cirrhosis predisposes to liver cancer. Liver cancer, when diagnosed early, can be treated or resected, or liver transplantation can be offered.[8] Early liver cancer produces no symptoms. For this reason we recommend a liver ultrasound examination and a blood test measuring levels of alfa-fetoprotein every six months. Elevated levels of alfa-fetoprotein or more advanced liver disease may require an abdominal CT scan (computerized tomography) or MRI (Magnetic Resonance Imaging) study to detect small liver cancers.

General Health Maintenance

When patients with liver disease see their physicians, their medical care is centered on the liver disease. Often, other preventive care issues are neglected. Patients with liver disease should see their primary care physician on a regular basis to be sure these items are taken care of. Screening for breast, uterine, prostate, and colon cancer in appropriate individuals should be regularly scheduled. Patients with hepatitis C and cirrhosis have a higher incidence of diabetes. Monitoring and treating diabetes is important to maintain good health.

Treatment of the Hepatitis C Infection

The presence of cirrhosis is not a contraindication to treating the hepatitis C infection. Most patients with early cirrhosis can be safely treated with interferon and ribavirin. Eradication of the virus results in improvement in liver function and is associated with a decreased risk of liver cancer and liver failure. Even if the virus is not eradicated with treatment, there is evidence that taking interferon and ribavirin reverses the liver disease and delays the onset of liver failure and liver cancer. For patients who were not able to clear the virus with treatment, long-term treatment with reduced-dose interferon may be beneficial in delaying the onset of complications of cirrhosis and is generally well tolerated.

Once advanced cirrhosis is present, treatment with interferon and ribavirin may not be possible. Patients with anemia, low platelet or white cell counts, or complications from cirrhosis such as ascites and encephalopathy may not be able to tolerate treatment. In those cases, evaluation for liver transplantation instead of treatment with interferon and ribavirin may be advised.

Summary

Only a minority of patients with hepatitis C infection progress to cirrhosis. Cirrhosis is usually diagnosed by performing a liver biopsy. Early cirrhosis is not associated with any specific symptoms or laboratory test abnormalities. Once cirrhosis develops, patients usually live for decades without complications. Successful treatment of the hepatitis C infection will decrease the chance of developing complications from cirrhosis. Patients with cirrhosis should take steps to maintain good health, and receive adequate immunizations and regular medical care. Close monitoring by their primary care physician as well as a gastroenterologist or hepatologist is important for the early detection of possible complications.

References

1. Rodger AJ, Roberts S, Lanigan A, Bowden S, Crofts N. Assessment of long-term outcomes of community-acquired hepatitis C infection in a cohort with sera stored from 1971–1975. *Hepatology* 2000; 32:58287.

2. Zarski JP, McHutchison J, Bronowicki JP, et al. Rate of natural disease progression in patients with chronic hepatitis C. *J Hepatol* 2003; 38:307–14.

3. Peters MG, Terrault N. Alcohol use and hepatitis C. *Hepatology* 2002; 36:S220–S225.

4. Erhardt A, Maschner-Olberg A, Mellenthin C, et al. HFE mutations and chronic hepatitis C: H63D and C282Y heterozygosity are independent risk factors for liver fibrosis and cirrhosis. *J Hepatol* 2003; 38:335–42.

5. Poynard T, Mathurin P, Lai CL, et al. A comparison of fibrosis progression in chronic liver diseases. *J Hepatol* 2003; 38:257–65.

6. Fattovich G, Giustina G, Degos F, et al. Morbidity and mortality in compensated cirrhosis type C: A retrospective follow up study of 384 patients. *Gastroenterology* 1997; 112:463–72.

7. Bosch J, Abraldes JG, Groszmann R. Current management of portal hypertension. *J Hepatol* 2003; 38:S54–S68.

8. Llovet JM, Beaugrand M. Hepatocellular carcinoma: present status and future prospects. *J Hepatol* 2003; 38:S136–S149.

Chapter 46

HCV and Cognitive Impairment

Cognitive impairment, or difficulty in thinking abilities, has long been recognized as a consequence of chronic liver disease. However, until recently, cognitive impairment was considered a complication of cirrhosis associated with hepatic encephalopathy (HE). Patients with HE may demonstrate subtle reversible cognitive difficulties, such as poor attention and concentration, or they may suffer severe cognitive deficits, such as disorientation and fluctuating consciousness that can result in coma and death.[1] HE originally was thought to be a metabolic disorder caused by the injured liver's inability to remove toxins effectively from the blood stream, which then were carried to the brain, altering its function. Current theories postulate that HE might also result from a variety of brain abnormalities, including vascular changes, brain cell (e.g., astrocyte) swelling, hemorrhage, and the deposition of certain metals in the brain stem.[2,3] New assessment techniques also have identified particular brain structures and functions that appear to be differentially affected by HE, resulting from both acute and chronic liver disease.[4,5]

With the epidemic of hepatitis C virus (HCV) infection came increasing numbers of patients without cirrhosis complaining of subtle cognitive impairment, most commonly difficulty in concentration and slowed thinking. These complaints led to investigations of possible

Reprinted from "Hepatitis C and Cognitive Impairment" by Robin C. Hilsabeck, Ph.D., and Tarek I. Hassanein, M.D., April 2003, with permission of the Hepatitis C Support Project, http://www.hcvadvocate.org, © 2003. All rights reserved.

cognitive impairment in patients with HCV presenting with mild (non-cirrhotic) liver disease. Using a neuroimaging technique called proton magnetic-resonance spectroscopy (MRS), Forton and colleagues were among the first to report cerebral metabolite abnormalities suggestive of frontal-subcortical dysfunction in patients with mild chronic HCV infection.[6,7] Specifically, they reported abnormalities in the white matter and basal ganglia of patients with chronic HCV that were not evident in patients with chronic hepatitis B or healthy volunteers.[6] These researchers later found that HCV-infected patients were impaired on more cognitive tasks than patients who had cleared HCV and healthy volunteers, with the most significant differences occurring on measures of concentration and information processing speed.[7] Moreover, HCV-infected patients who were impaired on two or more cognitive tasks exhibited greater cerebral metabolite abnormalities in the white matter and basal ganglia than unimpaired HCV patients and healthy volunteers. Depression, fatigue, and history of intravenous drug use (IVDU) could not account for the group differences in cognitive functioning. However, patients who had cleared the HCV infection with treatment did not show these neuroimaging abnormalities.

The prevalence of cognitive dysfunction in patients with chronic HCV was investigated by Hilsabeck and colleagues, who found that the proportion of impaired performances ranged from 0 percent on a design copy task to 49 percent on a measure of sustained attention and concentration.[8] Cognitive performances of patients with HCV did not differ significantly from patients with other types of chronic liver diseases. However, patients with HCV plus a second chronic medical condition, such as alcoholic hepatitis or human immunodeficiency virus (HIV), demonstrated greater levels of cognitive dysfunction. In addition, patients with more advanced liver disease and increasing levels of fibrosis were more likely to show greater cognitive impairment. The pattern of cognitive deficits was suggestive of frontal-subcortical dysfunction. These findings were replicated in a separate sample of HCV-infected patients using slightly different cognitive tests.[9] Prevalence of cognitive impairment was found to range from 9 percent on a figure copy task to 38 percent on a measure of complex attention, visual scanning and tracking, and psychomotor speed. As before, greater severity of liver disease and fibrosis was associated with poorer cognitive functioning. Performances on cognitive tests were not related to perceived cognitive dysfunction, depression, anxiety, or fatigue, replicating and extending the findings of Forton and colleagues.[7]

An independent group of researchers recently replicated the prevalence rate of cognitive impairment in patients with hepatitis C, reporting that 39 percent of their sample were cognitively impaired on at least four of twelve cognitive tests.[10] They also found no association between cognitive impairment and history of IVDU, history of psychiatric disorder, and depressive symptoms. In contrast to findings of Hilsabeck and colleagues,[8] these investigators reported no relationship between cognitive impairment and fibrosis stage, which may be due to their exclusion of patients with advanced liver disease (i.e., exclusion of patients with severe fibrosis and cirrhosis). Predictors of cognitive impairment in their sample were lower pre-illness intelligence and use of antidepressant medication. These findings suggest that HCV-infected patients with lower cognitive reserve may be more susceptible to cognitive impairment associated with HCV infection. The association between greater cognitive impairment and antidepressant medication usage is unclear, and the investigators did not report which antidepressants were used by their sample. Replication of these findings is needed to establish the validity of these relationships before firm conclusions can be drawn.

The etiology of cognitive dysfunction exhibited by patients with HCV is unknown. Increasing evidence suggests that there may be a direct effect of the virus on brain functioning via a "Trojan horse" mechanism, similar to that hypothesized to occur in HIV-infected patients.[7,11] The "Trojan horse" hypothesis suggests that cerebral dysfunction occurs secondary to infection of monocytes, which are believed to replace microglial cells. Microglial cells are located predominantly in the cerebral white matter and are known to release excitatory amino acids that can induce neuronal cell death. Moreover, microglia can produce neurotoxins and other neurochemicals that can influence cognitive functioning.[12] The possibility of a "Trojan horse" mechanism in HCV is suggested by data showing selective distribution of HCV quasi-species in cells of monocytic lineage.[13–15]

Indirect effects of HCV on brain functioning also are possible via production of secondary cytokines (e.g., interferons, interleukins). Cytokines may cross the blood brain barrier or interact with the cerebral vascular endothelium and generate secondary messengers, which can affect cognitive functioning via multiple mechanisms that can influence arousal, initiation, working memory, psychomotor movements, and mood.[15–19] The possibility that cognitive dysfunction may be related to personality characteristics or psychiatric disturbances appears unlikely given the consistent reports of no association between these variables and cognitive impairment. More likely is the possibility that psychiatric symptoms, in part, are manifestations of the cerebral effect of HCV.

The cognitive dysfunction evidenced by patients with chronic HCV is important to note as it may affect quality of life. Poor attention and concentration and problems with working memory can interfere with one's ability to learn new information, focus on a single task for a prolonged length of time, or perform multiple tasks simultaneously without error. Slowed thinking and psychomotor speed, especially in combination with impaired attention and concentration, can result in prolonged periods of time needed to complete even routine tasks. Cognitive problems such as these may influence medical care, as cognitively impaired patients may fail to remember (or remember incorrectly) important details about their liver disease, treatment regimen, or physicians' recommendations. They may experience difficulties performing household and job duties as efficiently and accurately as before. Ultimately, many patients may experience frustration and mood problems, such as depression and anxiety, which can exacerbate cognitive deficits.

In summary, cognitive impairment has long been associated with chronic liver disease, although it was believed to occur only in cirrhotic patients with HE. Recent research has demonstrated that cognitive dysfunction is apparent in patients with HCV with and without cirrhosis. Approximately one-third of HCV-infected patients exhibit cognitive impairment, with the likelihood of impairment increasing with the presence of greater levels of fibrosis or a comorbid chronic medical condition. Attention and concentration, working memory, and psychomotor speed are the cognitive functions most likely to be impaired, suggesting a proclivity for frontal-subcortical systems, which is consistent with metabolite abnormalities found in studies using MRS techniques. The etiology of cognitive impairments associated with HCV is unclear at this time, but evidence for both direct and indirect mechanisms has been presented. Further research to confirm these observations in larger numbers of patients and in all possible etiologies of chronic liver disease is needed so that treatment options can be identified and tested. Future research also could address predictors of cognitive impairment in HCV patients, as well as the effect of antiviral therapy on cognitive functioning.

References

1. Ferenci P, Lockwood A, Mullen K et al. Hepatic encephalopathy—definition, nomenclature, diagnosis, and quantification:

final report of the working party at the 11th World Congresses of Gastroenterology, Vienna, 1998. *Hepatology* 2002; 35:716–21.

2. Boon AP, Adams DH, Buckels JAC, McMaster P. Neuropathological findings in autopsies after liver transplantation. *Transplant Proc* 1991; 23:1471–72.

3. Rovira A, Cordoba J, Raguer N, Alonso J. Magnetic resonance imaging measurement of brain edema in patients with liver disease: resolution after transplantation. *Curr Opin Neurol* 2002; 15:731–37.

4. Catafau AM, Kulisevsky J, Berna L, et al. Relationship between cerebral perfusion in frontal-limbic-basal ganglia circuits and neuropsychologic impairment in patients with subclinical hepatic encephalopathy. *J Nucl Med* 2000; 41:405–10.

5. Huda A, Guze BH, Thomas MA, et al. Clinical correlation of neuropsychological test with 1H Magnetic resonance spectroscopy in hepatic encephalopathy. *Psychosomatic Med* 1998; 60:550–56.

6. Forton DM, Allsop JM, Main J, Foster GR, Thomas HC, Taylor-Robinson SD. Evidence for a cerebral effect of the hepatitis C virus. *Lancet* 2000; 358:38–39.

7. Forton DM, Thomas HC, Murphy CA, et al. Hepatitis C and cognitive impairment in a cohort of patients with mild liver disease. *Hepatology* 2002; 35:433–39.

8. Hilsabeck RC, Perry W, Hassassein TI. Neuropsychological impairment in patients with chronic hepatitis C. *Hepatology* 2002; 35:440–46.

9. Hilsabeck RC, Hassanein TI, Carlson MD, Ziegler EA, Perry W. Cognitive functioning and psychiatric symptomatology in patients with chronic hepatitis C. *J Inter Neuropsychol Soc* 2003; 9:847–854.

10. Back-Madruga C, Fontana R, Bieliauskas L, et al. Predictors of cognitive impairment in chronic hepatitis C patients entering the HALT-C trial. *J Inter Neuropsychol Soc* 2003; 9 (2): 245–46.

11. Meyerhoff DJ, Bloomer C, Cardenas V, Norman D, Weiner MW, Fein G. Elevated subcortical choline metabolites in cognitively

and clinically asymptomatic HIV+ patients. *Neurology* 1999; 52:995–1003.

12. Peterson PK, Hu S, Salak-Johnson J, Molitor TW, Chao CC. Differential production of and migratory response to beta chemokines by human microglia and astrocytes. *J Infect Dis* 1997; 175:478–81.

13. Afonso AM, Jiang J, Penin F, et al. Non-random distribution of hepatitis C virus quasispecies in plasma and peripheral blood mononuclear cell subsets. *J Virol* 1999; 73:9213–21.

14. Okuda M, Hino K, Korenaga M, Yamaguchi Y, Katoh Y, Okita K. Differences in hypervariable region 1 quasispecies of hepatitis C virus in human serum, peripheral blood mononuclear cells, and liver. *Hepatology* 1999; 29:217–22.

15. Forton DM, Taylor-Robinson SD, Thomas HC. Reduced quality of life in hepatitis C—Is it all in the head? *J Hepatology* 2002; 36:435–38.

16. Hurlock EC. Interferons: potential roles in affect. *Med Hypotheses* 2001; 56:558–66.

17. Dunn AJ. Cytokine activation of the HPA axis. *Annals of New York Academy of Sciences* 2000; 917:608–17.

18. Shimizu H, Ohtani K, Sato N, et al. Increase in serum interleukin-6, plasma ACTH and serum cortisol levels after systemic interferon-a administration. *Endocrine J* 1995; 42:551–56.

19. Blumenfeld H. *Neuroanatomy through clinical cases*. Sunderland, Mass.: Sinauer Associates, Inc., 2002.

Chapter 47

Frequently Asked Questions about Co-Infection with Human Immunodeficiency Virus (HIV) and HCV

Why should HIV-infected persons be concerned about co-infection with HCV?

About one-quarter of HIV-infected persons in the United States are also infected with hepatitis C virus (HCV). HCV is one of the most important causes of chronic liver disease in the United States, and HCV infection progresses more rapidly to liver damage in HIV-infected persons. HCV infection may also impact the course and management of HIV infection.

The latest U.S. Public Health Service/Infectious Diseases Society of America (USPHS/IDSA) guidelines recommend that all HIV-infected persons should be screened for HCV infection. Prevention of HCV infection for those not already infected and reducing chronic liver disease in those who are infected are important concerns for HIV-infected individuals and their health care providers.

Who is likely to have HIV-HCV co-infection?

The hepatitis C virus (HCV) is transmitted primarily by large or repeated direct percutaneous (i.e., passage through the skin by puncture) exposures to contaminated blood. Therefore, co-infection with HIV and HCV is common (50 percent to 90 percent) among HIV-infected

Reprinted from "Frequently Asked Questions and Answers about Co-infection with HIV and Hepatitis C Virus," Centers for Disease Control, January 2002.

injection drug users (IDUs). Co-infection is also common among persons with hemophilia who received clotting factor concentrates before concentrates were effectively treated to inactivate both viruses (i.e., products made before 1987). The risk for acquiring infection through perinatal or sexual exposures is much lower for HCV than for HIV. For persons infected with HIV through sexual exposure (e.g., male-to-male sexual activity), co-infection with HCV is no more common than among similarly aged adults in the general population (3 percent to 5 percent).

What are the effects of co-infection on disease progression of HCV and HIV?

Chronic HCV infection develops in 75 percent to 85 percent of infected persons and leads to chronic liver disease in 70 percent of these chronically infected persons. HIV-HCV co-infection has been associated with higher titers of HCV, more rapid progression to HCV-related liver disease, and an increased risk for HCV-related cirrhosis (scarring) of the liver. Because of this, HCV infection has been viewed as an opportunistic infection in HIV-infected persons and was included in the 1999 USPHS/IDSA Guidelines for the Prevention of Opportunistic Infections in Persons Infected with Human Immunodeficiency Virus. It is not, however, considered an AIDS-defining illness. As highly active antiretroviral therapy (HAART) and prophylaxis of opportunistic infections increase the life span of persons living with HIV, HCV-related liver disease has become a major cause of hospital admissions and deaths among HIV-infected persons.

The effects of HCV co-infection on HIV disease progression are less certain. Some studies have suggested that infection with certain HCV genotypes is associated with more rapid progression to AIDS or death. However, the subject remains controversial. Since co-infected patients are living longer on HAART, more data are needed to determine if HCV infection influences the long-term natural history of HIV infection.

How can co-infection with HCV be prevented?

Persons living with HIV who are not already co-infected with HCV can adopt measures to prevent acquiring HCV. Such measures will also reduce the chance of transmitting their HIV infection to others.

Not injecting or stopping injection drug use would eliminate the chief route of HCV transmission; substance-abuse treatment and relapse-prevention programs should be recommended. If patients continue to inject, they should be counseled about safer injection practices; that is, to use new, sterile syringes every time they inject drugs and never reuse or share syringes, needles, water, or drug preparation equipment.

Toothbrushes, razors, and other personal care items that might be contaminated with blood should not be shared. Although there are no data from the United States indicating that tattooing and body piercing place persons at increased risk for HCV infection, these procedures may be a source for infection with any blood-borne pathogen if proper infection control practices are not followed.

Although consistent data are lacking regarding the extent to which sexual activity contributes to HCV transmission, persons having multiple sex partners are at risk for other sexually transmitted diseases (STDs) as well as for transmitting HIV to others. They should be counseled accordingly.

How should patients co-infected with HIV and HCV be managed?

General Guidelines

Patients co-infected with HIV and HCV should be encouraged to adopt safe behaviors (as described in the previous section) to prevent transmission of HIV and HCV to others.

Individuals with evidence of HCV infection should be given information about prevention of liver damage, undergo evaluation for chronic liver disease, and, if indicated, be considered for treatment. Persons co-infected with HIV and HCV should be advised not to drink excessive amounts of alcohol. Avoiding alcohol altogether might be wise because the effects of even moderate or low amounts of alcohol (e.g., 12 oz. of beer, 5 oz. of wine or 1.5 oz. hard liquor per day) on disease progression are unknown. When appropriate, referral should be made to alcohol treatment and relapse-prevention programs. Because of possible effects on the liver, HCV- infected patients should consult with their health care professional before taking any new medicines, including over-the-counter, alternative, or herbal medicines.

Susceptible co-infected patients should receive hepatitis A vaccine because the risk for fulminant hepatitis associated with hepatitis A is increased in persons with chronic liver disease. Susceptible patients should receive hepatitis B vaccine because most HIV-infected persons are at risk for HBV infection. The vaccines appear safe for these patients and more than two-thirds of those vaccinated develop antibody responses. Prevaccination screening for antibodies against hepatitis A and hepatitis B in this high-prevalence population is generally cost-effective. Postvaccination testing for hepatitis A is not recommended, but testing for antibody to hepatitis B surface antigen (anti-HBs) should be performed one to two months after completion of the primary series of hepatitis B vaccine. Persons who fail to respond should be revaccinated with up to three additional doses.

HAART has no significant effect on HCV. However, co-infected persons may be at increased risk for HAART-associated liver toxicity and should be closely monitored during antiretroviral therapy. Data suggest that the majority of these persons do not appear to develop significant or symptomatic hepatitis after initiation of antiretroviral therapy.

Treatment for HCV Infection

A Consensus Development Conference Panel convened by the National Institutes of Health in 1997 recommended antiviral therapy for patients with chronic hepatitis C who are at the greatest risk for progression to cirrhosis. These persons include anti-HCV positive patients with persistently elevated liver enzymes, detectable HCV RNA, and a liver biopsy that indicates either portal or bridging fibrosis or at least moderate degrees of inflammation and necrosis. Patients with less severe histological disease should be managed on an individual basis.

In the United States, two different regimens have been approved as therapy for chronic hepatitis C: monotherapy with alpha interferon and combination therapy with alpha interferon and ribavirin. Among HIV-negative persons with chronic hepatitis C, combination therapy consistently yields higher rates (30 percent to 40 percent) of sustained response than monotherapy (10 percent to 20 percent). Combination therapy is more effective against viral genotypes 2 and 3, and requires a shorter course of treatment; however, viral genotype 1 is the most common among U.S. patients. Combination therapy is associated with more side effects than monotherapy, but, in most situations, it is preferable. At present, interferon monotherapy is reserved for patients who have contraindications to the use of ribavirin.

Studies thus far, although not extensive, have indicated that response rates in HIV-infected patients to alpha interferon monotherapy for HCV were lower than in non-HIV-infected patients, but the differences were not statistically significant. Monotherapy appears to be reasonably well tolerated in co-infected patients. There are no published

458

articles on the long-term effect of combination therapy in co-infected patients, but studies currently underway suggest it is superior to monotherapy. However, the side effects of combination therapy are greater in co-infected patients. Thus, combination therapy should be used with caution until more data are available.

The decision to treat people co-infected with HIV and HCV must also take into consideration their concurrent medications and medical conditions. If CD4 counts are normal or minimally abnormal (> 400/µl), there is little difference in treatment success rates between those who are co-infected and those who are infected with HCV alone.

Other Treatment Considerations

Persons with chronic hepatitis C who continue to abuse alcohol are at risk for ongoing liver injury, and antiviral therapy may be ineffective. Therefore, strict abstinence from alcohol is recommended during antiviral therapy, and interferon should be given with caution to a patient who has only recently stopped alcohol abuse. Typically, a six-month abstinence is recommended for alcohol abusers before starting therapy; such patients should be treated with the support and collaboration of alcohol abuse treatment programs.

Although there is limited experience with antiviral treatment for chronic hepatitis C of persons who are recovering from long-term injection drug use, there are concerns that interferon therapy could be associated with relapse into drug use, both because of its side effects and because it is administered by injection. There is even less experience with treatment of persons who are active injection drug users, and an additional concern for this group is the risk for reinfection with HCV. Although a six-month abstinence before starting therapy also has been recommended for injection drug users, additional research is needed on the benefits and drawbacks of treating these patients. Regardless, when patients with past or continuing problems of substance abuse are being considered for treatment, such patients should be treated only in collaboration with substance abuse specialists or counselors. Patients can be successfully treated while on methadone maintenance treatment of addiction.

Because many co-infected patients have conditions or factors (such as major depression or active illicit drug or alcohol use) that may prevent or complicate antiviral therapy, treatment for chronic hepatitis C in HIV-infected patients should be coordinated by health care providers with experience in treating co-infected patients or in clinical trials. It is not known if maintenance therapy is needed after successful therapy, but patients should be counseled to avoid injection drug use and other behaviors that could lead to reinfection with HCV and should continue to abstain from alcohol.

Infections in Infants and Children

The average rate of HCV infection among infants born to women co-infected with HCV and HIV is 14 percent to 17 percent, higher than among infants born to women infected with HCV alone. Data are limited on the natural history of HCV infection in children, and antiviral drugs for chronic hepatitis C are not FDA-approved for use in children under age eighteen years. Therefore, children should be referred to a pediatric hepatologist or similar specialist for management and for determination for eligibility in clinical trials.

What research is needed on HIV-HCV co-infection?

Many important questions remain about HIV-HCV co-infection:

- By what mechanism does HIV infection affect the natural history of hepatitis C?

- Does HAART affect the impact of HIV on the natural history of HCV infection?

- Does HCV affect the natural history of HIV and, if so, by what mechanism?

- How can we effectively and safely treat chronic hepatitis C in HIV-infected patients?

- How can we distinguish between liver toxicity caused by antiretrovirals and that caused by HCV infection?

- What is the best protocol for treating both HIV and chronic hepatitis C in the co-infected patient?

Chapter 48

Living with Chronic HCV Infection

Chapter Contents

Section 48.1

Coping with Your HCV Diagnosis

Reprinted from "Coping with Your Diagnosis of Hepatitis C,"
VA National Hepatitis C Program, Department of Veterans Affairs (VA),
June 2004.

Hepatitis C can have a major impact on many parts of your life.
Many people are surprised to learn that they have been diagnosed
with hepatitis C. Some people feel overwhelmed by the changes that
they will need to make in their lives. Having hepatitis C can also make
you feel very tired and drained emotionally. In addition, some hepatitis C medicines can make you feel more anxious, irritable, or sad.
There are many things you can do to deal with the emotional aspects
of having hepatitis C. Some of the most common feelings associated
with a diagnosis of hepatitis C are listed in the following, as well as
some suggestions on how to cope with these feelings.

Sadness or Depression

It is normal to feel sad when you learn you have hepatitis C. Some
people also feel guilty about getting the virus. Symptoms of depression may include the following:

- Feeling sad, anxious, irritable, or hopeless
- Gaining or losing weight
- Sleeping more or less than usual
- Moving slower than usual or finding it is hard to sit still
- Losing interest in the things you usually enjoy
- Feeling tired all the time
- Feeling worthless or guilty
- Having a hard time concentrating
- Thinking about death or giving up

Many people have these feelings at times, but if you find that these feelings don't go away or are getting worse, talk with your doctor or someone else you trust. You may also want to:

- Get involved with a support group.
- Spend time with supportive people.
- Talk with your doctor about medicines for depression.

Anger

Anger is another common feeling. Many people are upset about how they got the virus or angry that they didn't know that they had the virus. Suggestions on how to deal with feelings of anger include the following:

- Talk about your feelings with others (such as in a support group or with a counselor or social worker).
- Try to get some exercise (such as gardening, walking, or dancing) to relieve some of the tension.
- Avoid situations or triggers (people, places, and events) that cause you to feel angry or stressed.

Fear and Anxiety

Fear and anxiety may be caused by not knowing what to expect or how others will treat you once they know you have hepatitis C. Fear can make your heart beat faster or make it hard for you to sleep. Anxiety can also make you feel nervous or agitated. Fear and anxiety might make you sweat, feel dizzy, or feel short of breath. Some ways to control your feelings of fear and anxiety include the following:

- Learn as much about hepatitis C as you can, and get your questions answered by a health care provider.
- Talk with your friends, family members, health care providers, or join a support group.
- Help others in the same situation, which may empower you and lessen your feelings of isolation and fear.
- Talk to your doctor about medicines for anxiety if the feelings don't lessen with time or if they get worse.

Taking Care of Yourself

There are many ways to help take care of your emotional needs. Here are just a few ideas:

- Talk about your feelings with your doctor, friends, family members, or other supportive people.

- Try to find activities that relieve your stress, such as exercise or hobbies you enjoy.

- Try to get enough sleep each night to help you feel rested.

- Learn relaxation methods like meditation, yoga, or deep breathing.

- Limit the amount of caffeine and nicotine you use.

- Eat small, healthy meals throughout the day.

- Join a support group.

There are many different kinds of support groups that provide a place where you can talk about your feelings, help others, and get the latest new information about hepatitis C. Check with your health care provider for a listing of local support groups.

Section 48.2

Good Nutrition for People with HCV Infection

Reprinted from "Coping with Hepatitis C: Diet and Nutrition,"
VA National Hepatitis C Program, Department of Veterans Affairs (VA),
June 2004.

You may feel that you cannot control many things about your hepatitis C infection. But you can control what you eat and drink, and how much. Good nutrition is an important part of your wellness plan. Healthy food and drinks give your body the energy it needs to work well. Eating well can also help decrease some of the symptoms of your hepatitis C infection, like feeling tired and sick.

Help Is on the Way

This section tells you how eating well may help you feel better if you have hepatitis C infection. In general, the best diet for people with the hepatitis C virus is one that includes a variety of healthy foods. If you need more specific information, or if you have nausea, vomiting, or diarrhea, speak with your health care provider. Your health care provider can give you suggestions that are specific to your own needs. If necessary, your health care provider can refer you to a dietitian or nutritionist.

If you make the right choices, good nutrition can make a difference. Here are some guidelines for healthy eating and drinking.

Don't Drink Alcohol

Alcohol can lead to serious liver damage in people with hepatitis. Alcohol is a direct toxin (poison) to your liver. It prevents your body from absorbing certain vitamins that it needs to work properly. Alcohol can also make your hepatitis C medicines less effective. If you feel that you cannot stop drinking, or feel that you may have a drinking problem, talk with your health care provider.

Avoid Crash Diets or Binges

If your goal is to lose weight, you should learn healthy ways to decrease the amount of calories you eat. Exercise is another important part of losing weight and it may also lessen some of the unpleasant side effects of hepatitis C treatment. Your doctor or nutritionist can help find a diet and exercise plan that is right for you.

If your goal is to gain weight, you should continue to eat a variety of healthy foods. You may need to eat more snacks between meals and more calories per day. Your doctor may be able to refer you to a nutritionist who can help you learn more about good food choices and combinations.

Avoid over-the-counter appetite suppressants or herbal medicines to lose weight. These may actually damage your liver.

Educate Yourself

Learning healthy eating habits takes time and practice. The USDA Food Guide Pyramid gives you some basic rules for choosing a balanced diet. Learn how to read labels on food packages.

Foods we think are healthy, such as canned vegetables, may contain more sodium or calories than we need. Your health care provider or nutritionist can help you to understand food labels better.

Eat a Variety of Foods

The food pyramid gives you a picture of the different food choices in each group. If you eat a variety of foods, you will be more likely to get the vitamins and minerals that your body needs to function at its best. Sometimes nausea, vomiting, or loss of appetite can make it hard for you to get the nutrients that you need. Talk with your health care provider or nutritionist to see if a vitamin supplement might help you.

Do not take vitamin or mineral supplements until you check with your health care provider. You may not need a vitamin supplement and some vitamin supplements could damage your liver.

Fluids

Drink plenty of water. If you are not on a fluid restriction diet, try to drink eight to twelve full glasses a day. If you vomit a lot, you should drink more clear liquids. Don't drink too many things that may dehydrate you, such as drinks that have a lot of caffeine, alcohol, or sugar.

If you want to give your water a twist, try it with a slice of lemon and a teaspoon of honey.

Overcoming Barriers to Eating Well

Hepatitis C and its treatment can make it hard to eat well. Nausea, vomiting, diarrhea, and loss of appetite can make you feel like not eating. Here are a few suggestions that may help lessen these side effects:

- *Learn your triggers.* The smell, taste, and even the thought of some foods may make you feel worse. Learn to recognize those foods and stay away from them.

- *Keep a journal of foods you eat.* Write down which foods make you feel better or worse. This can also help you to keep track of both the calories and nutrients that you are getting each day.

- *Try to eat small, healthy meals.* Frequent, yet small meals may be easier for you to digest and may decrease feelings of bloating or fullness.

- *Try not to eat greasy or fatty foods.* These may upset your stomach. Try baking your favorite foods instead of frying them.

- *Do not buy unhealthy foods.* It will be easier to resist eating these foods if they are not in your house.

- *If you feel nauseous, eat foods that make your stomach feel better.* These may include crackers, toast, and mild carbonated drinks, such as ginger ale. If you feel nauseous when you first get up in the morning, keep these foods or beverages by your bed. It may help to eat them before you get up.

- *Eat regularly even if you are not very hungry.* If you have cirrhosis (or scarring of the liver), speak with your health care provider. You may need to make specific changes to your diet, such as eating less protein, salt, or iron, or drinking fewer fluids. Always check with your doctor before you start a new exercise or diet program.

Section 48.3

Telling People You Have HCV Infection

Reprinted from "Telling People You Have Hepatitis C,"
VA National Hepatitis C Program, Department of Veterans Affairs (VA),
June 2004.

Why should I tell people that I have hepatitis C?

If you share your diagnosis with people in your life, they might be able to:

- offer you support and understanding;

- provide you with assistance, such as running errands and helping with child care, doctor visits, and work;

- understand better how hepatitis C is spread and work with you to prevent the virus from spreading.

Who should I tell?

Sharing your diagnosis with others is an important personal decision. It can make a big difference in how you cope with the disease. It can also affect your relationships with people. If you decide to share your diagnosis, it is best to tell people you trust or people directly affected, such as people you have shared needles with to inject drugs, household members, or sex partner(s). You may want to ask that the information you share be kept private.

People you may want to share your diagnosis with include

- sex partner(s);

- past or present needle-sharing partners;

- roommates or family members;

- people who you spend a lot of time with, such as good friends;

- all your health care providers, such as doctors, nurses, and dentists.

What sorts of things should I say?

You may want to begin with when and how you found out that you have hepatitis C. You may want to give information on how the virus is spread and how the virus is *not* spread. Explain that hepatitis C is spread through blood-to-blood contact. Inform the person that hepatitis C is not spread through casual contact, such as hugging or shaking hands. In particular, you should discuss:

- *Any shared risk factors:* If you got hepatitis C through an activity that involved other people, discuss the risk related to that activity. For example, if you shared needles to inject drugs, inform past and present needle-sharing partners that they may need to get tested for hepatitis C.

- *The risk of getting hepatitis C through sex and sexual contact:* Inform your sex partner(s) that though it is hard to get the virus through sexual contact, the two of you might want to practice safer sex. You may want to encourage your sex partner(s) to get tested for hepatitis C.

- *Medicines you are taking for hepatitis C:* Talk about the side effects you may have from the medicines.

- *Lifestyle changes:* Discuss lifestyle changes that you have made and will continue to make, such as avoiding alcohol and high-risk activities, including injection drug use and unsafe sex.

When should I tell them?

Many people share their diagnosis as soon as they find out. Others wait for some time to adjust to the news and get more information. You should share your diagnosis as soon as possible with people who may be directly affected by your diagnosis, such as sex partners or needle-sharing partners. Encourage sex partners and past or present needle-sharing partners to get tested for hepatitis C. When you decide to tell someone, choose a quiet moment when you will have time to talk and ask each other questions.

Part Six

Other Types of Hepatitis

Chapter 49

Hepatitis E (HEV)

What is hepatitis E?

Hepatitis E, known as enteric non-A, non-B, is a viral hepatitis that is most commonly found in geographical areas lacking clean water and sanitation.

How common is hepatitis E?

It is not common or typical in countries or areas with clean drinking water and adequate environmental sanitation. Typically, people diagnosed with hepatitis E have become infected during travels to or stays in geographical areas lacking clean water or sanitation.

How can I get hepatitis E?

Hepatitis E is transmitted through oral contact with feces. This is primarily through contaminated water sources and a lack of sanitation. Transmission from person to person appears to be uncommon.

What are the signs or symptoms of hepatitis E?

Symptoms of hepatitis E resemble those of hepatitis A:

- Low-grade fever
- Malaise (feeling of ill-health)
- Anorexia (lack of appetite)
- Nausea
- Abdominal discomfort
- Dark-colored urine
- Jaundice

Hepatitis E is not known to cause chronic infection.

How can I find out if I have hepatitis E?

There are no specific blood tests commercially available for detecting HEV antigen or antibodies. There are diagnostic tests available in research laboratories. Talk to your health care provider about testing.

What can I do to reduce my risk of getting hepatitis E?

When traveling to geographical areas where the water supply is doubtful:

- Avoid drinking the water unless it is sealed bottled water.
- Avoid using local ice.
- Avoid uncooked shellfish.
- Avoid uncooked fruits or vegetables that are not peeled or prepared by the traveler.

What is the treatment for hepatitis E?

Most people with hepatitis E experience a self-limited illness (one that runs a defined, limited course) and go on to recover completely. There is no accepted therapy, nor restrictions on diet or activity.

In most cases, hospitalization should be considered for people who are severely ill for provision of supportive care.

Why worry about hepatitis E?

Pregnant women who become infected with HEV are at greater risk of death. The fatality rate may reach 15 to 20 percent among women during pregnancy.

Epidemics have occurred in Asia, Africa, and Mexico; travelers to developing nations might be at risk, but this virus is not likely to be a problem in the United States.

Do I need to talk to my partner about hepatitis E?

No. Hepatitis E is primarily transmitted by contaminated drinking water and is not thought to be sexually transmitted.

Should I talk to my health care provider about hepatitis E?

Outbreaks of hepatitis E have occurred in Asia, Africa, and Mexico, as well as in other geographical areas lacking a clean water source and sanitation. If you think you may be infected with hepatitis E, talk to your health care provider about testing.

There is no vaccine to prevent hepatitis E, therefore the only way to protect yourself is to avoid contaminated food or water.

Where can I get more information?

If you have additional questions about hepatitis E, call the National STD and AIDS Hotlines at 800-342-2437 or 800-227-8922. The hotlines are open twenty-four hours a day, seven days a week. For information in Spanish call 800-344-7432, 8:00 a.m. to 2:00 a.m. Eastern Time, seven days a week. For the deaf and hard-of-hearing call 800-243-7889, 10:00 a.m. to 10:00 p.m. Eastern Time, Monday through Friday. The hotlines provide referrals and more answers to your questions.

Chapter 50

Hepatitis G (HGV)

Definition

Hepatitis G is a newly discovered form of liver inflammation caused by hepatitis G virus (HGV), a distant relative of the hepatitis C virus.

Description

HGV, also called hepatitis GB virus, was first described early in 1996. Little is known about the frequency of HGV infection, the nature of the illness, or how to prevent it. What is known is that transfused blood containing HGV has caused some cases of hepatitis. For this reason, patients with hemophilia and other bleeding conditions who require large amounts of blood or blood products are at risk of hepatitis G. HGV has been identified in between 1 and 2 percent of blood donors in the United States. Also at risk are patients with kidney disease who have blood exchange by hemodialysis, and those who inject drugs into their veins. It is possible that an infected mother can pass on the virus to her newborn infant. Sexual transmission also is a possibility.

Often patients with hepatitis G are infected at the same time by the hepatitis B or C virus, or both. In about three of every thousand patients with acute viral hepatitis, HGV is the only virus present.

From *Gale Encyclopedia of Medicine, 2nd Edition*, by David A. Cramer, Volume 3. © 2002 Gale Group. Reprinted by permission of the Gale Group.

There is some indication that patients with hepatitis G may continue to carry the virus in their blood for many years, and so might be a source of infection in others.

Causes and Symptoms

Some researchers believe that there may be a group of GB viruses, rather than just one. Others remain doubtful that HGV actually causes illness. If it does, the type of acute or chronic (long-lasting) illness that results is not clear. When diagnosed, acute HGV infection has usually been mild and brief. There is no evidence of serious complications, but it is possible that, like other hepatitis viruses, HGV can cause severe liver damage resulting in liver failure. The virus has been identified in as many as 20 percent of patients with long-lasting viral hepatitis, some of whom also have hepatitis C.

Diagnosis

The only method of detecting HGV is a complex and costly DNA test that is not widely available. Efforts are under way, however, to develop a test for the HGV antibody, which is formed in response to invasion by the virus. Once antibody is present, however, the virus itself generally has disappeared, making the test too late to be of use.

Treatment

There is no specific treatment for any form of acute hepatitis. Patients should rest in bed as needed, avoid alcohol, and be sure to eat a balanced diet.

Prognosis

What little is known about the course of hepatitis G suggests that illness is mild and does not last long. When more patients have been followed up after the acute phase, it will become clear whether HGV can cause severe liver damage.

Prevention

Since hepatitis G is a blood-borne infection, prevention relies on avoiding any possible contact with contaminated blood. Drug users should not share needles, syringes, or other equipment.

Chapter 51

Neonatal Hepatitis

What is neonatal hepatitis?

Neonatal hepatitis is an inflammation of the liver that occurs in early infancy, usually one to two months after birth. About 20 percent of infants who develop neonatal hepatitis were infected with a virus causing inflammation of the liver either before birth through their mother, or shortly after birth. Viruses which can cause neonatal hepatitis in infants include cytomegalovirus, rubella (measles), and hepatitis A, B, and C. In the remaining 80 percent of affected infants, no specific cause can be identified, but many experts suspect a virus is to blame.

What are the symptoms of neonatal hepatitis?

An infant with neonatal hepatitis usually has jaundice (yellow eyes and skin) that appears at one to two months of age. Jaundice occurs when the flow of bile from the liver is blocked due to an inflammation or obstruction of the bile ducts. Since bile is essential in the digestion of fats and absorption of fat-soluble vitamins, a child with neonatal hepatitis may fail to gain weight and grow normally. The infant will also have an enlarged liver and spleen.

How is neonatal hepatitis diagnosed?

The diagnosis of neonatal hepatitis is initially based on blood tests aimed at identifying possible viral infections leading to the disease. In cases where no virus is identified, a liver biopsy is performed. This involves the removal of a small piece of the liver using a special syringe for examination under a microscope.

Biopsy results will often show that groups of four or five liver cells have joined together to form larger cells. Although these large cells continue to function, they do so at a lesser rate than normal liver cells. This type of neonatal hepatitis is sometimes called giant cell hepatitis.

The symptoms of neonatal hepatitis are similar to those associated with another infant liver disease called biliary atresia. In infants with biliary atresia, however, bile ducts are progressively destroyed for reasons that are poorly understood. Although an infant with biliary atresia is also jaundiced with an enlarged liver, there is generally normal growth and the spleen is not inflamed. In addition to symptoms, a liver biopsy and blood tests are needed to distinguish biliary atresia from neonatal hepatitis.

What complications are associated with neonatal hepatitis?

Infants with neonatal hepatitis caused by rubella or cytomegalovirus are at risk of developing an infection of the brain that could lead to mental retardation or cerebral palsy. Many of these infants will also have permanent liver disease due to the destruction of liver cells and the resulting scarring (cirrhosis).

The majority of infants with giant cell hepatitis will recover with little or no scarring to the liver. Their growth pattern will also normalize as bile flow improves. However, about 20 percent of affected infants will go on to develop chronic (ongoing) liver disease and cirrhosis. In these children, the liver becomes very hard due to scarring, and the jaundice does not dissipate by six months of age. Infants who reach this point in the disease eventually require a liver transplant.

Infants with chronic neonatal hepatitis will not be able to digest fats and absorb fat-soluble vitamins (A, D, E, and K) as a result of insufficient bile flow and the damage caused to liver cells. The lack of vitamin D will lead to poor bone and cartilage development (rickets). A deficiency in vitamin A may affect normal growth and vision. Vitamin K deficiency is associated with easy bruising and a tendency to bleed, whereas the lack of vitamin E results in poor coordination. Since bile is responsible for the elimination of many toxins in the body, chronic neonatal hepatitis can also lead to a buildup of toxins in the blood, which in turn may result in itching, skin eruptions, and irritability.

How is neonatal hepatitis treated?

There is no specific treatment for neonatal hepatitis. Vitamin supplements are usually prescribed and many infants are given medications which improve bile flow. Formulas containing fats more easily digested by the body are also given.

Can neonatal hepatitis be spread to others?

Infants with neonatal hepatitis caused by the cytomegalovirus, rubella, or viral hepatitis may transmit the infection to others who come in close contact with them. These infected infants should not come into contact with pregnant women because of the possibility that the woman could transmit the virus to her unborn child.

Chapter 52

Autoimmune Hepatitis

Autoimmune hepatitis is a disease in which the body's immune system attacks liver cells. This causes the liver to become inflamed (hepatitis). Researchers think a genetic factor may predispose some people to autoimmune diseases. About 70 percent of those with autoimmune hepatitis are women, most between the ages of fifteen and forty.

The disease is usually quite serious and, if not treated, gets worse over time. It's usually chronic, meaning it can last for years, and can lead to cirrhosis (scarring and hardening) of the liver and eventually liver failure.

Autoimmune hepatitis is classified as either type I or II. Type I is the most common form in North America. It occurs at any age and is more common among women than men. About half of those with type I have other autoimmune disorders, such as type 1 diabetes, proliferative glomerulonephritis, thyroiditis, Graves disease, Sjögren syndrome, autoimmune anemia, and ulcerative colitis. Type II autoimmune hepatitis is less common, typically affecting girls ages two to fourteen, although adults can have it too.

Autoimmune Disease

One job of the immune system is to protect the body from viruses, bacteria, and other living organisms. Usually, the immune system does

Reprinted from "Autoimmune Hepatitis," National Institute of Diabetes and Digestive and Kidney Diseases, National Institutes of Health, NIH Publication No. 04-4761, March 2004.

not react against the body's own cells. However, sometimes it mistakenly attacks the cells it is supposed to protect. This response is called autoimmunity. Researchers speculate that certain bacteria, viruses, toxins, and drugs trigger an autoimmune response in people who are genetically susceptible to developing an autoimmune disorder.

Symptoms

Fatigue is probably the most common symptom of autoimmune hepatitis. Other symptoms include

- enlarged liver
- jaundice
- itching
- skin rashes
- joint pain
- abdominal discomfort
- fatigue
- spider angiomas (abnormal blood vessels) on the skin
- nausea
- vomiting
- loss of appetite
- dark urine
- pale or gray-colored stools

People in advanced stages of the disease are more likely to have symptoms such as fluid in the abdomen (ascites) or mental confusion. Women may stop having menstrual periods.

Symptoms of autoimmune hepatitis range from mild to severe. Because severe viral hepatitis or hepatitis caused by a drug—for example, certain antibiotics—has the same symptoms, tests may be needed for an exact diagnosis. Your doctor should also review and rule out all your medicines before diagnosing autoimmune hepatitis.

Diagnosis

Your doctor will make a diagnosis based on your symptoms, blood tests, and liver biopsy.

- *Blood tests.* A routine blood test for liver enzymes can help reveal a pattern typical of hepatitis, but further tests, especially for autoantibodies, are needed to diagnose autoimmune hepatitis. Antibodies are proteins made by the immune system to fight off bacteria and viruses. In autoimmune hepatitis, the immune system makes antinuclear antibodies (ANA), antibodies against smooth muscle cells (SMA), or liver and kidney microsomes (anti-LKM). The pattern and level of these antibodies help define the type of autoimmune hepatitis (type I or type II). Blood tests also help distinguish autoimmune hepatitis from viral hepatitis (such as hepatitis B or C) or a metabolic disease (such as Wilson disease).

- *Liver biopsy.* A tiny sample of your liver tissue, examined under a microscope, can help your doctor accurately diagnose autoimmune hepatitis and tell how serious it is. You will go to a hospital or outpatient surgical facility for this procedure.

Treatment

Treatment works best when autoimmune hepatitis is diagnosed early. With proper treatment, autoimmune hepatitis can usually be controlled. In fact, recent studies show that sustained response to treatment not only stops the disease from getting worse, but also may actually reverse some of the damage.

The primary treatment is medicine to suppress (slow down) an overactive immune system.

Both types of autoimmune hepatitis are treated with daily doses of a corticosteroid called prednisone. Your doctor may start you on a high dose (20 to 60 mg per day) and lower the dose to 5 to 15 mg/day as the disease is controlled. The goal is to find the lowest possible dose that will control your disease.

Another medicine, azathioprine (Imuran) is also used to treat autoimmune hepatitis. Like prednisone, azathioprine suppresses the immune system, but in a different way. It helps lower the dose of prednisone needed, thereby reducing its side effects. Your doctor may prescribe azathioprine, in addition to prednisone, once your disease is under control.

Most people will need to take prednisone, with or without azathioprine, for years. Some people take it for life. Corticosteroids may slow down the disease, but everyone is different. In about one out of every three people, treatment can eventually be stopped. After stopping, it is important to carefully monitor your condition and promptly report any new symptoms to your doctor because the disease may return and be even more severe, especially during the first few months after stopping treatment.

In about seven out of ten people, the disease goes into remission, with a lessening of severity of symptoms, within two years of starting treatment. A portion of persons with a remission will see the disease return within three years, so treatment may be necessary on and off for years, if not for life.

Side Effects

Both prednisone and azathioprine have side effects. Because high doses of prednisone are needed to control autoimmune hepatitis, managing side effects is very important. However, most side effects appear only after a long period of time.

Some possible side effects of prednisone include the following:

- weight gain
- anxiety and confusion
- thinning of the bones (osteoporosis)
- thinning of the hair and skin
- diabetes
- high blood pressure
- cataracts
- glaucoma

Azathioprine can lower your white blood cell count and sometimes causes nausea and poor appetite. Rare side effects are allergic reaction, liver damage, and pancreatitis (inflammation of the pancreas gland with severe stomach pain).

Other Treatments

People who do not respond to standard immune therapy or who have severe side effects may benefit from other immunosuppressive agents like mycophenolate mofetil, cyclosporine, or tacrolimus. People who progress to end-stage liver disease (liver failure) or cirrhosis may need a liver transplant. Transplantation has a one-year survival rate of 90 percent and a five-year survival rate of 70 to 80 percent.

Hope through Research

Scientists are studying various aspects of autoimmune hepatitis to find out who gets it and why and to discover better ways to treat it. Basic research on the immune system will expand knowledge of autoimmune diseases in general. Epidemiologic research will help doctors understand what triggers autoimmune hepatitis in some people. Research on different steroids, alternatives to steroids, and other immunosuppressants will eventually lead to more effective treatments.

Points to Remember

- Autoimmune hepatitis is a long-term disease in which your body's immune system attacks liver cells.

- The disease is diagnosed using various blood tests and a liver biopsy.

- With proper treatment, autoimmune hepatitis can usually be controlled. The main treatment is medicine that suppresses the body's overactive immune system.

Chapter 53

Alcoholic Hepatitis

Introduction

Background

Alcoholic hepatitis is a syndrome of progressive inflammatory liver injury associated with long-term heavy intake of ethanol. The pathogenesis is incompletely understood.

Patients who are severely affected present with subacute onset of fever, hepatomegaly, leukocytosis, marked impairment of liver function (e.g., jaundice, coagulopathy), and manifestations of portal hypertension (e.g., ascites, hepatic encephalopathy, variceal hemorrhage). However, milder forms of alcoholic hepatitis are often completely asymptomatic.

On microscopic examination, the liver characteristically exhibits centrilobular ballooning necrosis of hepatocytes, neutrophilic infiltration, megamitochondria, and Mallory hyaline inclusions. Steatosis (fatty liver) and cirrhosis frequently accompany alcoholic hepatitis.

Disease that is sufficiently severe to cause acute development of encephalopathy is associated with substantial early mortality, which may be ameliorated by treatment with glucocorticoids.

Alcoholic hepatitis usually persists and progresses to cirrhosis if heavy alcohol use continues. If alcohol use ceases, alcoholic hepatitis resolves slowly over weeks to months, sometimes without permanent sequelae and often with residual cirrhosis.

Pathophysiology

Although the association of alcohol and liver disease has been known since antiquity, the precise mechanism of alcoholic liver disease remains in dispute. Genetic, environmental, nutritional, metabolic, and, more recently, immunologic factors and cytokines have been invoked.

Ethanol Metabolism

Most tissues of the body, including the skeletal muscles, contain the necessary enzymes for the oxidative or nonoxidative metabolism of ethanol. However, the major site of ethanol metabolism is the liver. Within the liver, the following three enzyme systems can oxidize ethanol:

- Cytosolic alcohol dehydrogenase (ADH) uses nicotinamide adenine dinucleotide (NAD) as an oxidizing agent. ADH exists in numerous isoenzyme forms in the human liver and is encoded by three separate genes, designated as ADH1, ADH2, and AD3. Variations in ADH isoforms may account for significant differences in ethanol elimination rates.

- The microsomal ethanol-oxidizing system (MEOS) uses nicotinamide adenine dinucleotide phosphate (NADPH) and molecular oxygen. The central enzyme of MEOS is cytochrome P450 2E1 (CYP2E1). This enzyme, in addition to catalyzing ethanol oxidation, is also responsible for the biotransformation of other drugs, such as acetaminophen, haloalkanes, and nitrosamines. Ethanol up-regulates CYP2E1, and the proportion of alcohol metabolized via this pathway increases with the severity and the duration of alcohol use.

- Peroxisomal catalase uses hydrogen peroxide as an oxidizing agent.

The product of all three reactions is acetaldehyde, which then is further metabolized to acetate by acetaldehyde dehydrogenase (ALDH). Acetaldehyde is a reactive metabolite that can produce injury in a variety of ways.

Mechanisms of Liver Injury

Genetic Factors

Although adequate evidence exists to prove a genetic predilection to alcoholism, the role of genetic factors in determining susceptibility to alcoholic liver injury is much less clear. Most people who are alcoholics do not develop severe or progressive liver injury. Attempts to link persons who are susceptible with specific human leukocyte antigen (HLA) groups have yielded inconsistent results, as have studies of genetic polymorphisms of collagen, ADH, ALDH, and CYP2E1. The genetic factor that most clearly affects susceptibility is sex. For a given level of ethanol intake, women are more susceptible than men to developing alcoholic liver disease (see Sex).

Malnutrition

Most patients with alcoholic hepatitis exhibit evidence of protein-energy malnutrition (PEM). In the past, nutritional deficiencies were assumed to play a major role in the development of liver injury. This assumption was supported by several animal models in which susceptibility to alcohol-induced cirrhosis could be produced by diets deficient in choline and methionine. This view changed in the early 1970s after key studies by Lieber and DiCarlo performed in baboons demonstrated that alcohol ingestion could lead to steatohepatitis and cirrhosis in the presence of a nutritionally complete diet. However, more recent studies suggest that enteral or parenteral nutritional supplementation in patients with alcoholic hepatitis may improve survival.

Toxic Effects on Cell Membranes

Ethanol and its metabolite, acetaldehyde, have been shown to damage liver cell membranes. Ethanol can alter the fluidity of cell membranes, thereby altering the activity of membrane-bound enzymes and transport proteins. Ethanol damage to mitochondrial membranes may be responsible for the giant mitochondria (megamitochondria) observed in patients with alcoholic hepatitis. Acetaldehyde-modified proteins and lipids on the cell surface may behave as neoantigens and trigger immunologic injury.

Hypermetabolic State of the Hepatocyte

Hepatic injury in alcoholic hepatitis is most prominent in the perivenular area (zone 3) of the hepatic lobule. This zone is known to be sensitive to hypoxic damage. Ethanol induces a hypermetabolic state in the hepatocytes, partially because ethanol metabolism via the MEOS does not result in energy capture via formation of ATP. Rather, this pathway leads to loss of energy in the form of heat. In some studies, antithyroid drugs, such as propylthiouracil, that reduce the basal metabolic rate of the liver, have shown to be beneficial in the treatment of alcoholic hepatitis.

Generation of Free Radicals and Oxidative Injury

Free radicals, superoxide and hydroperoxides, are generated as byproducts of ethanol metabolism via the microsomal and peroxisomal pathways. In addition, acetaldehyde reacts with glutathione and depletes this key element of the hepatocytic defense against free radicals. Other antioxidant defenses, including selenium, zinc, and vitamin E, are often reduced in individuals with alcoholism. Peroxidation of membrane lipids accompanies alcoholic liver injury and may be involved in cell death and inflammation.

Steatosis

Oxidation of ethanol requires conversion of NAD to the reduced form NADH. Because NAD is required for the oxidation of fat, its depletion inhibits fatty acid oxidation, thus causing accumulation of fat within the hepatocytes (steatosis). Some of the excess NADH may be reoxidized in the conversion of pyruvate to lactate. Accumulation of fat in hepatocytes may occur within days of alcohol ingestion; with abstinence from alcohol, the normal redox state is restored, the lipid is mobilized, and steatosis resolves. Although steatosis has generally been considered a benign and reversible condition, rupture of lipid-laden hepatocytes may lead to focal inflammation, granuloma formation, and fibrosis, and it may contribute to progressive liver injury. Nonoxidative metabolism of ethanol may lead to the formation of fatty acid ethyl esters, which may also be implicated in the pathogenesis of alcohol-induced liver damage.

Formation of Acetaldehyde Adducts

Acetaldehyde may be the principal mediator of alcoholic liver injury. The deleterious effects of acetaldehyde include impairment of the mitochondrial beta-oxidation of fatty acids, formation of oxygen-free radicals, and depletion of mitochondrial glutathione. In addition, acetaldehyde may bind covalently with several hepatic macromolecules, such as amines and thiols, in cell membranes, enzymes, and microtubules to form acetaldehyde adducts. This binding may trigger an immune response through formation of neoantigens, impair function of intracellular transport through precipitation of intermediate filaments and other cytoskeletal elements, and stimulate hepatic stellate cells to produce collagen.

Levels of acetaldehyde in the liver represent a balance between its rate of formation (determined by the alcohol load and activities of the three alcohol-dehydrogenating enzymes) and its rate of degradation by ALDH. ALDH is down-regulated by long-term ethanol abuse, with resultant acetaldehyde accumulation.

Role of the Immune System

Active alcoholic hepatitis often persists for months after cessation of drinking. In fact, its severity may worsen during the first few weeks of abstinence. This observation suggests that an immunologic mechanism may be responsible for the perpetuation of the injury. Levels of serum immunoglobulins, especially the immunoglobulin A class, are increased in alcoholic hepatitis. Antibodies directed against acetaldehyde-modified cytoskeletal proteins can be demonstrated in some individuals. Autoantibodies, including antinuclear and anti–single-stranded or anti–double-stranded DNA antibodies, have also been detected in some patients with alcoholic liver disease.

B and T lymphocytes are noted in the portal and periportal areas, and natural killer lymphocytes are noted around hyalin-containing hepatocytes. The peripheral lymphocyte count in patients is decreased, with an associated increase in the ratio of helper cells to suppressor cells, signifying that lymphocytes are involved in a cell-mediated inflammatory process. Lymphocyte activation on exposure to liver extracts has been demonstrated in patients with alcoholic hepatitis. Immunosuppressive therapy with glucocorticoids appears to improve survival and accelerate recovery in patients with severe alcoholic hepatitis.

Cytokines

Tumor necrosis factor-a (TNF-a) can induce programmed cellular death (apoptosis) in liver cells. Several studies have demonstrated extremely high levels of TNF and several TNF-inducible cytokines, such as interleukin 1 (IL-1), interleukin 6 (IL-6), and interleukin 8 (IL-8), in the sera of patients with alcoholic hepatitis. Both inflammatory (TNF, IL-1, IL-8) cytokines and hepatic acute-phase (IL-6) cytokines have been postulated to play a significant role in modulating certain metabolic complications in alcoholic hepatitis, and they are probably instrumental in the liver injury of alcoholic hepatitis and cirrhosis.

Role of Concomitant Viral Disease

Alcohol consumption may exacerbate injury caused by other pathogenic factors, including hepatitis viruses. Extensive epidemiologic studies suggest that the risk of cirrhosis in patients with chronic hepatitis C infection is exacerbated greatly by heavy alcohol ingestion. Possible mechanisms include the impairment of immune-mediated viral killing or enhanced virus gene expression due to the interaction of alcohol and hepatitis C virus (HCV).

Acetaminophen-Alcohol Interactions

Long-term alcohol abuse has been established as potentiating acetaminophen toxicity via induction of CYP2E1 and depletion of glutathione. Patients who are alcoholics may develop severe, even fatal, toxic liver injury after ingestion of standard therapeutic doses of acetaminophen.

Frequency

- In the United States: Alcohol abuse is the most common cause of serious liver disease in Western societies. In the United States alone, alcoholic liver disease affects more than two million people (i.e., approximately 1 percent of the population). The true incidence of alcoholic hepatitis, especially of its milder forms, is unknown because patients may be asymptomatic and never seek medical attention.

- Internationally: The prevalence appears to differ widely among different countries. In the Western hemisphere, when liver biopsies were performed in people who drank moderate to heavy amounts of alcohol and were asymptomatic, the prevalence of alcoholic hepatitis was found to be approximately 25 to 30 percent.

Mortality/Morbidity

Mild alcoholic hepatitis is a benign disorder with negligible short-term mortality. However, when alcoholic hepatitis is of sufficient severity to cause hepatic encephalopathy, jaundice, or coagulopathy, mortality can be substantial.

- The overall thirty-day mortality rate in patients hospitalized with alcoholic hepatitis is approximately 15 percent; however, in patients with severe liver disease, the rate approaches or exceeds 50 percent. In those lacking encephalopathy, jaundice, or coagulopathy, the thirty-day mortality rate is less than 5 percent. Overall, the one-year mortality rate after hospitalization for alcoholic hepatitis is approximately 40 percent.

- The long-term prognosis depends heavily on whether patients have established cirrhosis and whether they continue to drink. With abstinence, patients with alcoholic hepatitis exhibit progressive improvement in liver function over months to years, and histologic features of active alcoholic hepatitis resolve. If alcohol abuse continues, alcoholic hepatitis invariably persists and progresses to cirrhosis over months to years.

Race

Although no genetic predilection for any particular race exists, the incidence of alcoholism and alcoholic liver disease is higher in minority groups, particularly among Native Americans. Likewise, since the 1960s, death rates of alcoholic hepatitis and cirrhosis have consistently been far greater for the nonwhite population than the white population. The nonwhite male rate of alcoholic hepatitis is 1.7 times the white male rate, 1.9 times the nonwhite female rate, and almost 4 times the white female rate.

Sex

Women are more susceptible than men to the adverse effects of alcohol. Women develop alcoholic hepatitis after a shorter period and smaller amounts of alcohol abuse than men, and alcoholic hepatitis progresses more rapidly in women than in men.

- The estimated minimum daily ethanol intake required for the development of cirrhosis is 40 g for men and 20 g for women older than fifteen to twenty years. Furthermore, for patients who continue to drink after diagnosis of alcoholic liver disease, the five-year survival rate is approximately 30 percent for women compared with 70 percent for men.

- To date, no single factor can account for this increased female susceptibility to alcoholic liver damage. Lower gastric mucosal ADH content in women has been suggested to possibly lead to less first-pass clearance of alcohol in the stomach. A higher incidence of autoantibodies has been found in the sera of females who are alcoholics compared with males who are alcoholics, but their clinical significance is questionable. Perhaps, hormonal influences on the metabolism of alcohol or the higher incidence of immunologic abnormalities are responsible for the differences described in the incidence of alcoholic liver damage between men and women.

Age

Alcoholic hepatitis can develop at any age. However, its prevalence parallels the prevalence of ethanol abuse in the population, with a peak incidence in individuals aged twenty to sixty years.

Clinical

History

Heavy alcohol use is a prerequisite for the development of alcoholic hepatitis. The history is usually apparent; however, in some patients, alcohol use may be covert.

- Clues to the presence of alcoholism include a history of multiple motor vehicle accidents, convictions for driving while intoxicated, and poor interpersonal relationships. Alcoholism exhibits a genetic predisposition, and a history of alcoholism in a close relative may also indicate that a patient is at risk.

- Patients with clinically symptomatic alcoholic hepatitis typically present with nonspecific symptoms of nausea, malaise, and low-grade fever.

- The clinical presentation may be precipitated by complications of impaired liver function or portal hypertension, such as upper gastrointestinal hemorrhage from esophageal varices, confusion and lethargy from hepatic encephalopathy, or increased abdominal girth from ascites.

- A person who heavily uses alcohol may come to medical attention because of an intercurrent medical illness that produces altered mental status or persistent vomiting, which, in turn, triggers alcohol withdrawal symptoms. In such instances, the physician must be alert to the presence of a precipitating illness (e.g., subdural hematoma, acute pancreatitis, gastrointestinal hemorrhage) and to the likelihood of alcohol withdrawal symptoms (e.g., seizures, delirium tremens) in addition to the problems associated with alcoholic hepatitis.

Physical

The diagnosis of alcoholic hepatitis is straightforward and requires no further diagnostic studies in patients presenting with a history of alcohol abuse, typical symptoms and physical findings, evidence of liver functional impairment, and compatible liver enzymes. In milder cases of alcoholic hepatitis, a mild elevation of aspartate aminotransferase (AST) level may be the only diagnostic clue.

- Patients with alcoholic hepatitis are commonly febrile with tachycardia. Mild tachypnea with primary respiratory alkalosis may be observed. The liver is usually enlarged, often with mild hepatic tenderness. Hepatomegaly results from both steatosis and swelling of injured hepatocytes.

- Manifestations of hepatic failure or portal hypertension may include scleral icterus with darkening of the urine, splenomegaly, asterixis (a flapping tremor characteristic of metabolic encephalopathies), peripheral edema, and bulging flanks with shifting abdominal dullness indicating the presence of ascites.

- Spider angiomata, proximal muscle wasting, altered hair distribution, and gynecomastia may be observed, although these findings most commonly reflect coexistent cirrhosis.

Causes

Alcoholic hepatitis is a syndrome of progressive inflammatory liver injury associated with long-term heavy intake of ethanol. Heavy alcohol use is a prerequisite for the development of alcoholic hepatitis.

Differentials

Other Problems to Be Considered

Other common considerations in patients who are alcoholics and have jaundice include chronic pancreatitis with biliary strictures and pancreaticobiliary neoplasms.

A disorder histologically resembling alcoholic hepatitis can occur in patients who do not use alcohol. This syndrome, termed nonalcoholic steatohepatitis (NASH), is being recognized with increasing frequency. It occurs most frequently in the setting of obesity, hyperlipidemia, or type 2 diabetes mellitus. It is also observed in the setting of chronic parenteral hyperalimentation and in individuals who undergo jejunoileal bypass surgery for treatment of obesity. In most cases, NASH is indolent; however, in some individuals, it may progress insidiously to cirrhosis. NASH is currently believed to be responsible for a large fraction of cases of what was previously termed cryptogenic cirrhosis. In most patients with NASH, the ratio of AST to alanine aminotransferase (ALT) is less than one, unless cirrhosis is present.

Workup

Lab Studies

- CBC count

  - A CBC count commonly reveals some degree of neutrophilic leukocytosis with bandemia. Usually, this is moderate; however, rarely, it is severe enough to provide a leukemoid picture.

  - Alcohol is a direct marrow suppressant, and moderate anemia may be observed. In addition, alcohol use characteristically produces a moderate increase in mean corpuscular volume.

  - Thrombocytosis may be observed as part of the inflammatory response; conversely, myelosuppression or portal hypertension with splenic sequestration may produce thrombocytopenia.

- Liver enzyme levels

  - Liver enzyme levels exhibit a characteristic pattern. In most patients, the AST level is elevated moderately, while the ALT level is in the reference range or only mildly elevated. This is the opposite of what is observed in most other liver diseases. An AST/ALT ratio greater than one is almost universal in alcoholic hepatitis. Even in severe disease, the elevations of aminotransferase levels are modest, and an AST level greater than 500 should raise suspicion of an alternative diagnosis. An AST/ALT ratio greater than one may accompany cirrhosis of any cause and, therefore, is less diagnostically specific in the setting of cirrhosis.

  - Alkaline phosphatase level elevations are typically mild in alcoholic hepatitis. Levels greater than 500 occur in a small percentage of patients, but abnormalities of this magnitude suggest a coexisting infiltrative or biliary obstructive process.

  - The gamma-glutamyl transpeptidase level is elevated markedly by alcohol use. While a normal value helps to exclude alcohol as a cause of liver disease, an elevated level is of no value in distinguishing between simple alcoholism and alcoholic hepatitis.

- Liver function tests
  - Common liver function tests include albumin level, prothrombin time (PT), and bilirubin level.
  - Hypoalbuminemia occurs because of decreased hepatic synthetic function and coexisting PEM.
  - Hyperbilirubinemia is typically a mixture of unconjugated and conjugated bilirubin, with the latter predominating. Bilirubinuria is normally present in patients who are icteric.
  - Coagulopathy predominantly affects the extrinsic pathway of coagulation (measured by PT). It is usually unresponsive to vitamin K.
  - The severity of hyperbilirubinemia and coagulopathy reflect the severity of alcoholic hepatitis and is of prognostic value.
- Electrolyte panel
  - Electrolyte disorders may reflect effects of vomiting, portal hypertension with decreased circulating volume, alcoholic ketoacidosis, or respiratory alkalosis.
  - Hypophosphatemia and hypomagnesemia are common consequences of coexistent malnutrition.
- Screening blood tests to exclude other conditions (appropriate in any patient with alcoholic hepatitis)
  - Hepatitis B surface antigen detects hepatitis B.
  - Anti-HCV by enzyme-linked immunosorbent assay detects hepatitis C.
  - Ferritin and transferrin saturation detect hemochromatosis.
  - Marked elevation of aminotransferase levels should raise the possibility of viral hepatitis or drug hepatotoxicity. In particular, people who are alcoholics may develop severe liver necrosis from standard therapeutic doses of acetaminophen.
  - Rapid deterioration of liver function should raise the possibility of hepatocellular carcinoma, which can be tested for by determination of alpha-fetoprotein.
  - Jaundice with fever can be caused by gallstones producing cholangitis and is suggested by a disproportionate elevation of alkaline phosphatase level.

Imaging Studies

- Imaging studies are rarely required for the diagnosis of alcoholic hepatitis, but they can be useful in excluding other causes of liver disease.

- Ultrasonography

  - In general, real-time ultrasonography is the preferred study because it is inexpensive, noninvasive, and widely available; it provides a good evaluation of the liver and other viscera; and it permits guided liver biopsy.

  - On sonograms, the liver in patients with alcoholic hepatitis appears enlarged and diffusely hyperechoic.

  - Features suggestive of coexistent portal hypertension or cirrhosis include the presence of varices, splenomegaly, and ascites.

  - Ultrasonography is also helpful in excluding gallstones, bile duct obstruction, and hepatic or biliary neoplasms. Jaundice with fever can be caused by gallstones producing cholangitis; ultrasonographic examination of the abdomen is usually sufficient to exclude this possibility. However, if stones are found or fever persists, cholangiography may be necessary.

  - Rapid deterioration of liver function should raise the possibility of hepatocellular carcinoma, which can be tested for by performing imaging studies (e.g., ultrasonography, CT scanning, MRI) of the liver.

- Other imaging tests

  - Similar and complementary information can be obtained by CT scanning or MRI of the abdomen.

  - These imaging studies are more expensive and are usually required only in atypical cases. They are more sensitive and accurate if cancer is suspected.

Procedures

- Liver biopsy: This is not always required in evaluation of alcoholic hepatitis, but it may be useful in establishing the diagnosis, in determining the presence or the absence of cirrhosis, and in excluding other causes of liver disease.

- Percutaneous liver biopsy

- Percutaneous biopsy can be performed at the bedside by an experienced practitioner, usually a gastroenterologist or a hepatologist.

- Real-time ultrasonographic guidance may be desirable to optimize biopsy site selection and to reduce the risk of complications.

- Usually, a biopsy should be avoided in the presence of severe thrombocytopenia or coagulopathy because of the risk of serious or fatal hemorrhage.

- Transjugular liver biopsy

  - If biopsy information is considered essential and the risk of percutaneous biopsy appears excessive, an alternative approach is to perform a biopsy angiographically via a catheter passed into the hepatic vein under fluoroscopic guidance. In principle, the risk of hemorrhage should be reduced because the puncture site is contained within the venous system.

  - At the time of transjugular liver biopsy, the angiographer can determine the transhepatic venous pressure gradient.

  - In alcoholic hepatitis and cirrhosis, the pressure measurement obtained with a catheter-wedged retrograde in a branch of the hepatic vein accurately reflects the portal venous pressure.

Histologic Findings

In alcoholic hepatitis, injury is characteristically most prominent in centrilobular (perivenular) areas (zone 3 of Rappaport). Hepatocytes exhibit ballooning with necrosis. Focal accumulation of polymorphonuclear leukocytes is noted in areas of injury. Lymphocytes may also be present, especially in portal tracts.

Ropy eosinophilic hyaline inclusions termed Mallory bodies may be observed in the perinuclear cytoplasm. On electron microscopy, Mallory bodies may be observed to be composed of fibril clumps that histochemically are identifiable as intermediate filaments. Mallory bodies are characteristic of alcoholic hepatitis, but they are not always present in this disease, and, occasionally, they can be observed in a variety of other disorders.

Macrovesicular steatosis, perivenular fibrosis, and frank cirrhosis commonly coexist with alcoholic hepatitis.

Treatment

Medical Care

In most patients with alcoholic hepatitis, the illness is mild. Their short-term prognosis is good, and no specific treatment is required. Hospitalization is not always necessary. Alcohol use must be stopped. Care should be taken to ensure good nutrition. Providing supplemental vitamins and minerals, including folate and thiamine, is reasonable.

- Patients who are coagulopathic should receive vitamin K parenterally. Anticipate symptoms of alcohol withdrawal, and manage them appropriately.

- In contrast, patients with severe acute alcoholic hepatitis are at high risk of early death, at a rate of 50 percent or greater within thirty days. In multiple studies, the strongest factor predictive of short-term mortality was hepatic encephalopathy. In some studies, a combination of hyperbilirubinemia and coagulopathy has also been found to independently predict a high short-term mortality. Individuals with these findings or with other complications, such as azotemia or gastrointestinal bleeding, should be hospitalized. Usually, observing the patient in an intensive care unit until liver function is stable and the patient is clinically improving is prudent.

- Patients with severe alcoholic hepatitis may benefit over the short term from specific therapies directed toward reducing liver injury, enhancing hepatic regeneration, and suppressing inflammation. Glucocorticosteroids are widely used for this purpose, although their benefits have not been proven unequivocally. Various other treatments remain experimental.

- For the long term, goals include improvement of liver function, prevention of progression to cirrhosis, and reduction of mortality. Only prolonged alcohol abstinence is of demonstrated benefit in all these areas.

Supportive Treatments

Supportive treatments include the following:

- Cessation of alcohol use is the mainstay of treatment of alcoholic hepatitis.

- In general, alcoholic hepatitis resolves or improves greatly following six to twelve months of alcohol abstinence, and continued improvement may be observed for several years. Mild alcoholic hepatitis often resolves completely, but, following severe alcoholic hepatitis, residual cirrhosis can usually be demonstrated. If alcohol abuse persists, alcoholic hepatitis invariably persists and progresses to cirrhosis, and the prognosis is dramatically worse.

- Some experts have questioned whether complete abstinence is necessary or whether reduced amounts of alcohol would be sufficient for recovery in most patients. Given the addictive nature of alcohol in most patients who heavily use it, counseling complete abstinence is prudent. Patients should be referred to a program of rehabilitation and support, and they should be strongly encouraged to attend. Also, patients should be fully informed regarding the serious potential health consequences of continued ethanol use.

- Additional treatment includes nutritional support.

  - Protein-energy malnutrition (PEM) is almost universal in patients hospitalized for alcoholic hepatitis. In a large Veterans Administration Cooperative Study of Alcoholic Hepatitis, the severity of PEM correlated with the severity of alcoholic hepatitis and the predicted mortality rate. In patients with alcoholic hepatitis and severe PEM, the mortality rate was 50 percent compared with a mortality rate of less than 10 percent in patients with mild PEM.

  - Some studies have suggested that improved energy and protein intake may improve the survival rate in patients with severe alcoholic hepatitis. However, complications associated with parenteral hyperalimentation (e.g., sepsis, hemothorax) or enteral hyperalimentation (e.g., aspiration pneumonia) may outweigh the benefits of these approaches. Thus, if patients are able to take food orally, this is the route of choice, and formal nutritional support can be reserved for those instances in which patients are unable to ingest enough by mouth to meet their needs. Calories should be carefully counted to ensure adequate intake. Use of nutritional supplements and appetite stimulants may be appropriate.

  - Except in severe encephalopathy, protein restriction is unnecessary and should be avoided, because a protein-deficient diet impairs liver regeneration and worsens liver function. Even in the presence of hepatic encephalopathy, patients are usually able to ingest a minimum of 60–100 g/d of dietary protein if other measures to control encephalopathy have been pursued aggressively. In rare instances, restricting dietary proteins may be necessary. In these cases, alternatives include provision of high-quality protein via the parenteral route or provision of oral amino acid supplements that are enriched selectively in branched-chain amino acids.

Use of Medication

Use of medications in alcoholic hepatitis remains controversial.

- Despite decades of research and multiple clinical trials, a consensus regarding effective therapy for alcoholic hepatitis has not been reached. At present, only glucocorticosteroid treatment can be considered of probable established benefit, and even this well-studied therapy continues to be a source of controversy.

- Treatments discussed in the "Medication" section have met with limited success in small clinical trials but have not been evaluated thoroughly and should be considered investigational.

Surgical Care

Patients with acute alcoholic hepatitis are at high risk of developing hepatic failure following general anesthesia and major surgery. Because postoperative mortality is high, surgery should be avoided in the setting of acute alcoholic hepatitis unless it is absolutely necessary. If patients remain abstinent, alcoholic hepatitis usually resolves over a period of time, permitting surgery to be undertaken with a substantially reduced risk.

- Orthotopic liver transplantation is widely used in patients with end-stage liver disease. Most patients with active alcoholic hepatitis are excluded from transplantation because of ongoing alcohol abuse. In most U.S. programs, patients must abstain from alcohol for at least six months before they can be considered for transplantation, and thorough psychosocial evaluation must demonstrate that patients have a low likelihood of reverting to alcohol abuse.

- Patients with alcoholic hepatitis may be informed that their liver injury can be expected to subside and liver function will improve following at least six months of abstinence. If they still develop cirrhosis and its complications, they can be considered for transplantation if they remain committed to sustained abstinence.

- The prospect of liver transplantation can be a powerful motivational tool for encouraging abstinence.

Consultations

Largely, mild and moderate alcoholic hepatitis can be managed on a hospital medical floor, requiring only a brief hospital stay. In fact, patients with the mildest forms of the disease may never seek medical attention, or they can be treated safely on an outpatient basis. By contrast, severe acute alcoholic hepatitis requires intensive medical care and often a multidisciplinary approach.

- Adequate nutritional support is of paramount importance for the survival and recovery of patients with alcoholic hepatitis. The complexity of the disease and the wide variation in nutritional regimens and modalities mandate a nutritional consultation. Customarily, the gastroenterology service of the hospital should be able to handle this issue and should be instrumental in the treatment of patients.

- The onset of acute renal failure may indicate the development of hepatorenal syndrome or, alternatively, an episode of acute tubular necrosis, resulting either from the use of nephrotoxic drugs or from acute intravascular volume changes. In these instances, obtaining a nephrologic consultation is advisable.

- If a patient with alcoholic hepatitis exhibits mental status changes, focal neurologic findings, or seizures, consider a neurologic consultation.

- The fever and leukocytosis that accompany alcoholic hepatitis often raise concerns regarding possible sepsis or other infectious processes. Routine evaluation with urinalysis, chest radiography, and cultures of blood and urine is appropriate, and findings from these tests are usually negative. If concerns persist, infectious disease consultation is appropriate.

- In patients with alcoholic hepatitis who have developed cirrhosis, especially those with coexistent chronic viral hepatitis B or C, consider periodic surveillance for hepatocellular carcinoma. A common algorithm includes determination of serum alpha-fetoprotein at six-month intervals with annual diagnostic ultrasonography. The finding of a liver nodule or an elevated alpha-fetoprotein level should lead to referral to a liver specialist and additional diagnostic studies.

- In general, for patients with severe alcoholic hepatitis or cirrhosis, observation by a gastroenterologist or a hepatologist is desirable, particularly if the illness is of sufficient severity or complexity to require intensive care.

Diet

- For patients with milder alcoholic hepatitis, a general diet containing 100 g/d of protein is appropriate.

- Provide supplemental multivitamins and minerals, including folate and thiamine.

- Salt restriction may be required in patients with ascites.

Medication

Pentoxifylline (Trental) is a hemorheologic agent that lowers blood viscosity and has been shown to decrease portal hypertension in experimental animals with cirrhosis. Recently, pentoxifylline was found to have inhibitory effects on TNF. Following two encouraging pilot studies in a small number of patients, a large, randomized, double-blind, placebo-controlled trial in 101 patients with acute alcoholic hepatitis was conducted and showed significant improvement in short-term survival (Akriviadis, 2000). The benefit of pentoxifylline appears to be related to a significant decrease in the risk of developing hepatorenal syndrome.

Anabolic steroids (e.g., oxandrolone) have been used to treat alcoholic hepatitis because of their ability to stimulate protein synthesis and cell repair. They may also enhance nutrition through increased appetite. In a recent, large study of 273 patients with severe alcoholic hepatitis, treatment with both oxandrolone and nutritional supplementation showed no benefit on survival when the results of all patients were analyzed. However, when patients were stratified according to their nutritional status on admission to the hospital, a significant improvement in short- and long-term survival was noted in those with moderate malnutrition. The survival rate in patients who were severely malnourished did not improve (Mendenhall, 1993).

Propylthiouracil (PTU) reduces the basal metabolic rate in the liver, thereby decreasing its requirement for oxygen. Only two randomized, double-blind, controlled trials are published in the English literature; however, no improvement in the survival of patients with alcoholic hepatitis could be demonstrated.

Insulin and glucagon are hepatatrophic hormones that may play an important role in promoting liver cell regeneration in response to injury. In two clinical trials, administration of insulin and glucagon along with glucose (to prevent hypoglycemia) led to a modest improvement of liver function in patients with alcoholic hepatitis; however, severe insulin-induced hypoglycemia resulted in several deaths. Other promoters of hepatic regeneration include prostaglandins and malotilate, which appeared to improve survival in a multicenter European trial. Peptide growth factors, such as hepatocyte growth factor, are candidates for future study.

Colchicine interferes with transcellular movement and transport of collagen from the cytoplasm to the extracellular space, thus inhibiting fibrogenesis. In the two randomized double-blind trials in the literature, colchicine was ineffective in treating patients with severe alcoholic hepatitis. By contrast, of seven studies on the use of colchicine in patients with cirrhosis (mostly alcoholic), four studies demonstrated improvement and three studies demonstrated a tendency toward improvement. D-Penicillamine inhibits collagen synthesis in vitro by decreasing cross-linking. D-Penicillamine has been used successfully in other liver diseases (e.g., Wilson disease) for its copper-chelating properties. No controlled trial with this agent has been performed in alcoholic hepatitis.

Sulfhydryl agents can act as free radical scavengers and promote formation of reduced glutathione, an important element of hepatic antioxidant defense. S-adenosyl-l-methionine (SAM) protects against alcoholic liver injury in animal models. A recent, randomized, double-blind, placebo-controlled trial in patients with alcoholic hepatitis resulted in improved survival of patients administered SAM compared with controls.

N-acetyl-L-cysteine (NAC) is widely used as an antidote to acetaminophen hepatotoxicity. Data from limited case-controlled studies suggest a beneficial effect of NAC in alcoholic liver disease. The beneficial effect is particularly apparent in patients who are alcoholics and also consume therapeutic doses of acetaminophen; however, preliminary evidence from prospective randomized trials did not show benefit. Vitamin E, a potent antioxidant substance, has been found to be hepatoprotective in both experimental animals and humans.

However, a double-blind trial among patients with alcoholic liver disease failed to improve liver chemistry, hospitalization rate, and cumulative mortality when the patients were administered 500 mg of vitamin E daily compared with the placebo-treated control group.

Polyunsaturated lecithin (phosphatidyl choline) has been studied because of the empiric observation that choline deficiency (which impairs endogenous lecithin synthesis) in rats increases sensitivity to alcoholic liver injury. The precise mechanism is unknown. Beneficial effects have been demonstrated in preventing alcoholic liver injury in baboons and, more recently, in a preliminary report of a Veterans Administration multicenter, cooperative, therapeutic trial among patients with alcoholic liver disease. Benefits were subtle, and the treatment appears to be more suited to long-term use for prevention of cirrhosis than for treatment of acute alcoholic hepatitis.

Several preliminary reports in alcoholic hepatitis have indicated a beneficial effect from calcium channel blockers (e.g., diltiazem, verapamil), although the only randomized double-blind trial of amlodipine failed to demonstrate any improvement in patients with alcoholic hepatitis.

Hepatoprotective bile acids include ursodeoxycholic acid (Ursodiol), a tertiary bile acid that has been used extensively either as monotherapy or as an adjuvant therapy in various cholestatic liver diseases, such as primary biliary cirrhosis and primary sclerosing cholangitis. Preliminary data from a small clinical trial in patients with alcoholic hepatitis showed a significant improvement in liver chemistry test results.

Herbal agents have been tried. Silymarin is the active ingredient in milk thistle and a member of the flavonoids with remarkable hepatoprotective effects in experimental toxic liver injury. The precise mechanism of its hepatoprotective mediation is not known, but it is probably related to its antioxidant properties. In humans with mild alcoholic hepatitis, silymarin improves liver chemistry tests. In a single controlled trial among 170 patients with alcoholic liver disease, silymarin reduced the liver-related deaths.

Cyanidanol-3 (catechin) is a naturally occurring flavonoid with antioxidant properties. As a hepatoprotective agent, it has been studied extensively in experimental toxic liver injury. Cyanidanol gained popularity in Europe in the mid-1980s and was used in a wide variety of liver diseases. Unfortunately, prospective randomized trials in alcoholic hepatitis failed to show any benefit. Moreover, the administration of cyanidanol was associated with adverse effects such as allergic hyperthermia and autoimmune hemolytic anemia.

Drug Category: Corticosteroids

Strong evidence of immunologic and inflammatory liver injury in alcoholic hepatitis provides the rationale for use of glucocorticosteroids. Over the past thirty years, more than fifty clinical trials have been published evaluating the use of glucocorticosteroids in treating alcoholic hepatitis. In most studies, treatment consists of the equivalent of 30–40 mg/d of prednisolone for thirty days, followed by a rapid taper and withdrawal over the subsequent two to four weeks. Study results have not been uniform. Larger studies demonstrate a significant benefit in severe alcoholic hepatitis, including reduction in mortality. Two meta-analyses of twelve randomized, prospective, placebo-controlled trials support the conclusion that glucocorticosteroid treatment reduces early mortality in patients with severe acute alcoholic hepatitis.

All studies conclude that in mild alcoholic hepatitis, no benefit can be demonstrated with glucocorticosteroid treatment; therefore, it is

Table 53.1. Methylprednisolone

Drug Name	Methylprednisolone (Solu-Medrol, Adlone, Medrol, Depo-Medrol): Decreases inflammation by suppressing migration of polymorphonuclear leukocytes and reversing increased capillary permeability. May be preferable to other glucocorticoids (e.g., prednisone) because hepatic metabolism is not required.
Adult Dose	32 mg/d PO/IV for 30 d; taper and discontinue over 2–4 wk
Pediatric Dose	Not established
Contraindications	Documented hypersensitivity; active sepsis; GI bleeding; acute pancreatitis
Interactions	Co-administration with digoxin may increase digitalis toxicity secondary to hypokalemia; estrogens may increase levels; phenobarbital, phenytoin, and rifampin may decrease levels (adjust dose); monitor for hypokalemia when taking concurrently with diuretics
Pregnancy	Safety for use during pregnancy has not been established.
Precautions	Only sodium succinate salt should be administered IV; commonly leads to impaired glucose tolerance and increases insulin requirements in diabetes; femoral osteonecrosis; increased susceptibility to fungal and other infections; impaired wound healing; increased risk of peptic ulcer hemorrhage or perforation; altered mental status with depression or psychosis

509

only appropriate in individuals with severe alcoholic hepatitis characterized by encephalopathy, hyperbilirubinemia, or coagulopathy.

Glucocorticosteroids may suppress inflammatory and immune-mediated hepatic destruction, but their marked antianabolic effect suppresses regeneration and may slow healing. They may increase complications and mortality associated with GI bleeding, pancreatitis, or sepsis, and they should be withheld or used judiciously if any of these are present.

Follow-Up

Further Inpatient Care

- In the absence of complications, patients generally can be discharged from acute medical inpatient care once alcohol withdrawal symptoms have cleared; liver function has begun to improve; and complications of liver failure, such as encephalopathy, have resolved with appropriate treatment.

- In patients who have a potential for rehabilitation, transferring them to an inpatient substance abuse treatment program rather than discharging them from the hospital may be appropriate.

Further Outpatient Care:

- Patients recently discharged from the hospital following an acute bout of alcoholic hepatitis should generally be observed within two weeks of their discharge. Subsequent periodic follow-up visits, at intervals ranging from weeks to several months, are appropriate to monitor patients' response to treatment, including obtaining electrolyte levels and liver tests, and to encourage sobriety.

- In patients with alcoholic hepatitis who have developed cirrhosis, especially those with coexistent chronic viral hepatitis B or C, consider periodic surveillance for hepatocellular carcinoma. A common algorithm includes determination of serum alpha-fetoprotein level at six-month intervals with annual diagnostic ultrasonography. The finding of a liver nodule or an elevated alpha-fetoprotein level should lead to referral to a liver specialist and additional diagnostic studies.

- Immunizing patients with alcoholic liver disease against common infectious pathogens, including hepatitis A, hepatitis B, pneumococcus, and influenza A, is prudent.

Transfer

- Patients with alcoholic hepatitis of mild to moderate severity can be treated in a primary care setting. In general, for patients with severe alcoholic hepatitis or cirrhosis, observation by a gastroenterologist or a hepatologist is desirable, particularly if the illness is of sufficient severity or complexity to require intensive care.

- If patients become comatose or have complications that may require surgical intervention, the treating physician should consider emergent transfer to a tertiary care center with experience in the treatment of liver failure. In selected cases, the use of novel liver-assist devices (artificial livers) may provide transient improvement in manifestations of liver failure.

Complications

- Most complications of alcoholic hepatitis are identical to those of cirrhosis.

  - *Variceal hemorrhage:* Acute variceal bleeding constitutes one of the most devastating emergencies, not only in gastroenterology but also in medicine at large. Resuscitation of the patient and protection of the airway are the two most important steps in the treatment of acute variceal bleeding. Cessation of the acute bleeding is usually achieved in more than 90 percent of patients, with the combination of interventional endoscopy (sclerotherapy or banding ligation) and the intravenous infusion of pharmaceutical agents that lower the pressure within the portal system (somatostatin or one of its long-acting analogues, e.g., octreotide). Alternatively and for patients who continue to bleed in spite of interventional endoscopy and drug therapy, more invasive options, such as balloon tamponade, transjugular intrahepatic portosystemic shunt, and emergency portal-caval shunt, may be used.

  - *Hepatic encephalopathy:* The development of encephalopathy in patients with alcoholic hepatitis is invariably associated with a grave prognosis. Treatment consists of close monitoring of the patient and the administration of lactulose or non-absorbable antibiotics. Low energy or protein intake is not indicated, except transiently in severe cases. The use of benzo-diazepine receptor antagonists (i.e., flumazenil [Romazicon]) is still at an experimental stage. Rarely, rapidly progressive worsening of encephalopathy leading to deep coma may be associated with cerebral edema, as observed in fulminant hepatic failure. In selected instances, aggressive treatment with intracranial pressure monitoring and liver-assist devices may be considered.

- *Coagulopathy and thrombocytopenia:* Profound hypoprothrombinemia may ensue in the course of severe alcoholic hepatitis, especially in patients with variceal bleeding. Administer fresh-frozen plasma to temporarily restore the depleted hepatic prothrombin stores. The value of parenteral administration of vitamin K is dubious because the hepatocytes are incapable of synthesizing new prothrombin. Platelet transfusions are not usually necessary to correct thrombocytopenia unless the patient is actively bleeding or undergoes an invasive procedure.

- *Ascites:* Acute onset of ascites may develop in patients with alcoholic hepatitis, even in the absence of overtly decompensated liver disease and portal hypertension. The ascites are typically transudative, with a very low albumin concentration (<1 g/dL). In patients who are hemodynamically stable with normal renal function, bed rest and salt restriction may be sufficient to mobilize fluid. The addition of diuretics (typically spironolactone and furosemide) permits clearing of fluid in most patients. In some individuals who fail to respond to these measures, periodic large-volume paracentesis with intravenous albumin supplementation may be required. With continued abstinence, the salt-retaining tendency may improve; in many instances, the diuretics can be withdrawn safely after a period of months without any reaccumulation of ascites.

- *Spontaneous bacterial peritonitis:* This condition may develop in patients with alcoholic hepatitis and ascites, especially in those with concomitant gastrointestinal bleeding. Following a confirmatory diagnostic paracentesis, broad-spectrum antibiotic therapy with a second- or third-generation cephalosporin is the treatment of choice.

- *Iron overload:* Several histopathologic studies have shown that as many as 50 percent of patients with alcoholic liver disease have increased hepatic iron content compared with healthy controls. This excess deposition of iron may play a significant role in the progression of the alcoholic liver damage. Portosystemic shunts, especially the side-to-side variety, increase enormously the deposition of iron to the liver. Occasionally, this excessive iron deposition leads to a clinical and pathologic entity that is analogous to primary hemochromatosis. Attempts to treat alcoholic liver disease with phlebotomy to reduce iron overload have been hampered by the development of anemia, and no clear benefit has been observed.

Prognosis

- During the past several decades, various formulas and algorithms have been proposed for predicting the outcome of severe alcoholic hepatitis. The single most reliable indicator of severity is the presence of hepatic encephalopathy.

- The discriminant function (DF) of Maddrey and coworkers is based on PT and bilirubin, and it is calculated as follows:

  - DF = (4.6 X PT prolongation) + total serum bilirubin in mg/dL

  - Values greater than 32 indicate severe disease and predict a thirty-day mortality rate of approximately 50 percent, assuming only supportive treatment.

  - Subsequent studies have found the DF to be an inexact predictor of mortality in alcoholic hepatitis, especially in patients receiving glucocorticoids.

- Other formulas have been proposed for the assessment of prognosis of alcoholic hepatitis, but none have become popular among clinicians. The Combined Clinical and Laboratory Index of the University of Toronto permits a linear estimate of acute mortality in alcoholic hepatitis. Its major disadvantages are the large number (fourteen) of variables that must be scored and the complexity of the calculation itself.

- In contrast to the Combined Clinical and Laboratory Index, a much simpler formula for assessing mortality was proposed in a large series of 142 patients with histologically proved alcoholic hepatitis based on PT, serum bilirubin level, and serum albumin level (Mihas, 1978).

  - According to this study, the mortality rate in patients with a serum bilirubin level greater than 2 mg/dL, a serum albumin level less than 2.5 g/dL, and a PT greater than 5 seconds was 75 percent.

513

- Conversely, patients who did not meet all three criteria had a much lower mortality rate (approximately 25 percent).

- Other factors that correlate with poor prognosis include older age, impaired renal function, encephalopathy, and a rise in the white blood cell count in the first two weeks of hospitalization.

Bibliography

Akriviadis E, Botla R, Briggs W, et al: Pentoxifylline improves short-term survival in severe acute alcoholic hepatitis: a double-blind, placebo-controlled trial. *Gastroenterology* 2000 Dec; 119(6): 1637–48.

Aleynik S, Lieber CS: Role of S-adenosylmethionine in hyperhomo-cysteinemia and in the treatment of alcoholic liver disease. *Nutrition* 2000 Nov–Dec; 16(11–12): 1104–8.

Aleynik SI, Leo MA, Aleynik MK, Lieber CS: Polyenylphosphatidyl-choline protects against alcohol but not iron-induced oxidative stress in the liver. *Alcohol Clin Exp Res* 2000 Feb; 24(2): 196–206.

Bird GL, Prach AT, McMahon AD, et al: Randomised controlled double-blind trial of the calcium channel antagonist amlodipine in the treatment of acute alcoholic hepatitis. *J Hepatol* 1998 Feb; 28(2): 194–98.

Bonet H, Manez R, Kramer D, et al: Liver transplantation for alcoholic liver disease: survival of patients transplanted with alcoholic hepatitis plus cirrhosis as compared with those with cirrhosis alone. *Alcohol Clin Exp Res* 1993 Oct; 17(5): 1102–6.

Carithers RL, Herlong HF, Diehl AM, et al: Methylprednisolone therapy in patients with severe alcoholic hepatitis. A randomized multicenter trial. *Ann Intern Med* 1989 May 1; 110(9): 685–90.

Christensen E, Gluud C: Glucocorticoids are ineffective in alcoholic hepatitis: a meta-analysis adjusting for confounding variables. *Gut* 1995 Jul; 37(1): 113–18.

Daures JP, Peray P, Bories P, et al: [Corticoid therapy in the treatment of acute alcoholic hepatitis. Results of a meta-analysis]. *Gastroenterol Clin Biol* 1991; 15(3): 223–28.

el-Newihi HM, Mihas AA: Alcoholic hepatitis. Recent advances in pathogenesis and therapy. *Postgrad Med* 1994 Dec; 96(8): 61–64, 68–70.

French SW, Nash J, Shitabata P, et al: Pathology of alcoholic liver disease. VA Cooperative Study Group 119. *Semin Liver Dis* 1993 May; 13(2): 154–69.

French SW: Mechanisms of alcoholic liver injury. *Can J Gastroenterol* 2000 Apr; 14(4): 327–32.

French SW, Burbige EJ: Alcoholic hepatitis: clinical, morphologic, pathogenic, and therapeutic aspects. *Prog Liver Dis* 1979; 6: 557–79.

Fujimoto M, Uemura M, Kojima H, et al: Prognostic factors in severe alcoholic liver injury. Nara Liver Study Group. *Alcohol Clin Exp Res* 1999 Apr; 23(4 Suppl): 33S–38S.

Galambos JT: Natural history of alcoholic hepatitis. 3. Histological changes. *Gastroenterology* 1972 Dec; 63(6): 1026–35.

Grant BF, Dufour MC, Harford TC: Epidemiology of alcoholic liver disease. *Semin Liver Dis* 1988 Feb; 8(1): 12–25.

Imperiale TF, McCullough AJ: Do corticosteroids reduce mortality from alcoholic hepatitis? A meta-analysis of the randomized trials. *Ann Intern Med* 1990 Aug 15; 113(4): 299–307.

Jensen K, Gluud C: The Mallory body: morphological, clinical and experimental studies (Part 1 of a literature survey). *Hepatology* 1994 Oct; 20(4 Pt 1): 1061–77.

Lieber CS: Metabolism of alcohol. *Clinics in Liver Disease* 1998; 2: 673–702.

Lieber CS: Alcoholic liver disease: new insights in pathogenesis lead to new treatments. *J Hepatol* 2000; 32(1 Suppl): 113–28.

Lieber CS: Ethanol metabolism, cirrhosis and alcoholism. *Clin Chim Acta* 1997 Jan 3; 257(1): 59–84.

Lieber CS, DeCarli LM: An experimental model of alcohol feeding and liver injury in the baboon. *J Med Primatol* 1974; 3(3): 153–63.

Maddrey WC: Alcohol-induced liver disease. *Clin Liver Dis* 2000 Feb; 4(1): 115–31, vii.

McCormick PA, Burroughs AK: Relation between liver pathology and prognosis in patients with portal hypertension. *World J Surg* 1994 Mar-Apr; 18(2): 171–75.

McCullough AJ, O'Connor JF: Alcoholic liver disease: proposed recommendations for the American College of Gastroenterology. *Am J Gastroenterol* 1998 Nov; 93(11): 2022–36.

Mendenhall C, Roselle GA, Gartside P, Moritz T: Relationship of protein calorie malnutrition to alcoholic liver disease: a reexamination of data from two Veterans Administration Cooperative Studies. *Alcohol Clin Exp Res* 1995 Jun; 19(3): 635–41.

Mendenhall CL, Moritz TE, Roselle GA, et al: A study of oral nutritional support with oxandrolone in malnourished patients with alcoholic hepatitis: results of a Department of Veterans Affairs cooperative study. *Hepatology* 1993 Apr; 17(4): 564–76.

Mihas AA, Doos WG, Spenney JG: Alcoholic hepatitis—a clinical and pathological study of 142 cases. *J Chronic Dis* 1978; 31(6–7): 461–72.

Mitchell RG, Michael M, Sandidge D: High mortality among patients with the leukemoid reaction and alcoholic hepatitis. *South Med J* 1991 Feb; 84(2): 281–82.

Morgan MY: The prognosis and outcome of alcoholic liver disease. *Alcohol* Alcohol Suppl 1994; 2: 335–43.

Nordmann R, Ribiere C, Rouach H: Implication of free radical mechanisms in ethanol-induced cellular injury. *Free Radic Biol Med* 1992; 12(3): 219–40.

Ramond MJ, Poynard T, Rueff B, et al: A randomized trial of prednisolone in patients with severe alcoholic hepatitis. *N Engl J Med* 1992 Feb 20; 326(8): 507–12.

Tilg H, Diehl AM: Cytokines in alcoholic and nonalcoholic steatohepatitis. *N Engl J Med* 2000 Nov 16; 343(20): 1467–76.

Zimmerman HJ, Maddrey WC: Acetaminophen (paracetamol) hepatotoxicity with regular intake of alcohol: analysis of instances of therapeutic misadventure. *Hepatology* 1995 Sep; 22(3): 767–73.

Chapter 54

Nonalcoholic Steatohepatitis

Nonalcoholic steatohepatitis or NASH is a common, often "silent" liver disease. It resembles alcoholic liver disease, but occurs in people who drink little or no alcohol. The major feature in NASH is fat in the liver, along with inflammation and damage. Most people with NASH feel well and are not aware that they have a liver problem. Nevertheless, NASH can be severe and can lead to cirrhosis, in which the liver is permanently damaged and scarred and no longer able to work properly.

NASH affects 2 to 5 percent of Americans. An additional 10 to 20 percent of Americans have fat in their liver, but no inflammation or liver damage, a condition called "fatty liver." Although having fat in the liver is not normal, by itself it probably causes little harm or permanent damage. If fat is suspected based on blood test results or scans of the liver, this problem is called nonalcoholic fatty liver disease (NAFLD). If a liver biopsy is performed in this case, it will show that some people have NASH while others have simple fatty liver.

Both NASH and NAFLD are becoming more common, possibly because of the greater number of Americans with obesity. In the past ten years, the rate of obesity has doubled in adults and tripled in children. Obesity also contributes to diabetes and high blood cholesterol, which can further complicate the health of someone with NASH. Diabetes and high blood cholesterol are also becoming more common among Americans.

Reprinted from "Nonalcoholic Steatohepatitis," National Institute of Diabetes and Digestive and Kidney Diseases, National Institutes of Health, NIH Publication No. 04-4921, February 2004.

Diagnosis

NASH is usually first suspected in a person who is found to have elevations in liver tests that are included in routine blood test panels, such as alanine aminotransferase (ALT) or aspartate aminotransferase (AST). When further evaluation shows no apparent reason for liver disease (such as medications, viral hepatitis, or excessive use of alcohol) and when x-rays or imaging studies of the liver show fat, NASH is suspected. The only means of proving a diagnosis of NASH and separating it from simple fatty liver is a liver biopsy. For a liver biopsy, a needle is inserted through the skin to remove a small piece of the liver. NASH is diagnosed when examination of the tissue under the microscope shows fat along with inflammation and damage to liver cells. If there is fat without inflammation and damage, simple fatty liver or NAFLD is diagnosed. An important piece of information learned from the biopsy is whether scar tissue has developed in the liver. Currently, no blood tests or scans can reliably provide this information.

Symptoms

NASH is usually a silent disease with few or no symptoms. Patients generally feel well in the early stages and only begin to have symptoms—such as fatigue, weight loss, and weakness—once the disease is more advanced or cirrhosis develops. The progression of NASH can take years, even decades. The process can stop and, in some cases, reverse on its own without specific therapy. Or NASH can slowly worsen, causing scarring or "fibrosis" to appear and accumulate in the liver. As fibrosis worsens, cirrhosis develops; the liver becomes seriously scarred, hardened, and unable to function normally. Not every person with NASH develops cirrhosis, but once serious scarring or cirrhosis is present, few treatments can halt the progression. A person with cirrhosis experiences fluid retention, muscle wasting, bleeding from the intestines, and liver failure. Liver transplantation is the only treatment for advanced cirrhosis with liver failure, and transplantation is increasingly performed in people with NASH. NASH ranks as one of the major causes of cirrhosis in America, behind hepatitis C and alcoholic liver disease.

Causes

Although NASH has become more common, its underlying cause is still not clear. It most often occurs in persons who are middle-aged and overweight or obese. Many patients with NASH have elevated blood lipids, such as cholesterol and triglycerides, and many have diabetes or pre-diabetes, but not every obese person or every patient with diabetes has NASH. Furthermore, some patients with NASH are not obese, do not have diabetes, and have normal blood cholesterol and lipids. NASH can occur without any apparent risk factor and can even occur in children. Thus, NASH is not simply obesity that affects the liver.

While the underlying reason for the liver injury that causes NASH is not known, several factors are possible candidates:

- insulin resistance
- release of toxic inflammatory proteins by fat cells (cytokines)
- oxidative stress (deterioration of cells) inside liver cells

Treatment

It is important to stress that there are currently no specific therapies for NASH. The following are the most important recommendations given to persons with this disease:

- reduce their weight (if obese or overweight)
- follow a balanced and healthy diet
- increase physical activity
- avoid alcohol
- avoid unnecessary medications

These are standard recommendations, but they can make a difference. They are also helpful for other conditions, such as heart disease, diabetes, and high cholesterol.

A major attempt should be made to lower body weight into the healthy range. Weight loss can improve liver tests in patients with NASH and may reverse the disease to some extent. Research at present is focusing on how much weight loss improves the liver in patients with NASH and whether this improvement lasts over a period of time.

People with NASH often have other medical conditions, such as diabetes, high blood pressure, or elevated cholesterol. These conditions should be treated with medication and adequately controlled; having NASH or elevated liver enzymes should not lead people to avoid treating these other conditions.

Experimental approaches under evaluation in patients with NASH include antioxidants, such as vitamin E, selenium, and betaine. These medications act by reducing the oxidative stress that appears to increase inside the liver in patients with NASH. Whether these substances actually help treat the disease is not known, but the results of clinical trials should become available in the next few years.

Another experimental approach to treating NASH is the use of newer antidiabetic medications—even in persons without diabetes. Most patients with NASH have insulin resistance, meaning that the insulin normally present in the bloodstream is less effective for them in controlling blood glucose and fatty acids in the blood than it is for people who do not have NASH. The newer antidiabetic medications make the body more sensitive to insulin and may help reduce liver injury in patients with NASH. Studies of these medications—including metformin, rosiglitazone, and pioglitazone—are being sponsored by the National Institutes of Health and should answer the question of whether these medications are beneficial in NASH.

Hope through Research

What is most needed in the management of NASH is more research to better understand the liver injury found in this disease. When the pathways that lead to the injury are fully known, safe and effective means can be developed to reverse these pathways and help patients with NASH. Recent breakthroughs in mapping the human genome and uncovering the individual steps by which insulin and other hormones regulate blood glucose and fat could provide the necessary clues.

Points to Remember

- Nonalcoholic steatohepatitis (NASH) is fat in the liver, with inflammation and damage.

- NASH occurs in people who drink little or no alcohol and affects 2 to 5 percent of Americans, especially people who are middle-aged and overweight or obese.

- NASH can occur in children.

- People who have NASH may feel well and may not know that they have a liver disease.

- NASH can lead to cirrhosis, a condition in which the liver is permanently damaged and cannot work properly.

- Fatigue can occur at any stage of NASH.

- Weight loss and weakness may begin once the disease is advanced or cirrhosis is present.

- NASH may be suspected if blood tests show high levels of liver enzymes or if scans show fatty liver.

- NASH is diagnosed by examining a small piece of the liver taken through a needle, a procedure called biopsy.

- People who have NASH should reduce their weight, eat a balanced diet, engage in physical activity, and avoid alcohol and unnecessary medications.

- There are no specific therapies for NASH. Experimental therapies being studied include antioxidants and antidiabetes medications.

Chapter 55

Toxic Hepatitis

What does the liver do?

The liver processes everything a person consumes. Among many complex functions the liver cleanses the blood, regulates the supply of body fuel, and manufactures many essential body proteins, including clotting factors.

What is toxic hepatitis?

Toxic hepatitis is an inflammation of the liver caused by chemicals. Many chemicals that are intentionally or unintentionally inhaled or consumed can have toxic effects on the liver. Among these chemicals are drugs, industrial solvents, and pollutants. Virtually every drug imaginable has at one time or another been indicated as a cause of toxic hepatitis.

Toxins can occasionally cause chronic liver disease and even cirrhosis if the use of the drug is not stopped.

Do all toxins affect the liver in the same manner?

Toxins that can damage the liver have been divided into two groups:

- *Predictable:* those that are known to cause toxic hepatitis and liver damage with sufficient exposure to one or more of these

---

chemicals. Examples of chemicals found in this group are cleaning solvents, carbon tetrachloride, and the pain reliever acetaminophen.

- *Unpredictable:* those toxins that damage the liver in a very small proportion of individuals exposed to the chemical. Unpredictable injury produced by most drugs is very poorly understood, but recent data suggest that a toxic response to a drug probably depends on the kind of enzyme a person inherits to metabolize the drug.

Why is the liver susceptible to injury by chemicals?

The liver is susceptible to injury by chemicals because it plays a fundamental role in chemical metabolism. The liver has the unique job of processing almost all chemicals and drugs that enter the blood stream and removing the chemicals that are difficult for the kidneys to excrete. The liver turns these chemicals into products that can be eliminated from the body through bile or urine. However, during this chemical process in the liver, unstable highly toxic products are sometimes produced; these highly toxic products can attack and injure the liver.

Regular alcohol consumption will likely enhance the chance of drug toxicity especially in the case of acetaminophen. Therefore, alcohol should not be consumed when using medications.

What are the symptoms of toxic hepatitis?

Clinically, toxic hepatitis can resemble any form of acute or chronic liver disease, such as viral hepatitis or bile-duct obstruction. Symptoms such as nausea, vomiting, fever, and jaundice as well as liver blood tests and liver biopsy findings are often identical to viral hepatitis. On the other hand, symptoms like fever, abdominal pain, and jaundice can mimic other liver conditions, such as stones blocking the bile ducts.

How is the diagnosis of toxic hepatitis made?

At present there is no clear test to prove the diagnosis. Therefore, the diagnosis is made based on a thorough assessment of a patient. First, the doctor must pay close attention to all drugs used (prescribed or over-the-counter ones including herbal remedies), as well as the environmental and occupational exposures to chemicals of each individual with liver disease.

The doctor must also consider the time of exposure. Some forms of chemical liver injury will occur within days to weeks of the exposure; however, sometimes it takes many months of regular ingestion of a drug before liver injury becomes apparent.

How is toxic hepatitis treated?

If an individual has toxic hepatitis, the drug(s) should be immediately discontinued and further exposure to the offending chemical prevented. Removal of the offending chemical or drug leads to rapid improvement, often within days, but sometimes several months may elapse before improvement is noted, even if chronic liver disease has already developed. No other specific therapy is needed.

Part Seven

Additional Help
and Information

Chapter 56

Glossary of Hepatitis-Related Terms

Abnormality: Deviation from normal.

Acquired Immune Deficiency Syndrome (AIDS): A severe disorder caused by the HIV retrovirus. It effects your immunity by making you more susceptible to infections and to certain rare cancers. It is mostly transmitted by exposure to contaminated blood and semen.

Active Immunity: See Immunity, Active.

Acute: A short-term, intense health effect.

Acute Hepatitis C: Newly acquired symptomatic hepatitis C virus (HCV) infection.

Adefovir Dipivoxil: FDA approved antiviral drug, given by mouth, for treatment of persons with chronic hepatitis B.

Adverse Events: Undesirable experiences occurring after immunization that may or may not be related to the vaccine.

The terms in this glossary were excerpted from "Viral Hepatitis: Glossary," Centers for Disease Control, December 2004; "Glossary of Terms," VA National Hepatitis C Program, Department of Veterans Affairs (VA), August 2003; and "What I Need to Know about Liver Transplantation," National Institute of Diabetes and Digestive and Kidney Diseases, National Institutes of Health, NIH Publication No. 03-4941, March 2003.

Alanine Aminotransferase (ALT): An enzyme released from liver cells. A blood test that reveals ALT levels above normal may indicate liver damage.

Albumin: A protein made in the liver that assists in maintaining blood volume in the arteries and veins. If albumin drops to very low levels, fluid may leak into tissues from the blood vessels, resulting in edema or swelling.

Alkaline Phosphatase: Elevated levels of this liver enzyme are not commonly seen with HBV, although modest elevations may occur with the development of cirrhosis.

Alpha-Fetoprotein (AFP): A substance produced by the fetus that is found in fetal serum, amniotic fluid, and the mother's bloodstream. Elevated levels of AFP may indicate that the baby has a neural tube defect such as spina bifida (incomplete closure of the spinal column) which can lead to paralysis of the lower limbs, repeated urinary tract infections, mental retardation, or hydrocephalus ("water on the brain"); it is also a useful nonspecific tumor-associated antigen (tumor marker) that, when elevated, can indicate liver cancer.

ALT: See Alanine Aminotransferase.

Antibiotic: A substance that fights bacteria.

Antibody: A protein found in the blood that is produced in response to foreign substances (e.g., bacteria or viruses) invading the body. Antibodies protect the body from disease by binding to these organisms and destroying them.

Antigens: Foreign substances (e.g., bacteria or viruses) in the body that are capable of causing disease. The presence of antigens in the body triggers an immune response, usually the production of antibodies.

Anti-HBc: See Hepatitis B Core Antibody.

Anti-HBe: See Hepatitis B e Antibody.

Anti-HBs: See Hepatitis B Surface Antibody.

Anti-HCV (Antibody to Hepatitis C Virus): The antibody directed against the hepatitis C virus (HCV). Its presence in the bloodstream often indicates HCV infection. This antibody has not been shown to protect people against hepatitis C.

Antiviral: Literally "against-virus"—any medicine capable of destroying or weakening a virus.

Ascites: A buildup of fluid in the abdomen.

Aspartate Aminotransferase (AST): An enzyme released from liver cells. A blood test that reveals AST levels above normal may indicate liver damage.

Assay: A test or analysis.

AST: See Aspartate Aminotransferase.

Asymptomatic: Presenting no symptoms of disease.

Autoimmune: A term that refers to a person's immune system attacking his or her own body.

Bacteria: Tiny one-celled organisms present throughout the environment that require a microscope to be seen. While not all bacteria are harmful, some cause disease.

bDNA (branched DNA) Assay: One of the two tests that reveal the presence in the bloodstream of minute quantities of DNA and RNA, such as RNA fragments from hepatitis C virus.

Benign: Not recurrent or progressive; nonmalignant; of a mild type or character that does not threaten health or life.

Biliary Atresia: A condition that results when the bile ducts inside or outside the liver don't have normal openings. Bile becomes trapped in the liver, causing jaundice and cirrhosis. This condition is present from birth and without surgery may cause death.

Bilirubin: A yellow pigment formed when red blood cells break down. Bilirubin levels may rise when liver function is impaired, leading to the development of jaundice, a yellowing of the eyes and skin.

Biochemical Response (BR): Refers to patient's response to interferon therapy by normalization of ALT.

Biopsy: Removing a small piece of tissue to view under a microscope.

Blood-Borne Substances: Those substances that are present in the blood and are carried by it throughout the body. Blood-borne substances, such as viruses, can be passed on to others through blood transfusions, needle sharing, and even sharing a toothbrush if both people have bleeding gums.

Booster Dose: An additional dose of an immunizing agent to increase the protection afforded by the original series of injections.

Breakthrough Response: A "breaking through" of the virus while on therapy. Detection of virus during therapy in those who had initially lost virus during treatment.

Carrier: A person in apparent good health, who has been infected with an organism and is capable of infecting or causing disease in others. Individuals persistently infected with hepatitis B and C without evidence of liver injury are considered "carriers."

Chronic Hepatitis B Virus Infection: The clinical definition for an individual for whom the hepatitis B surface antigen test is positive (indicates HBV in the blood and infectiousness) for more than six months; in the past, such a person was referred to as a hepatitis B carrier.

Chronic Hepatitis C Virus Infection: Liver inflammation in patients with chronic HCV infection; characterized by abnormal levels of liver enzymes.

Chronic Infection: An infection that persists and that returns after it had seemed to be cured. Disease is defined as evidence of liver injury by abnormality in serum ALT or liver histology.

CIA: Enhanced chemiluminescence immunoassay; FDA licensed and approved laboratory screening test that detects HCV antibody.

Cirrhosis: A chronic liver condition caused by scar tissue and damage to cells. Cirrhosis makes it hard for the liver to remove poisons (toxins) like alcohol and drugs from the blood. These toxins build up in the blood and may affect the brain.

Clotting Factors: Proteins made in the liver that are important in maintaining normal blood clotting. Disruption in the blood's ability to clot may indicate that the liver is not creating enough clotting factors. A severe shortage in clotting factors may indicate that a liver transplant is needed.

Coinfection: The condition of an organism or individual cells being infected simultaneously by two different pathological microorganisms, such as infection with both HIV and hepatitis C virus (HCV).

Combination Vaccine: Two or more vaccines combined and administered at once in order to reduce the number of shots given. For example, the MMR (measles, mumps, rubella) vaccine.

Communicable: Capable of spreading disease. Also known as infectious.

Concomitant Event: An event, such as a medical condition, that occurs at the same time as another.

Contact: One who has been recently exposed to an infectious agent.

Contagious: Capable of being transmitted from one person to another by contact or close proximity.

Contaminate: To make unfit for use through the introduction of a substance that is harmful or injurious; to make impure or unclean.

Contraindication: Any circumstance or symptom that makes a method of treatment inadvisable in a particular case.

Controlled Clinical Trials: Trials in which the outcome of a group given one treatment is compared with the outcome of a group given no treatment or given a different treatment.

Cyclosporine: An immunosuppressant used after transplantation to prevent rejection.

Decompensated Cirrhosis: A late-stage cirrhosis accompanied by abnormal blood tests and other complications. At this stage of the disease, evaluation for liver transplant becomes an option.

DNA: Deoxyribonucleic acid; DNA molecules carry the genetic information necessary for the organization and functioning of most living cells and control the inheritance of characteristics.

DNA Polymerase: An enzyme essential to the replication of HBV DNA.

Edema: The puffiness that occurs from abnormal amounts of fluid in the spaces between cells in the body, especially just below the skin.

EIA: See Enzyme Immunoassay.

ELISA: See Enzyme-Linked Immunosorbent assay.

Encephalopathy: A variety of brain function abnormalities experienced by some patients with liver disease. These most commonly include confusion, disorientation, and insomnia, and may progress to coma.

End Treatment Response (ETR): Refers to response to medications at the end of therapy regime.

Enteric: Relating to, or being within the small intestine.

Enzyme Immunoassay (EIA): A test that provides information on the presence or amount of antibodies in the bloodstream. This test is sometimes referred to as an "ELISA."

Enzyme-Linked Immunosorbent Assay: This is a test that provides information on the presence or amount of antibodies in the bloodstream. This test is sometimes referred to as an "EIA."

Enzymes: Naturally occurring chemical substances in the human body that help a chemical reaction take place. High levels of these enzymes in blood may be a marker of disease.

Epidemic: The occurrence of disease within a specific geographical area or population that is in excess of what is normally expected.

Epidemiology: The study of the spread of diseases. Epidemiologists are often sent to investigate outbreaks.

Exposure: Coming in direct contact with an agent that might cause a disease or infectious process.

False Negative: Test result that indicates that an abnormality or disease is not present when, in fact, it is.

False Positive: Test result that indicates that an abnormality or disease is present when, in fact, it is not.

Fecal-Oral: Mode of transmission of an infectious agent from person to person by putting something in the mouth that has been contaminated with the stool of an infected person.

Fibrosis: Scar tissue developed as a result of chronic infection and inflammation. The presence of fibrosis usually means several years of active infection have taken place.

Flavivirus: A group of related viruses, including the viruses that cause yellow fever. Hepatitis C is a hepacivirus related to flavivirus.

Fulminant: Occurring suddenly, with lightning-like rapidity, and with great intensity or severity.

Gamma-Glutamyl Transferase: A liver enzyme that may be elevated in patients with hepatitis.

Genotype: A pattern of genetic information that is unique to a group of organisms or viruses. Doctors may determine the genotype of hepatitis C to help decide the best treatment.

GGT: See Gamma-Glutamyl Transferase.

HBeAb: See Hepatitis B e Antibody.

HBeAg: See Hepatitis B e Antigen.

HBIG: See Hepatitis B Immune Globulin.

HBsAg: See Hepatitis B Surface Antigen.

HBV DNA: See Hepatitis B Virus DNA (Deoxyribonucleic Acid).

HCV RNA: See Hepatitis C Virus RNA (Ribonucleic Acid).

Hemodialysis: The use of a machine to clean wastes from the blood after the kidneys have failed; the blood travels through tubes to a dialyzer, a machine that removes wastes and extra fluid; the cleaned blood then goes back into the body.

Hemophilia: A sex-linked hereditary blood defect that occurs almost exclusively in males and is characterized by delayed clotting of the blood and consequent difficulty in controlling hemorrhage even after minor injuries.

Hepatic: Related to the liver.

Hepatitis: An inflammation of the liver; the most common cause is infection with one of the five hepatitis viruses; hepatitis can also be caused by other viruses, bacteria, parasites, and toxic reactions to drugs, alcohol, and chemicals.

Hepatitis A: A liver disease caused by the hepatitis A virus (HAV). HAV is a 27-nm agent classified as a picornavirus and does not cause a chronic (long-lasting) illness. The virus is transmitted through close intimate contact with an infected person or through ingestion of contaminated food or water.

Hepatitis B: A liver disease caused by the Hepatitis B virus (HBV). HBV is found in the blood of infected persons and is most commonly transmitted through unprotected sex.

Hepatitis B Core Antibody (anti-HBc): Appears at the onset of symptoms in acute hepatitis B and persists for life. The presence of anti-HBc indicates previous or ongoing infection with HBV.

Hepatitis B e Antibody (HBeAb or anti-HBe): The corresponding antibody to hepatitis B e antigen. The presence indicates low levels of virus in the blood of an hepatitis B virus (HBV)-infected person; its presence also can indicate a good response to the treatment of chronic hepatitis B.

Hepatitis B e Antigen (HBeAg): A secreted product of the nucleocapsid gene of HBV and is found in serum during acute and chronic hepatitis B. Its presence indicates that the virus is replicating and the infected individual is potentially infectious.

Hepatitis B Immune Globulin (HBIG): A product available for prophylaxis against hepatitis B virus infection. HBIG is prepared from plasma containing high titers of anti-HBs and provides short-term protection (three to six months).

Hepatitis B Surface Antibody (anti-HBs): The presence of anti-HBs is generally interpreted as indicating recovery and immunity from HBV infection.

Hepatitis B Surface Antigen (HBsAg): A serologic marker on the surface of HBV. It can be detected in high levels in serum during acute or chronic hepatitis. The body normally produces antibodies to surface antigen as part of the normal immune response to infection.

Hepatitis B Virus DNA (Deoxyribonucleic Acid): Controls the manufacture of the hepatitis B virus. Presence of HBV DNA indicates active viral replication, with high levels of HBV DNA correlated with high rates of replication. HBV DNA levels are used to determine response to antiviral therapy.

Hepatitis C: A liver disease caused by the Hepatitis C virus (HCV), which is found in the blood of persons who have the disease. HCV is spread by contact with the blood of an infected person, most commonly through injection drug use.

Hepatitis C Virus RNA (Ribonucleic Acid): Fragments of the replicating hepatitis C virus (HCV). These can be detected using sophisticated testing to determine the level of hepatitis C virus present in the serum.

Hepatitis D: A liver disease caused by Hepatitis Delta virus (HDV). HDV is a defective virus that needs HBV to exist. HDV is found in the blood of persons infected with the virus and is transmitted in much the same way as HBV is transmitted; however the case fatality rate with HDV infection is higher than with Hepatitis B.

Hepatitis E: A disease of the liver caused by the Hepatitis E virus (HEV). HEV is transmitted in much the same way as HAV. Hepatitis E, however, does not often originate in the United States. Mortality is high among pregnant women who have hepatitis E.

Hepatocellular Carcinoma (HCC): Cancer of the liver cells that has progressed into a tumor.

HIV: Human immunodeficiency virus.

IDU: Injection Drug User.

IgM anti-HBc: Detected at onset of acute hepatitis B and persists for three to twelve months if the disease resolves. In patients who develop chronic hepatitis B, IgM anti-HBc persists at low levels as long as viral replication persists.

Immune Globulin (IG): Proteins found in the blood that function as antibodies that fight infection. Previously known as gamma globulin.

Immune System: The complex system in the body responsible for fighting disease. Its primary function is to identify foreign substances in the body (bacteria, viruses, fungi or parasites) and develop a defense against them. This defense is known as the immune response. It involves production of protein molecules called antibodies to eliminate foreign organisms that invade the body.

Immunity: Protection against a disease. There are two types of immunity, passive and active. Immunity is indicated by the presence of antibodies in the blood and can usually be determined with a laboratory test.

Immunity, Active: Resistance developed in response to an antigen (infecting agent or vaccine) and usually characterized by the presence of antibody produced by the host.

Immunity, Passive: Immunity conferred by an antibody produced in another host. This type of immunity can be acquired naturally by an infant from its mother or artificially by administration of an antibody-containing preparation (antiserum or immune globulin).

Immunization: The process by which a person or animal becomes protected against a disease.

Immunocompromised: Any condition in which the immune system functions in an abnormal or incomplete manner; such conditions are more frequent in the young, the elderly, and individuals undergoing extensive drug or radiation therapy.

Immunogenic: Producing immunity; capable of inducing an immune response; for example, hepatitis B vaccine produces a protective immune response in 90 to 95 percent of young healthy adults.

Immunoprophylaxis: Preventing the spread of disease by providing physiological immunity.

Immunosuppressants: Medicines that stop your immune system from attacking bacteria, viruses, and transplanted organs.

Immunosuppression: When the immune system is unable to protect the body from disease. This condition can be caused by disease (like AIDS) or by certain drugs (like those used in chemotherapy). Individuals whose immune systems are compromised should not receive live, attenuated vaccines.

Incidence: The number of new disease cases reported in a population over a certain period of time.

Incubation Period: The time from contact with infectious agents (bacteria or viruses) to onset of disease.

Infection: An invasion of an organism by a pathogen such as bacteria or viruses. Some infections lead to disease.

Infectious: Capable of spreading disease. Also known as communicable.

Infectious Agents: Organisms capable of spreading disease (e.g., bacteria or viruses).

Interferon: A protein produced naturally by the cells of our bodies; interferon increases the resistance of surrounding cells to attacks by viruses; one type of interferon, alpha interferon, is effective against certain types of cancer and is used in the treatment of chronic hepatitis B and chronic hepatitis C; others might prove effective in treating autoimmune diseases.

Intravenous Drug Abuse (IVDA): Acquiring an addiction to narcotic-type drugs that require intravenous administration. The intravenous use and abuse of recreational and other illegal drugs is a common route of transmission for hepatitis C infection.

Jaundice: A symptom of many disorders. Jaundice causes the skin and the whites of the eyes to turn yellow.

Lamivudine: FDA approved antiviral drug, administered by mouth, for use in treating chronic hepatitis B.

Liver: A large reddish-brown glandular organ located in the upper right portion of the abdominal cavity; secretes bile and functions in metabolism of protein, carbohydrate, and fat; synthesizes substances involved in the clotting of the blood; synthesizes vitamin A; detoxifies poisonous substances and breaks down worn-out erythrocytes; the liver is capable of repairing itself in some instances, but a person must have some liver function to survive; liver damage caused by HCV infection is the primary cause for liver transplantation.

Liver Enzymes: Proteins that catalyze chemical reactions needed for bodily functions. Levels of certain enzymes, such as ALT and AST, are higher when the liver is injured, as they leak into the bloodstream when the cell is injured or destroyed.

Marker: A device or substance used to indicate or mark something; an identifying characteristic or trait that allows apparently similar materials or disease conditions to be differentiated; this term is often used when discussing blood tests; for example, the hepatitis B surface antigen test is a serologic marker for current infectiousness with hepatitis B virus.

Microbes: Tiny organisms (including viruses and bacteria) that can be seen only with a microscope.

Morbidity: Any departure, subjective or objective, from a state of physiological or psychological well-being.

Mortality: The number of deaths in a given time or place.

MSM: Men who have sex with men.

Mycophenolate Mofetil: An immunosuppressant used after transplantation to prevent rejection.

Nosocomial: Referring to an infection acquired by a patient while in a hospital.

Onset: Beginning of the disease.

Organism: Any living thing. Organisms include humans, animals, plants, bacteria, protozoa, and fungi.

Outbreak: Sudden appearance of a disease in a specific geographic area (e.g., neighborhood or community) or population (e.g., adolescents).

Pandemic: An epidemic occurring over a very large area.

Parenteral: A route through which medicine can be taken into the body or given in a manner other than through the digestive tract (e.g., intravenous or intramuscular injection).

Passive Immunity: See Immunity, Passive.

Pathogens: Bacteria, viruses, parasites, or fungi that can cause disease.

Pegylated interferon: FDA approved antiviral drug for treatment of chronic hepatitis C in persons eighteen years and older; pegylated interferon remains active in the bloodstream longer and at a more constant level than standard interferon and can be given less often than standard interferon; combination therapy using pegylated interferon and ribavirin is the treatment of choice for chronic hepatitis C.

Percutaneous: Passed through the skin.

Pharmaceutical Clinical Trial: A carefully designed and executed investigation of the effects of a drug administered to human subjects; the goal is to define the clinical efficacy and pharmacological effects (toxicity, side effects, incompatibilities or interactions); the federal government requires strict testing of all new drugs before their approval for use as therapeutic agents.

Post-Exposure Prophylaxis (PEP): Prevention or treatment of disease after a possible exposure.

Prevalence: The number of disease cases (new and existing) within a population at a given time.

Prophylaxis: Measures designed to preserve health (as of an individual or of society) and prevent the spread of disease (e.g., HBIG and hepatitis B vaccine given to a baby born to an HBV infected mother is a prophylactic treatment to prevent perinatal HBV transmission).

Recombinant DNA: Genetic material that has been altered and recombined through insertion of new DNA sequences using bioengineering. Many drugs are now produced using recombinant DNA methods.

Recombinant Immunoblot Assay (RIBA): A test that provides detailed information on the level of HCV antibodies in the bloodstream.

Recreational Drugs: Illegal drugs, such as marijuana, cocaine, and heroin, that are used by people addicted to the drugs, or, if not addicted, who feel the effects of the drugs outweigh the risk factors associated with them.

Remission: Partial or complete disappearance—or a lessening of the severity—of symptoms of a disease. Remission may happen on its own or occur as a result of a medical treatment.

RIBA: See Recombinant immunoblot assay.

Ribavirin: An oral antiviral medication; when combined with interferon improves the effectiveness of interferon in treating chronic hepatitis C; combination therapy that includes pegylated interferon and ribavirin is the current treatment of choice for chronic hepatitis C.

Risk Factors: Certain behaviors (such as intravenous drug use or transfusions) linked to the development of an infection such as hepatitis.

RNA (Ribonucleic Acid): Molecules, found in all cells, that translate DNA genetic information into proteins.

Seroconversion: Development of antibodies in the blood of an individual who previously did not have detectable antibodies.

Serology: Measurement of antibodies, and other immunological properties, in the blood serum.

Seronegative: When the suspected substance being searched for, such as hepatitis C virus, does not show up in a blood test.

Seropositive: When the suspected substance being searched for, such as hepatitis C, does show up in a blood test.

Seroprevalence: The rate at which a given population tests positive for certain diseases or conditions at a certain point in time.

Serotype: An antigenic property of a cell (e.g., bacteria, RBC) or virus identified by serological methods.

Sexually Transmitted Disease (STD): A communicable disease transmitted by sexual intercourse or genital contact.

Side Effect: Undesirable reaction resulting from immunization or other medication or treatment.

Sirolimus: An immunosuppressant used after transplantation to prevent rejection.

Specimen: A portion or quantity of material for use in testing, examination, or study (e.g., stool specimen).

Sporadic: Occurring occasionally or in scattered instances.

STD: See Sexually transmitted disease.

Steroids: A group of immunosuppressants used after transplantation to prevent rejection.

Superinfection: A new infection caused by an organism different from that which caused the initial infection; the microbe responsible is usually resistant to the treatment given for the initial infection; for example, this term is used when a person with chronic hepatitis B contracts a superinfection with hepatitis Delta virus.

Susceptible: Unprotected against a certain disease.

Sustained Response (SR): Refers to the absence of virus in follow-up period six months after end of medication therapy.

Tacrolimus: An immunosuppressant used after transplantation to prevent rejection.

Thimerosal: A mercury-containing preservative used in some vaccines and other products since the 1930s. No harmful effects have been reported from thimerosal at doses used in vaccines, except for minor reactions like redness and swelling at the injection site. However, in July 1999, the Public Health Service (PHS) agencies, the American Academy of Pediatrics (AAP), and vaccine manufacturers agreed that thimerosal should be reduced or eliminated in vaccines as a precautionary measure. Today, all routinely recommended pediatric vaccines manufactured for the U.S. market contain no thimerosal or only trace amounts.

Transaminase: An older term for alanine aminotransferase (ALT) and aminotransferases (AST).

Transmission: Passing an infection or disease from one person to another.

True-Positive: A test result that accurately gives a positive reading.

Twinrix: Combined hepatitis A and hepatitis B vaccine manufactured by Glaxo-SmithKline.

Vaccination: Injection of a killed or weakened infectious organism in order to prevent the disease.

Vaccine: A product that produces immunity therefore protecting the body from the disease. Vaccines are administered through needle injections, by mouth, and by aerosol.

Viral Load: Measurement of the actual amount of virus in the bloodstream.

Viremia: The presence of a given virus in the bloodstream.

Virologic Response (VR): Refers to patients' loss of detectable HCV RNA during or after medication therapy.

Virus: A tiny organism that multiplies within cells and causes disease such as chickenpox, measles, mumps, rubella, pertussis, and hepatitis. Viruses are not affected by antibiotics, the drugs used to kill bacteria.

Chapter 57

Hepatitis Resources

General Information

American Liver Foundation (ALF)
75 Maiden Lane, Suite 603
New York, NY 10038-4810
Toll-Free: 800-GO-LIVER (465-4837) or 888-4HEP-USA (443-7872)
Phone: 212-668-1000
Fax: 212-483-8179
Website: www.liverfoundation.org
E-mail: info@liverfoundation.org

American Liver Society
952 Wemberton Drive
Nashville TN 37214
Phone: 615-210-4174
Website: http://liversociety.org
E-mail: info@liversociety.org

American Social Health Association
P.O. Box 13827
Research Triangle Park
NC 27709
Phone: 919-361-8400
Fax: 919-361-8425
Website: http://www.ashastd.org

Asian Liver Center at Stanford University
300 Pasteur Drive, H3680
Stanford, CA 94305
Toll-Free: 1-888-311-3331
Phone: 650-72-LIVER (650-725-4837)
Fax: 650-723-0006
Website: http://liver.stanford.edu

The information in this chapter was compiled from various sources deemed accurate. All contact information was verified and updated in May 2005. Inclusion does not imply endorsement. This list is intended to serve as a starting point for information gathering; it is not comprehensive.

Canadian Liver Foundation
2235 Sheppard Avenue East,
Suite 1500
Toronto, Ontario, M2J 5B5
Canada
Toll-Free: 800-563-5483
Phone: 416-491-3353
Fax: 416-491-4952
Website: http://www.liver.ca
E-mail: clf@liver.ca

Centers for Disease Control and Prevention (CDC)
Division of Viral Hepatitis
1600 Clifton Road
Mail Stop C-14
Atlanta, GA 30333
Toll-Free: 800-443-7232
Phone: 404-371-5900
Website: http://www.cdc.gov/hepatitis
E-mail: ncid@cdc.gov

Hepatitis Education Project
4603 Aurora Avenue N.
Seattle, WA 98103
Phone: 206-732-0311
Fax: 206-732-0312
Website: http://www.scn.org/health/hepatitis
E-mail: hep@scn.org

Hepatitis Foundation International (HFI)
504 Blick Drive
Silver Spring, MD 20904-2901
Toll-Free: 800-891-0707
Phone: 301-622-4200
Fax: 301-622-4702
Website: http://www.hepfi.org
E-mail: hfi@comcast.net

Hepatitis Information Network
Website: http://www.hepnet.com

National Digestive Diseases Information Clearinghouse (NDDIC)
2 Information Way
Bethesda, MD 20892-3570
Toll-Free: 800-891-5389
Fax: 703-738-4929
Website: http://digestive.niddk.nih.gov
E-mail: nddic@info.niddk.nih.gov

National Center for Complementary and Alternative Medicine (NCCAM)
P.O. Box 7923
Gaithersburg, MD 20898
Toll-Free: 888-644-6226
Phone: 301-519-3153
TTY: 866-464-3615
Fax: 866-464-3616
Website: http://nccam.nih.gov
E-mail: info@nccam.nih.gov

Parents of Kids with Infectious Diseases (PKIDS)
P.O. Box 5666
Vancouver, WA 98668
Toll-Free: 877-55-PKIDS
Phone: 360-695-0293
Fax: 360-695-6941
Website: http://www.pkids.org
E-mail: pkids@pkids.org

Clinical Trials

National Institutes of Health (NIH)

Clinical Center Communications
6100 Executive Blvd.
Suite 3C01
Bethesda, MD 20892
Toll-Free: 800-411-1222
Website: http://
www.clinicaltrials.gov

Food and Drug Administration (FDA)

Office of Special Health Issues
Parklawn Building, HF-12
5600 Fishers Lane
Rockville, MD 20857
Toll-Free: 888-463-6332
Website: http://www.fda.gov

Hepatitis and AIDS

National AIDS Treatment Advocacy Project (NATAP)

580 Broadway, Suite 1010
New York, NY 10012
Toll-Free: 888-26-NATAP
Phone: 212-219-0106
Fax: 212-219-8473
Website: http://www.natap.org
E-mail: info@natap.org

Hepatitis B

Hepatitis B Foundation

700 East Butler Avenue
Doylestown, PA 18901-2697
Phone: 215-489-4900
Fax: 215-489-4920
Website: http://www.hepb.org
E-mail: info@hepb.org

HPB Research Archive

Website: http://archive.mail-list.com/hbv_research

Hepatitis C

Hep C Connection

1177 Grant Street
Suite 200
Denver, CO 80203
Toll-Free: 800-522-HEPC
Phone: 303-860-0800
Website: http://www.
hepc-connection.org
E-mail: info@hepc-connection.org

Hepatitis C Foundation

1502 Russett Drive
Warminster, PA 18974
Phone: 215-672-2606
Website: http://
www.hepcfoundation.org

Hepatitis C Support Project

P.O. Box 427037
San Francisco, CA 94142-7037
Website: http://
www.hcvadvocate.org
E-mail:
alanfranciscus@hcvadvocate.org

Veterans Affairs National Hepatitis C Program

Toll-Free: 877-222-8387
Website: http://
www.hepatitis.va.gov

Liver Cancer

National Cancer Institute
Public Inquiries Office
Building 31, Room 10A31
31 Center Drive, MSC 2580
Bethesda, Maryland 20892-2580
Toll-Free: 800-4-CANCER (800-
422-6237)
Website: http://www.nci.nih.gov
E-mail: cancergovstaff@mail
.nih.gov

Liver Transplant

**United Network for Organ
Sharing (UNOS)**
Toll-Free: 888-TX-INFO-1 (888-
894-6361)
Website: http://www
.transplantliving.org

Index

Index

Page numbers followed by 'n' indicate a footnote. Page numbers in *italics* indicate a table or illustration.

A

abnormality, defined 529
"About Hepatitis B: Transmission and Symptoms" (Hepatitis B Foundation) 207n
acetaldehyde *see* alcoholic hepatitis
acetaminophen
    alcoholic hepatitis 62, 494
    alcohol use 13, 18
    chronic hepatitis C 444
    hepatitis 94
    hepatitis B immune globulin 216
    liver function 11, 22–25
    liver toxicity 26–27
acquired immune deficiency syndrome (AIDS), defined 529n
active immunity, defined 537
acute, defined 529
acute hepatitis, described 60
acute hepatitis B, described 67
acute hepatitis C
    defined 529
    described 76, 273

acute viral hepatitis, outlook 92
A.D.A.M., Inc., publications
    alanine transaminase test 38n
    albumin-serum test 46n
    alkaline phosphatase test 43n
    aspartate aminotransferase test 40n
    bilirubin test 48n
    hepatitis 59n
    hepatitis test 155n
"Additional Blood Tests" (Hepatitis B Foundation) 219n
adefovir 73, 234
adefovir dipivoxil
    defined 529
    described 203
    hepatitis B 151–52, *226*, 255
adenomas, oral contraceptives 33
adolescents
    alkaline phosphatase test 37
    hepatitis A vaccine 143, *144*
    hepatitis B vaccine 144, *145*
adverse events, defined 529
AFP *see* alpha-fetoprotein
African Americans, hepatitis 116–21
age factor
    alcoholic hepatitis 496
    hepatitis A 187
    immune globulin 195

Health Reference Series

COMPLETE CATALOG

List price $87 per volume. **School and library price $78 per volume.**

Adolescent Health Sourcebook

Basic Consumer Health Information about Common Medical, Mental, and Emotional Concerns in Adolescents, Including Facts about Acne, Body Piercing, Mononucleosis, Nutrition, Eating Disorders, Stress, Depression, Behavior Problems, Peer Pressure, Violence, Gangs, Drug Use, Puberty, Sexuality, Pregnancy, Learning Disabilities, and More

Along with a Glossary of Terms and Other Resources for Further Help and Information

Edited by Chad T. Kimball. 658 pages. 2002. 0-7808-0248-9.

"It is written in clear, nontechnical language aimed at general readers. . . . Recommended for public libraries, community colleges, and other agencies serving health care consumers."
— *American Reference Books Annual, 2003*

"Recommended for school and public libraries. Parents and professionals dealing with teens will appreciate the easy-to-follow format and the clearly written text. This could become a 'must have' for every high school teacher." — *E-Streams, Jan '03*

"A good starting point for information related to common medical, mental, and emotional concerns of adolescents." — *School Library Journal, Nov '02*

"This book provides accurate information in an easy to access format. It addresses topics that parents and caregivers might not be aware of and provides practical, useable information." — *Doody's Health Sciences Book Review Journal, Sep-Oct '02*

"Recommended reference source."
— *Booklist, American Library Association, Sep '02*

AIDS Sourcebook, 3rd Edition

Basic Consumer Health Information about Acquired Immune Deficiency Syndrome (AIDS) and Human Immunodeficiency Virus (HIV) Infection, Including Facts about Transmission, Prevention, Diagnosis, Treatment, Opportunistic Infections, and Other Complications, with a Section for Women and Children, Including Details about Associated Gynecological Concerns, Pregnancy, and Pediatric Care

Along with Updated Statistical Information, Reports on Current Research Initiatives, a Glossary, and Directories of Internet, Hotline, and Other Resources

Edited by Dawn D. Matthews. 664 pages. 2003. 0-7808-0631-X.

ALSO AVAILABLE: AIDS Sourcebook, 1st Edition. Edited by Karen Bellenir and Peter D. Dresser. 831 pages. 1995. 0-7808-0031-1.

AIDS Sourcebook, 2nd Edition. Edited by Karen Bellenir. 751 pages. 1999. 0-7808-0225-X.

"The 3rd edition of the *AIDS Sourcebook*, part of Omnigraphics' *Health Reference Series*, is a welcome update. . . . This resource is highly recommended for academic and public libraries."
— *American Reference Books Annual, 2004*

"Excellent sourcebook. This continues to be a highly recommended book. There is no other book that provides as much information as this book provides."
— *AIDS Book Review Journal, Dec-Jan 2000*

"Recommended reference source."
— *Booklist, American Library Association, Dec '99*

"A solid text for college-level health libraries."
— *The Bookwatch, Aug '99*

Cited in *Reference Sources for Small and Medium-Sized Libraries, American Library Association, 1999*

Alcoholism Sourcebook

Basic Consumer Health Information about the Physical and Mental Consequences of Alcohol Abuse, Including Liver Disease, Pancreatitis, Wernicke-Korsakoff Syndrome (Alcoholic Dementia), Fetal Alcohol Syndrome, Heart Disease, Kidney Disorders, Gastrointestinal Problems, and Immune System Compromise and Featuring Facts about Addiction, Detoxification, Alcohol Withdrawal, Recovery, and the Maintenance of Sobriety

Along with a Glossary and Directories of Resources for Further Help and Information

Edited by Karen Bellenir. 613 pages. 2000. 0-7808-0325-6.

"This title is one of the few reference works on alcoholism for general readers. For some readers this will be a welcome complement to the many self-help books on the market. Recommended for collections serving general readers and consumer health collections."
— *E-Streams, Mar '01*

"This book is an excellent choice for public and academic libraries."
— *American Reference Books Annual, 2001*

"Recommended reference source."
— *Booklist, American Library Association, Dec '00*

"Presents a wealth of information on alcohol use and abuse and its effects on the body and mind, treatment, and prevention." — *SciTech Book News, Dec '00*

"Important new health guide which packs in the latest consumer information about the problems of alcoholism." — *Reviewer's Bookwatch, Nov '00*

SEE ALSO Drug Abuse Sourcebook, Substance Abuse Sourcebook

Allergies Sourcebook, 2nd Edition

Basic Consumer Health Information about Allergic Disorders, Triggers, Reactions, and Related Symptoms, Including Anaphylaxis, Rhinitis, Sinusitis, Asthma, Dermatitis, Conjunctivitis, and Multiple Chemical Sensitivity

Along with Tips on Diagnosis, Prevention, and Treatment, Statistical Data, a Glossary, and a Directory of Sources for Further Help and Information

Edited by Annemarie S. Muth. 598 pages. 2002. 0-7808-0376-0.

ALSO AVAILABLE: Allergies Sourcebook, 1st Edition. Edited by Allan R. Cook. 611 pages. 1997. 0-7808-0036-2.

"This book brings a great deal of useful material together. . . . This is an excellent addition to public and consumer health library collections."
— American Reference Books Annual, 2003

"This second edition would be useful to laypersons with little or advanced knowledge of the subject matter. This book would also serve as a resource for nursing and other health care professions students. It would be useful in public, academic, and hospital libraries with consumer health collections." *— E-Streams, Jul '02*

Alternative Medicine Sourcebook, 2nd Edition

Basic Consumer Health Information about Alternative and Complementary Medical Practices, Including Acupuncture, Chiropractic, Herbal Medicine, Homeopathy, Naturopathic Medicine, Mind-Body Interventions, Ayurveda, and Other Non-Western Medical Traditions

Along with Facts about such Specific Therapies as Massage Therapy, Aromatherapy, Qigong, Hypnosis, Prayer, Dance, and Art Therapies, a Glossary, and Resources for Further Information

Edited by Dawn D. Matthews. 618 pages. 2002. 0-7808-0605-0.

ALSO AVAILABLE: Alternative Medicine Sourcebook, 1st Edition. Edited by Allan R. Cook. 737 pages. 1999. 0-7808-0200-4.

"Recommended for public, high school, and academic libraries that have consumer health collections. Hospital libraries that also serve the public will find this to be a useful resource." *— E-Streams, Feb '03*

"Recommended reference source."
— Booklist, American Library Association, Jan '03

"An important alternate health reference."
— MBR Bookwatch, Oct '02

"A great addition to the reference collection of every type of library." *— American Reference Books Annual, 2000*

Alzheimer's Disease Sourcebook, 3rd Edition

Basic Consumer Health Information about Alzheimer's Disease, Other Dementias, and Related Disorders, Including Multi-Infarct Dementia, AIDS Dementia Complex, Dementia with Lewy Bodies, Huntington's Disease, Wernicke-Korsakoff Syndrome (Alcohol-Reated Dementia), Delirium, and Confusional States

Along with Information for People Newly Diagnosed with Alzheimer's Disease and Caregivers, Reports Detailing Current Research Efforts in Prevention, Diagnosis, and Treatment, Facts about Long-Term Care Issues, and Listings of Sources for Additional Information

Edited by Karen Bellenir. 645 pages. 2003. 0-7808-0666-2.

ALSO AVAILABLE: Alzheimer's, Stroke & 29 Other Neurological Disorders Sourcebook, 1st Edition. Edited by Frank E. Bair. 579 pages. 1993. 1-55888-748-2.

ALSO AVAILABLE: Alzheimer's Disease Sourcebook, 2nd Edition. Edited by Karen Bellenir. 524 pages. 1999. 0-7808-0223-3.

"This very informative and valuable tool will be a great addition to any library serving consumers, students and health care workers."
— American Reference Books Annual, 2004

"This is a valuable resource for people affected by dementias such as Alzheimer's. It is easy to navigate and includes important information and resources."
— Doody's Review Service, Feb. 2004

"Recommended reference source."
— Booklist, American Library Association, Oct '99

SEE ALSO Brain Disorders Sourcebook

Arthritis Sourcebook, 2nd Edition

Basic Consumer Health Information about Osteoarthritis, Rheumatoid Arthritis, Other Rheumatic Disorders, Infectious Forms of Arthritis, and Diseases with Symptoms Linked to Arthritis, Featuring Facts about Diagnosis, Pain Management, and Surgical Therapies

Along with Coping Strategies, Research Updates, a Glossary, and Resources for Additional Help and Information

Edited by Amy L. Sutton. 593 pages. 2004. 0-7808-0667-0.

ALSO AVAILABLE: Arthritis Sourcebook, 1st Edition. Edited by Allan R. Cook. 550 pages. 1998. 0-7808-0201-2.

". . . accessible to the layperson."
— Reference and Research Book News, Feb '99

Asthma Sourcebook

Basic Consumer Health Information about Asthma, Including Symptoms, Traditional and Nontraditional Remedies, Treatment Advances, Quality-of-Life Aids,

Medical Research Updates, and the Role of Allergies, Exercise, Age, the Environment, and Genetics in the Development of Asthma

Along with Statistical Data, a Glossary, and Directories of Support Groups, and Other Resources for Further Information

Edited by Annemarie S. Muth. 628 pages. 2000. 0-7808-0381-7.

"A worthwhile reference acquisition for public libraries and academic medical libraries whose readers desire a quick introduction to the wide range of asthma information." *— Choice, Association of College & Research Libraries, Jun '01*

"Recommended reference source." *— Booklist, American Library Association, Feb '01*

"Highly recommended." *— The Bookwatch, Jan '01*

"There is much good information for patients and their families who deal with asthma daily." *— American Medical Writers Association Journal, Winter '01*

"This informative text is recommended for consumer health collections in public, secondary school, and community college and the libraries of universities with a large undergraduate population." *— American Reference Books Annual, 2001*

Attention Deficit Disorder Sourcebook

Basic Consumer Health Information about Attention Deficit/Hyperactivity Disorder in Children and Adults, Including Facts about Causes, Symptoms, Diagnostic Criteria, and Treatment Options Such as Medications, Behavior Therapy, Coaching, and Homeopathy

Along with Reports on Current Research Initiatives, Legal Issues, and Government Regulations, and Featuring a Glossary of Related Terms, Internet Resources, and a List of Additional Reading Material

Edited by Dawn D. Matthews. 470 pages. 2002. 0-7808-0624-7.

"Recommended reference source." *— Booklist, American Library Association, Jan '03*

"This book is recommended for all school libraries and the reference or consumer health sections of public libraries." *— American Reference Books Annual, 2003*

Back & Neck Sourcebook, 2nd Edition

Basic Consumer Health Information about Spinal Pain, Spinal Cord Injuries, and Related Disorders, Such as Degenerative Disk Disease, Osteoarthritis, Scoliosis, Sciatica, Spina Bifida, and Spinal Stenosis, and Featuring Facts about Maintaining Spinal Health, Self-Care, Pain Management, Rehabilitative Care, Chiropractic Care, Spinal Surgeries, and Complementary Therapies

Along with Suggestions for Preventing Back and Neck Pain, a Glossary of Related Terms, and a Directory of Resources

Edited by Amy L. Sutton. 633 pages. 2004. 0-7808-0738-3

ALSO AVAILABLE: *Back & Neck Disorders Sourcebook, 1st Edition.* Edited by Karen Bellenir. 548 pages. 1997. 0-7808-0202-0.

"The strength of this work is its basic, easy-to-read format. Recommended." *— Reference and User Services Quarterly, American Library Association, Winter '97*

Blood & Circulatory Disorders Sourcebook, 2nd Edition

Basic Consumer Health Information about the Blood and Circulatory System and Related Disorders, Such as Anemia and Other Hemoglobin Diseases, Cancer of the Blood and Associated Bone Marrow Disorders, Clotting and Bleeding Problems, and Conditions That Affect the Veins, Blood Vessels, and Arteries, Including Facts about the Donation and Transplantation of Bone Marrow, Stem Cells, and Blood and Tips for Keeping the Blood and Circulatory System Healthy

Along with a Glossary of Related Terms and Resources for Additional Help and Information

Edited by Amy L. Sutton. 659 pages. 2005. 0-7808-0746-4.

ALSO AVAILABLE: *Blood and Circulatory Disorders Sourcebook, 1st Edition.* Edited by Karen Bellenir and Linda M. Shin. 554 pages. 1998. 0-7808-0203-9.

"Recommended reference source." *— Booklist, American Library Association, Feb '99*

"An important reference sourcebook written in simple language for everyday, non-technical users." *— Reviewer's Bookwatch, Jan '99*

Brain Disorders Sourcebook, 2nd Edition

Basic Consumer Health Information about Acquired and Traumatic Brain Injuries, Infections of the Brain, Epilepsy and Seizure Disorders, Cerebral Palsy, and Degenerative Neurological Disorders, Including Amyotrophic Lateral Sclerosis (ALS), Dementias, Multiple Sclerosis, and More

Along with Information on the Brain's Structure and Function, Treatment and Rehabilitation Options, Reports on Current Research Initiatives, a Glossary of Terms Related to Brain Disorders and Injuries, and a Directory of Sources for Further Help and Information

Edited by Sandra J. Judd. 625 pages. 2005. 0-7808-0744-8.

ALSO AVAILABLE: *Brain Disorders Sourcebook, 1st Edition.* Edited by Karen Bellenir. 481 pages. 1999. 0-7808-0229-2.

"Belongs on the shelves of any library with a consumer health collection." *— E-Streams, Mar '00*

SEE ALSO *Alzheimer's Disease Sourcebook*

■

Breast Cancer Sourcebook, 2nd Edition

Basic Consumer Health Information about Breast Cancer, Including Facts about Risk Factors, Prevention, Screening and Diagnostic Methods, Treatment Options, Complementary and Alternative Therapies, Post-Treatment Concerns, Clinical Trials, Special Risk Populations, and New Developments in Breast Cancer Research

Along with Breast Cancer Statistics, a Glossary of Related Terms, and a Directory of Resources for Additional Help and Information

Edited by Sandra J. Judd. 595 pages. 2004. 0-7808-0668-9.

ALSO AVAILABLE: *Breast Cancer Sourcebook, 1st Edition.* Edited by Edward J. Prucha and Karen Bellenir. 580 pages. 2001. 0-7808-0244-6.

"It would be a useful reference book in a library or on loan to women in a support group."
—*Cancer Forum, Mar '03*

"Recommended reference source."
—*Booklist, American Library Association, Jan '02*

"This reference source is highly recommended. It is quite informative, comprehensive and detailed in nature, and yet it offers practical advice in easy-to-read language. It could be thought of as the 'bible' of breast cancer for the consumer." —*E-Streams, Jan '02*

"The broad range of topics covered in lay language make the *Breast Cancer Sourcebook* an excellent addition to public and consumer health library collections."
—*American Reference Books Annual 2002*

"From the pros and cons of different screening methods and results to treatment options, *Breast Cancer Sourcebook* provides the latest information on the subject."
—*Library Bookwatch, Dec '01*

"This thoroughgoing, very readable reference covers all aspects of breast health and cancer. . . . Readers will find much to consider here. Recommended for all public and patient health collections."
—*Library Journal, Sep '01*

SEE ALSO *Cancer Sourcebook for Women, Women's Health Concerns Sourcebook*

■

Breastfeeding Sourcebook

Basic Consumer Health Information about the Benefits of Breastmilk, Preparing to Breastfeed, Breastfeeding as a Baby Grows, Nutrition, and More, Including Information on Special Situations and Concerns Such as Mastitis, Illness, Medications, Allergies, Multiple Births, Prematurity, Special Needs, and Adoption

Along with a Glossary and Resources for Additional Help and Information

Edited by Jenni Lynn Colson. 388 pages. 2002. 0-7808-0332-9.

SEE ALSO *Pregnancy & Birth Sourcebook*

"Particularly useful is the information about professional lactation services and chapters on breastfeeding when returning to work. . . . *Breastfeeding Sourcebook* will be useful for public libraries, consumer health libraries, and technical schools offering nurse assistant training, especially in areas where Internet access is problematic."
—*American Reference Books Annual, 2003*

■

Burns Sourcebook

Basic Consumer Health Information about Various Types of Burns and Scalds, Including Flame, Heat, Cold, Electrical, Chemical, and Sun Burns

Along with Information on Short-Term and Long-Term Treatments, Tissue Reconstruction, Plastic Surgery, Prevention Suggestions, and First Aid

Edited by Allan R. Cook. 604 pages. 1999. 0-7808-0204-7.

"This is an exceptional addition to the series and is highly recommended for all consumer health collections, hospital libraries, and academic medical centers."
—*E-Streams, Mar '00*

"This key reference guide is an invaluable addition to all health care and public libraries in confronting this ongoing health issue."
—*American Reference Books Annual, 2000*

"Recommended reference source."
—*Booklist, American Library Association, Dec '99*

SEE ALSO *Skin Disorders Sourcebook*

■

Cancer Sourcebook, 4th Edition

Basic Consumer Health Information about Major Forms and Stages of Cancer, Featuring Facts about Head and Neck Cancers, Lung Cancers, Gastrointestinal Cancers, Genitourinary Cancers, Lymphomas, Blood Cell Cancers, Endocrine Cancers, Skin Cancers, Bone Cancers, Sarcomas, and Others, and Including Information about Cancer Treatments and Therapies, Identifying and Reducing Cancer Risks, and Strategies for Coping with Cancer and the Side Effects of Treatment

Along with a Cancer Glossary, Statistical and Demographic Data, and a Directory of Sources for Additional Help and Information

Edited by Karen Bellenir. 1,119 pages. 2003. 0-7808-0633-6.

ALSO AVAILABLE: *Cancer Sourcebook, 1st Edition.* Edited by Frank E. Bair. 932 pages. 1990. 1-55888-888-8.

New Cancer Sourcebook, 2nd Edition. Edited by Allan R. Cook. 1,313 pages. 1996. 0-7808-0041-9.

Cancer Sourcebook, 3rd Edition. Edited by Edward J. Prucha. 1,069 pages. 2000. 0-7808-0227-6.

"With cancer being the second leading cause of death for Americans, a prodigious work such as this one, which locates centrally so much cancer-related information, is clearly an asset to this nation's citizens and others."
— *Journal of the National Medical Association, 2004*

"This title is recommended for health sciences and public libraries with consumer health collections."
— *E-Streams, Feb '01*

". . . can be effectively used by cancer patients and their families who are looking for answers in a language they can understand. Public and hospital libraries should have it on their shelves."
— *American Reference Books Annual, 2001*

"Recommended reference source."
—*Booklist, American Library Association, Dec '00*

Cited in *Reference Sources for Small and Medium-Sized Libraries, American Library Association, 1999*

"The amount of factual and useful information is extensive. The writing is very clear, geared to general readers. Recommended for all levels." — *Choice, Association of College & Research Libraries, Jan '97*

SEE ALSO *Breast Cancer Sourcebook, Cancer Sourcebook for Women, Pediatric Cancer Sourcebook, Prostate Cancer Sourcebook*

Cancer Sourcebook for Women, 2nd Edition

Basic Consumer Health Information about Gynecologic Cancers and Related Concerns, Including Cervical Cancer, Endometrial Cancer, Gestational Trophoblastic Tumor, Ovarian Cancer, Uterine Cancer, Vaginal Cancer, Vulvar Cancer, Breast Cancer, and Common Non-Cancerous Uterine Conditions, with Facts about Cancer Risk Factors, Screening and Prevention, Treatment Options, and Reports on Current Research Initiatives

Along with a Glossary of Cancer Terms and a Directory of Resources for Additional Help and Information

Edited by Karen Bellenir. 604 pages. 2002. 0-7808-0226-8.

ALSO AVAILABLE: Cancer Sourcebook for Women, 1st Edition. Edited by Allan R. Cook and Peter D. Dresser. 524 pages. 1996. 0-7808-0076-1.

"An excellent addition to collections in public, consumer health, and women's health libraries."
— *American Reference Books Annual, 2003*

"Overall, the information is excellent, and complex topics are clearly explained. As a reference book for the consumer it is a valuable resource to assist them to make informed decisions about cancer and its treatments." — *Cancer Forum, Nov '02*

"Highly recommended for academic and medical reference collections." — *Library Bookwatch, Sep '02*

"This is a highly recommended book for any public or consumer library, being reader friendly and containing accurate and helpful information."
— *E-Streams, Aug '02*

"Recommended reference source."
— *Booklist, American Library Association, Jul '02*

SEE ALSO *Breast Cancer Sourcebook, Women's Health Concerns Sourcebook*

Cardiovascular Diseases & Disorders Sourcebook, 3rd Edition

Basic Consumer Health Information about Heart and Vascular Diseases and Disorders, Such as Angina, Heart Attacks, Arrhythmias, Cardiomyopathy, Valve Disease, Atherosclerosis, and Aneurysms, with Information about Managing Cardiovascular Risk Factors and Maintaining Heart Health, Medications and Procedures Used to Treat Cardiovascular Disorders, and Concerns of Special Significance to Women

long with Reports on Current Research Initiatives, a Glossary of Related Medical Terms, and a Directory of Sources for Further Help and Information

Edited by Sandra J. Judd. 713 pages. 2005. 0-7808-0739-1.

ALSO AVAILABLE: Heart Diseases & Disorders Sourcebook, 2nd Edition. Edited by Karen Bellenir. 612 pages. 2000. 0-7808-0238-1.

Cardiovascular Diseases & Disorders Sourcebook, 1st Edition. Edited by Karen Bellenir and Peter D. Dresser. 683 pages. 1995. 0-7808-0032-X.

"This work stands out as an imminently accessible resource for the general public. It is recommended for the reference and circulating shelves of school, public, and academic libraries."
—*American Reference Books Annual, 2001*

"Recommended reference source."
—*Booklist, American Library Association, Dec '00*

"Provides comprehensive coverage of matters related to the heart. This title is recommended for health sciences and public libraries with consumer health collections."
— *E-Streams, Oct '00*

SEE ALSO *Healthy Heart Sourcebook for Women*

Caregiving Sourcebook

Basic Consumer Health Information for Caregivers, Including a Profile of Caregivers, Caregiving Responsibilities and Concerns, Tips for Specific Conditions, Care Environments, and the Effects of Caregiving

Along with Facts about Legal Issues, Financial Information, and Future Planning, a Glossary, and a Listing of Additional Resources

Edited by Joyce Brennfleck Shannon. 600 pages. 2001. 0-7808-0331-0.

"Essential for most collections."
— *Library Journal, Apr 1, 2002*

"An ideal addition to the reference collection of any public library. Health sciences information professionals may also want to acquire the *Caregiving Source-*

575

book for their hospital or academic library for use as a ready reference tool by health care workers interested in aging and caregiving."   —*E-Streams, Jan '02*

"Recommended reference source."
—*Booklist, American Library Association, Oct '01*

Child Abuse Sourcebook

Basic Consumer Health Information about the Physical, Sexual, and Emotional Abuse of Children, with Additional Facts about Neglect, Munchausen Syndrome by Proxy (MSBP), Shaken Baby Syndrome, and Controversial Issues Related to Child Abuse, Such as Withholding Medical Care, Corporal Punishment, and Child Maltreatment in Youth Sports, and Featuring Facts about Child Protective Services, Foster Care, Adoption, Parenting Challenges, and Other Abuse Prevention Efforts

Along with a Glossary of Related Terms and Resources for Additional Help and Information

Edited by Dawn D. Matthews. 620 pages. 2004. 0-7808-0705-7.

Childhood Diseases & Disorders Sourcebook

Basic Consumer Health Information about Medical Problems Often Encountered in Pre-Adolescent Children, Including Respiratory Tract Ailments, Ear Infections, Sore Throats, Disorders of the Skin and Scalp, Digestive and Genitourinary Diseases, Infectious Diseases, Inflammatory Disorders, Chronic Physical and Developmental Disorders, Allergies, and More

Along with Information about Diagnostic Tests, Common Childhood Surgeries, and Frequently Used Medications, with a Glossary of Important Terms and Resource Directory

Edited by Chad T. Kimball. 662 pages. 2003. 0-7808-0458-9.

"This is an excellent book for new parents and should be included in all health care and public libraries."
—*American Reference Books Annual, 2004*

Colds, Flu & Other Common Ailments Sourcebook

Basic Consumer Health Information about Common Ailments and Injuries, Including Colds, Coughs, the Flu, Sinus Problems, Headaches, Fever, Nausea and Vomiting, Menstrual Cramps, Diarrhea, Constipation, Hemorrhoids, Back Pain, Dandruff, Dry and Itchy Skin, Cuts, Scrapes, Sprains, Bruises, and More

Along with Information about Prevention, Self-Care, Choosing a Doctor, Over-the-Counter Medications, Folk Remedies, and Alternative Therapies, and Including a Glossary of Important Terms and a Directory of Resources for Further Help and Information

Edited by Chad T. Kimball. 638 pages. 2001. 0-7808-0435-X.

"A good starting point for research on common illnesses. It will be a useful addition to public and consumer health library collections."
—*American Reference Books Annual 2002*

"Will prove valuable to any library seeking to maintain a current, comprehensive reference collection of health resources. . . . Excellent reference."
—*The Bookwatch, Aug '01*

"Recommended reference source."
—*Booklist, American Library Association, July '01*

Communication Disorders Sourcebook

Basic Information about Deafness and Hearing Loss, Speech and Language Disorders, Voice Disorders, Balance and Vestibular Disorders, and Disorders of Smell, Taste, and Touch

Edited by Linda M. Ross. 533 pages. 1996. 0-7808-0077-X.

"This is skillfully edited and is a welcome resource for the layperson. It should be found in every public and medical library."   —*Booklist Health Sciences Supplement, American Library Association, Oct '97*

Congenital Disorders Sourcebook

Basic Information about Disorders Acquired during Gestation, Including Spina Bifida, Hydrocephalus, Cerebral Palsy, Heart Defects, Craniofacial Abnormalities, Fetal Alcohol Syndrome, and More

Along with Current Treatment Options and Statistical Data

Edited by Karen Bellenir. 607 pages. 1997. 0-7808-0205-5.

"Recommended reference source."
—*Booklist, American Library Association, Oct '97*

SEE ALSO Pregnancy & Birth Sourcebook

Consumer Issues in Health Care Sourcebook

Basic Information about Health Care Fundamentals and Related Consumer Issues, Including Exams and Screening Tests, Physician Specialties, Choosing a Doctor, Using Prescription and Over-the-Counter Medications Safely, Avoiding Health Scams, Managing Common Health Risks in the Home, Care Options for Chronically or Terminally Ill Patients, and a List of Resources for Obtaining Help and Further Information

Edited by Karen Bellenir. 618 pages. 1998. 0-7808-0221-7.

"Both public and academic libraries will want to have a copy in their collection for readers who are interested in self-education on health issues."
—*American Reference Books Annual, 2000*

Contagious Diseases Sourcebook

Basic Consumer Health Information about Infectious Diseases Spread by Person-to-Person Contact through Direct Touch, Airborne Transmission, Sexual Contact, or Contact with Blood or Other Body Fluids, Including Hepatitis, Herpes, Influenza, Lice, Measles, Mumps, Pinworm, Ringworm, Severe Acute Respiratory Syndrome (SARS), Streptococcal Infections, Tuberculosis, and Others

Along with Facts about Disease Transmission, Antimicrobial Resistance, and Vaccines, with a Glossary and Directories of Resources for More Information

Edited by Karen Bellenir. 643 pages. 2004. 0-7808-0736-7.

Contagious & Non-Contagious Infectious Diseases Sourcebook

Basic Information about Contagious Diseases like Measles, Polio, Hepatitis B, and Infectious Mononucleosis, and Non-Contagious Infectious Diseases like Tetanus and Toxic Shock Syndrome, and Diseases Occurring as Secondary Infections Such as Shingles and Reye Syndrome

Along with Vaccination, Prevention, and Treatment Information, and a Section Describing Emerging Infectious Disease Threats

Edited by Karen Bellenir and Peter D. Dresser. 566 pages. 1996. 0-7808-0075-3.

Death & Dying Sourcebook

Basic Consumer Health Information for the Layperson about End-of-Life Care and Related Ethical and Legal Issues, Including Chief Causes of Death, Autopsies, Pain Management for the Terminally Ill, Life Support Systems, Insurance, Euthanasia, Assisted Suicide, Hospice Programs, Living Wills, Funeral Planning, Counseling, Mourning, Organ Donation, and Physician Training

Along with Statistical Data, a Glossary, and Listings of Sources for Further Help and Information

Edited by Annemarie S. Muth. 641 pages. 1999. 0-7808-0230-6.

Dental Care & Oral Health Sourcebook, 2nd Edition

Basic Consumer Health Information about Dental Care, Including Oral Hygiene, Dental Visits, Pain Management, Cavities, Crowns, Bridges, Dental Implants, and Fillings, and Other Oral Health Concerns, Such as Gum Disease, Bad Breath, Dry Mouth, Genetic and Developmental Abnormalities, Oral Cancers, Orthodontics, and Temporomandibular Disorders

Along with Updates on Current Research in Oral Health, a Glossary, a Directory of Dental and Oral Health Organizations, and Resources for People with Dental and Oral Health Disorders

Edited by Amy L. Sutton. 609 pages. 2003. 0-7808-0634-4.

ALSO AVAILABLE: Oral Health Sourcebook, 1st Edition. Edited by Allan R. Cook. 558 pages. 1997. 0-7808-0082-6.

Depression Sourcebook

Basic Consumer Health Information about Unipolar Depression, Bipolar Disorder, Postpartum Depression, Seasonal Affective Disorder, and Other Types of Depression in Children, Adolescents, Women, Men, the Elderly, and Other Selected Populations

Along with Facts about Causes, Risk Factors, Diagnostic Criteria, Treatment Options, Coping Strategies, Suicide Prevention, a Glossary, and a Directory of Sources for Additional Help and Information

Edited by Karen Belleni. 602 pages. 2002. 0-7808-0611-5.

Dermatological Disorders Sourcebook, 2nd Edition

Basic Consumer Health Information about Conditions and Disorders Affecting the Skin, Hair, and Nails, Such as Acne, Rosacea, Rashes, Dermatitis, Pigmentation Disorders, Birthmarks, Skin Cancer, Skin Injuries, Psoriasis, Scleroderma, and Hair Loss, Including Facts about Medications and Treatments for Dermatological Disorders and Tips for Maintaining Healthy Skin, Hair, and Nails

Along with Information about How Aging Affects the Skin, a Glossary of Related Terms, and a Directory of Resources for Additional Help and Information

Edited by Amy L. Sutton. 600 pages. 2005. 0-7808-0795-2.

ALSO AVAILABLE: *Skin Disorders Sourcebook, 1st Edition.* Edited by Allan R. Cook. 647 pages. 1997. 0-7808-0080-X.

". . . comprehensive, easily read reference book."
—*Doody's Health Sciences Book Reviews, Oct '97*

■

Diabetes Sourcebook, 3rd Edition

Basic Consumer Health Information about Type 1 Diabetes (Insulin-Dependent or Juvenile-Onset Diabetes), Type 2 Diabetes (Noninsulin-Dependent or Adult-Onset Diabetes), Gestational Diabetes, Impaired Glucose Tolerance (IGT), and Related Complications, Such as Amputation, Eye Disease, Gum Disease, Nerve Damage, and End-Stage Renal Disease, Including Facts about Insulin, Oral Diabetes Medications, Blood Sugar Testing, and the Role of Exercise and Nutrition in the Control of Diabetes

Along with a Glossary and Resources for Further Help and Information

Edited by Dawn D. Matthews. 622 pages. 2003. 0-7808-0629-8.

ALSO AVAILABLE: *Diabetes Sourcebook, 1st Edition.* Edited by Karen Bellenir and Peter D. Dresser. 827 pages. 1994. 1-55888-751-2.

Diabetes Sourcebook, 2nd Edition. Edited by Karen Bellenir. 688 pages. 1998. 0-7808-0224-1.

"This edition is even more helpful than earlier versions. . . . It is a truly valuable tool for anyone seeking readable and authoritative information on diabetes."
—*American Reference Books Annual, 2004*

"An invaluable reference." —*Library Journal, May '00*

Selected as one of the 250 "Best Health Sciences Books of 1999." —*Doody's Rating Service, Mar-Apr 2000*

"Provides useful information for the general public."
—*Healthlines, University of Michigan Health Management Research Center, Sep/Oct '99*

". . . provides reliable mainstream medical information . . . belongs on the shelves of any library with a consumer health collection." —*E-Streams, Sep '99*

"Recommended reference source."
—*Booklist, American Library Association, Feb '99*

Diet & Nutrition Sourcebook, 2nd Edition

Basic Consumer Health Information about Dietary Guidelines, Recommended Daily Intake Values, Vitamins, Minerals, Fiber, Fat, Weight Control, Dietary Supplements, and Food Additives

Along with Special Sections on Nutrition Needs throughout Life and Nutrition for People with Such Specific Medical Concerns as Allergies, High Blood Cholesterol, Hypertension, Diabetes, Celiac Disease, Seizure Disorders, Phenylketonuria (PKU), Cancer, and Eating Disorders, and Including Reports on Current Nutrition Research and Source Listings for Additional Help and Information

Edited by Karen Bellenir. 650 pages. 1999. 0-7808-0228-4.

ALSO AVAILABLE: *Diet & Nutrition Sourcebook, 1st Edition.* Edited by Dan R. Harris. 662 pages. 1996. 0-7808-0084-2.

"This book is an excellent source of basic diet and nutrition information." —*Booklist Health Sciences Supplement, American Library Association, Dec '00*

"This reference document should be in any public library, but it would be a very good guide for beginning students in the health sciences. If the other books in this publisher's series are as good as this, they should all be in the health sciences collections."
—*American Reference Books Annual, 2000*

"This book is an excellent general nutrition reference for consumers who desire to take an active role in their health care for prevention. Consumers of all ages who select this book can feel confident they are receiving current and accurate information." —*Journal of Nutrition for the Elderly, Vol. 19, No. 4, '00*

"Recommended reference source."
—*Booklist, American Library Association, Dec '99*

SEE ALSO *Digestive Diseases & Disorders Sourcebook, Eating Disorders Sourcebook, Gastrointestinal Diseases & Disorders Sourcebook, Vegetarian Sourcebook*

■

Digestive Diseases & Disorders Sourcebook

Basic Consumer Health Information about Diseases and Disorders that Impact the Upper and Lower Digestive System, Including Celiac Disease, Constipation, Crohn's Disease, Cyclic Vomiting Syndrome, Diarrhea, Diverticulosis and Diverticulitis, Gallstones, Heartburn, Hemorrhoids, Hernias, Indigestion (Dyspepsia), Irritable Bowel Syndrome, Lactose Intolerance, Ulcers, and More

Along with Information about Medications and Other Treatments, Tips for Maintaining a Healthy Digestive Tract, a Glossary, and Directory of Digestive Diseases Organizations

Edited by Karen Bellenir. 335 pages. 2000. 0-7808-0327-2.

"This title would be an excellent addition to all public or patient-research libraries."
—*American Reference Books Annual, 2001*

"This title is recommended for public, hospital, and health sciences libraries with consumer health collections." — *E-Streams, Jul-Aug '00*

"Recommended reference source." —*Booklist, American Library Association, May '00*

SEE ALSO *Diet & Nutrition Sourcebook, Eating Disorders Sourcebook, Gastrointestinal Diseases & Disorders Sourcebook*

■

Disabilities Sourcebook

Basic Consumer Health Information about Physical and Psychiatric Disabilities, Including Descriptions of Major Causes of Disability, Assistive and Adaptive Aids, Workplace Issues, and Accessibility Concerns

Along with Information about the Americans with Disabilities Act, a Glossary, and Resources for Additional Help and Information

Edited by Dawn D. Matthews. 616 pages. 2000. 0-7808-0389-2.

"It is a must for libraries with a consumer health section." — *American Reference Books Annual 2002*

"A much needed addition to the Omnigraphics *Health Reference Series*. A current reference work to provide people with disabilities, their families, caregivers or those who work with them, a broad range of information in one volume, has not been available until now. . . . It is recommended for all public and academic library reference collections." —*E-Streams, May '01*

"An excellent source book in easy-to-read format covering many current topics; highly recommended for all libraries." — *Choice, Association of College and Research Libraries, Jan '01*

"Recommended reference source." —*Booklist, American Library Association, Jul '00*

■

Domestic Violence Sourcebook, 2nd Edition

Basic Consumer Health Information about the Causes and Consequences of Abusive Relationships, Including Physical Violence, Sexual Assault, Battery, Stalking, and Emotional Abuse, and Facts about the Effects of Violence on Women, Men, Young Adults, and the Elderly, with Reports about Domestic Violence in Selected Populations, and Featuring Facts about Medical Care, Victim Assistance and Protection, Prevention Strategies, Mental Health Services, and Legal Issues

Along with a Glossary of Related Terms and Resources for Additional Help and Information

Edited by Dawn D. Matthews. 628 pages. 2004. 0-7808-0669-7.

ALSO AVAILABLE: *Domestic Violence & Child Abuse Sourcebook, 1st Edition.* Edited by Helene Henderson. 1,064 pages. 2001. 0-7808-0235-7.

"Interested lay persons should find the book extremely beneficial. . . . A copy of *Domestic Violence and Child*

Abuse Sourcebook should be in every public library in the United States." — *Social Science & Medicine, No. 56, 2003*

"This is important information. The Web has many resources but this sourcebook fills an important societal need. I am not aware of any other resources of this type." — *Doody's Review Service, Sep '01*

"Recommended for all libraries, scholars, and practitioners." — *Choice, Association of College & Research Libraries, Jul '01*

"Recommended reference source." — *Booklist, American Library Association, Apr '01*

"Important pick for college-level health reference libraries." — *The Bookwatch, Mar '01*

"Because this problem is so widespread and because this book includes a lot of issues within one volume, this work is recommended for all public libraries." — *American Reference Books Annual, 2001*

■

Drug Abuse Sourcebook, 2nd Edition

Basic Consumer Health Information about Illicit Substances of Abuse and the Misuse of Prescription and Over-the-Counter Medications, Including Depressants, Hallucinogens, Inhalants, Marijuana, Stimulants, and Anabolic Steroids

Along with Facts about Related Health Risks, Treatment Programs, Prevention Programs, a Glossary of Abuse and Addiction Terms, a Glossary of Drug-Related Street Terms, and a Directory of Resources for More Information

Edited by Catherine Ginther. 607 pages. 2004. 0-7808-0740-5.

ALSO AVAILABLE: *Drug Abuse Sourcebook, 1st Edition.* Edited by Karen Bellenir. 629 pages. 2000. 0-7808-0242-X.

"Containing a wealth of information . . . . This resource belongs in libraries that serve a lower-division undergraduate or community college clientele as well as the general public." — *Choice, Association of College and Research Libraries, Jun '01*

"Recommended reference source." — *Booklist, American Library Association, Feb '01*

"Highly recommended." — *The Bookwatch, Jan '01*

"Even though there is a plethora of books on drug abuse, this volume is recommended for school, public, and college libraries." — *American Reference Books Annual, 2001*

SEE ALSO *Alcoholism Sourcebook, Substance Abuse Sourcebook*

Ear, Nose & Throat Disorders Sourcebook

Basic Information about Disorders of the Ears, Nose, Sinus Cavities, Pharynx, and Larynx, Including Ear Infections, Tinnitus, Vestibular Disorders, Allergic and Non-Allergic Rhinitis, Sore Throats, Tonsillitis, and Cancers That Affect the Ears, Nose, Sinuses, and Throat

Along with Reports on Current Research Initiatives, a Glossary of Related Medical Terms, and a Directory of Sources for Further Help and Information

Edited by Karen Bellenir and Linda M. Shin. 576 pages. 1998. 0-7808-0206-3.

"Overall, this sourcebook is helpful for the consumer seeking information on ENT issues. It is recommended for public libraries."
— *American Reference Books Annual, 1999*

"Recommended reference source."
— *Booklist, American Library Association, Dec '98*

■

Eating Disorders Sourcebook

Basic Consumer Health Information about Eating Disorders, Including Information about Anorexia Nervosa, Bulimia Nervosa, Binge Eating, Body Dysmorphic Disorder, Pica, Laxative Abuse, and Night Eating Syndrome

Along with Information about Causes, Adverse Effects, and Treatment and Prevention Issues, and Featuring a Section on Concerns Specific to Children and Adolescents, a Glossary, and Resources for Further Help and Information

Edited by Dawn D. Matthews. 322 pages. 2001. 0-7808-0335-3.

"Recommended for health science libraries that are open to the public, as well as hospital libraries. This book is a good resource for the consumer who is concerned about eating disorders." — *E-Streams, Mar '02*

"This volume is another convenient collection of excerpted articles. Recommended for school and public library patrons; lower-division undergraduates; and two-year technical program students." — *Choice, Association of College & Research Libraries, Jan '02*

"Recommended reference source." — *Booklist, American Library Association, Oct '01*

SEE ALSO *Diet & Nutrition Sourcebook, Digestive Diseases & Disorders Sourcebook, Gastrointestinal Diseases & Disorders Sourcebook*

■

Emergency Medical Services Sourcebook

Basic Consumer Health Information about Preventing, Preparing for, and Managing Emergency Situations, When and Who to Call for Help, What to Expect in the Emergency Room, the Emergency Medical Team, Patient Issues, and Current Topics in Emergency Medicine

Along with Statistical Data, a Glossary, and Sources of Additional Help and Information

Edited by Jenni Lynn Colson. 494 pages. 2002. 0-7808-0420-1.

"Handy and convenient for home, public, school, and college libraries. Recommended."
— *Choice, Association of College and Research Libraries, Apr '03*

"This reference can provide the consumer with answers to most questions about emergency care in the United States, or it will direct them to a resource where the answer can be found."
— *American Reference Books Annual, 2003*

"Recommended reference source."
— *Booklist, American Library Association, Feb '03*

■

Endocrine & Metabolic Disorders Sourcebook

Basic Information for the Layperson about Pancreatic and Insulin-Related Disorders Such as Pancreatitis, Diabetes, and Hypoglycemia; Adrenal Gland Disorders Such as Cushing's Syndrome, Addison's Disease, and Congenital Adrenal Hyperplasia; Pituitary Gland Disorders Such as Growth Hormone Deficiency, Acromegaly, and Pituitary Tumors; Thyroid Disorders Such as Hypothyroidism, Graves' Disease, Hashimoto's Disease, and Goiter; Hyperparathyroidism; and Other Diseases and Syndromes of Hormone Imbalance or Metabolic Dysfunction

Along with Reports on Current Research Initiatives

Edited by Linda M. Shin. 574 pages. 1998. 0-7808-0207-1.

"Omnigraphics has produced another needed resource for health information consumers."
— *American Reference Books Annual, 2000*

"Recommended reference source."
— *Booklist, American Library Association, Dec '98*

■

Environmental Health Sourcebook, 2nd Edition

Basic Consumer Health Information about the Environment and Its Effect on Human Health, Including the Effects of Air Pollution, Water Pollution, Hazardous Chemicals, Food Hazards, Radiation Hazards, Biological Agents, Household Hazards, Such as Radon, Asbestos, Carbon Monoxide, and Mold, and Information about Associated Diseases and Disorders, Including Cancer, Allergies, Respiratory Problems, and Skin Disorders

Along with Information about Environmental Concerns for Specific Populations, a Glossary of Related Terms, and Resources for Further Help and Information

Edited by Dawn D. Matthews. 673 pages. 2003. 0-7808-0632-8.

ALSO AVAILABLE: *Environmentally Induced Disorders Sourcebook, 1st Edition.* Edited by Allan R. Cook. 620 pages. 1997. 0-7808-0083-4.

"This recently updated edition continues the level of quality and the reputation of the numerous other volumes in Omnigraphics' *Health Reference Series*."
— *American Reference Books Annual, 2004*

"Recommended reference source."
— *Booklist, American Library Association, Sep '98*

"This book will be a useful addition to anyone's library." — *Choice Health Sciences Supplement, Association of College and Research Libraries, May '98*

". . . a good survey of numerous environmentally induced physical disorders . . . a useful addition to anyone's library."
— *Doody's Health Sciences Book Reviews, Jan '98*

". . . provide[s] introductory information from the best authorities around. Since this volume covers topics that potentially affect everyone, it will surely be one of the most frequently consulted volumes in the *Health Reference Series*." — *Rettig on Reference, Nov '97*

Environmentally Induced Disorders Sourcebook, 1st Edition

SEE *Environmental Health Sourcebook, 2nd Edition*

Ethnic Diseases Sourcebook

Basic Consumer Health Information for Ethnic and Racial Minority Groups in the United States, Including General Health Indicators and Behaviors, Ethnic Diseases, Genetic Testing, the Impact of Chronic Diseases, Women's Health, Mental Health Issues, and Preventive Health Care Services

Along with a Glossary and a Listing of Additional Resources

Edited by Joyce Brennfleck Shannon. 664 pages. 2001. 0-7808-0336-1.

"Recommended for health sciences libraries where public health programs are a priority."
— *E-Streams, Jan '02*

"Not many books have been written on this topic to date, and the *Ethnic Diseases Sourcebook* is a strong addition to the list. It will be an important introductory resource for health consumers, students, health care personnel, and social scientists. It is recommended for public, academic, and large hospital libraries."
— *American Reference Books Annual 2002*

"Recommended reference source."
— *Booklist, American Library Association, Oct '01*

"Will prove valuable to any library seeking to maintain a current, comprehensive reference collection of health resources. . . . An excellent source of health information about genetic disorders which affect particular ethnic and racial minorities in the U.S."
— *The Bookwatch, Aug '01*

Eye Care Sourcebook, 2nd Edition

Basic Consumer Health Information about Eye Care and Eye Disorders, Including Facts about the Diagnosis, Prevention, and Treatment of Common Refractive Problems Such as Myopia, Hyperopia, Astigmatism, and Presbyopia, and Eye Diseases, Including Glaucoma, Cataract, Age-Related Macular Degeneration, and Diabetic Retinopathy

Along with a Section on Vision Correction and Refractive Surgeries, Including LASIK and LASEK, a Glossary, and Directories of Resources for Additional Help and Information

Edited by Amy L. Sutton. 543 pages. 2003. 0-7808-0635-2.

ALSO AVAILABLE: Ophthalmic Disorders Sourcebook, 1st Edition. Edited by Linda M. Ross. 631 pages. 1996. 0-7808-0081-8.

". . . a solid reference tool for eye care and a valuable addition to a collection."
— *American Reference Books Annual, 2004*

Family Planning Sourcebook

Basic Consumer Health Information about Planning for Pregnancy and Contraception, Including Traditional Methods, Barrier Methods, Hormonal Methods, Permanent Methods, Future Methods, Emergency Contraception, and Birth Control Choices for Women at Each Stage of Life

Along with Statistics, a Glossary, and Sources of Additional Information

Edited by Amy Marcaccio Keyzer. 520 pages. 2001. 0-7808-0379-5.

"Recommended for public, health, and undergraduate libraries as part of the circulating collection."
— *E-Streams, Mar '02*

"Information is presented in an unbiased, readable manner, and the sourcebook will certainly be a necessary addition to those public and high school libraries where Internet access is restricted or otherwise problematic." — *American Reference Books Annual 2002*

"Recommended reference source."
— *Booklist, American Library Association, Oct '01*

"Will prove valuable to any library seeking to maintain a current, comprehensive reference collection of health resources. . . . Excellent reference."
— *The Bookwatch, Aug '01*

SEE ALSO *Pregnancy & Birth Sourcebook*

Fitness & Exercise Sourcebook, 2nd Edition

Basic Consumer Health Information about the Fundamentals of Fitness and Exercise, Including How to Begin and Maintain a Fitness Program, Fitness as a Lifestyle, the Link between Fitness and Diet, Advice for Specific Groups of People, Exercise as It Relates to Specific Medical Conditions, and Recent Research in Fitness and Exercise

Along with a Glossary of Important Terms and Resources for Additional Help and Information

Edited by Kristen M. Gledhill. 646 pages. 2001. 0-7808-0334-5.

ALSO AVAILABLE: Fitness & Exercise Sourcebook, 1st Edition. Edited by Dan R. Harris. 663 pages. 1996. 0-7808-0186-5.

"This work is recommended for all general reference collections."
— *American Reference Books Annual 2002*

"Highly recommended for public, consumer, and school grades fourth through college."
— *E-Streams, Nov '01*

"Recommended reference source." — *Booklist, American Library Association, Oct '01*

"The information appears quite comprehensive and is considered reliable. . . . This second edition is a welcomed addition to the series."
— *Doody's Review Service, Sep '01*

"This reference is a valuable choice for those who desire a broad source of information on exercise, fitness, and chronic-disease prevention through a healthy lifestyle."
— *American Medical Writers Association Journal, Fall '01*

"Will prove valuable to any library seeking to maintain a current, comprehensive reference collection of health resources. . . . Excellent reference."
— *The Bookwatch, Aug '01*

■

Food & Animal Borne Diseases Sourcebook

Basic Information about Diseases That Can Be Spread to Humans through the Ingestion of Contaminated Food or Water or by Contact with Infected Animals and Insects, Such as Botulism, E. Coli, Hepatitis A, Trichinosis, Lyme Disease, and Rabies

Along with Information Regarding Prevention and Treatment Methods, and Including a Special Section for International Travelers Describing Diseases Such as Cholera, Malaria, Travelers' Diarrhea, and Yellow Fever, and Offering Recommendations for Avoiding Illness

Edited by Karen Bellenir and Peter D. Dresser. 535 pages. 1995. 0-7808-0033-8.

"Targeting general readers and providing them with a single, comprehensive source of information on selected topics, this book continues, with the excellent caliber of its predecessors, to catalog topical information on health matters of general interest. Readable and thorough, this valuable resource is highly recommended for all libraries."
— *Academic Library Book Review, Summer '96*

"A comprehensive collection of authoritative information."
— *Emergency Medical Services, Oct '95*

Food Safety Sourcebook

Basic Consumer Health Information about the Safe Handling of Meat, Poultry, Seafood, Eggs, Fruit Juices, and Other Food Items, and Facts about Pesticides, Drinking Water, Food Safety Overseas, and the Onset, Duration, and Symptoms of Foodborne Illnesses, Including Types of Pathogenic Bacteria, Parasitic Protozoa, Worms, Viruses, and Natural Toxins

Along with the Role of the Consumer, the Food Handler, and the Government in Food Safety; a Glossary, and Resources for Additional Help and Information

Edited by Dawn D. Matthews. 339 pages. 1999. 0-7808-0326-4.

"This book is recommended for public libraries and universities with home economic and food science programs."
— *E-Streams, Nov '00*

"Recommended reference source."
— *Booklist, American Library Association, May '00*

"This book takes the complex issues of food safety and foodborne pathogens and presents them in an easily understood manner. [It does] an excellent job of covering a large and often confusing topic."
— *American Reference Books Annual, 2000*

■

Forensic Medicine Sourcebook

Basic Consumer Information for the Layperson about Forensic Medicine, Including Crime Scene Investigation, Evidence Collection and Analysis, Expert Testimony, Computer-Aided Criminal Identification, Digital Imaging in the Courtroom, DNA Profiling, Accident Reconstruction, Autopsies, Ballistics, Drugs and Explosives Detection, Latent Fingerprints, Product Tampering, and Questioned Document Examination

Along with Statistical Data, a Glossary of Forensics Terminology, and Listings of Sources for Further Help and Information

Edited by Annemarie S. Muth. 574 pages. 1999. 0-7808-0232-2.

"Given the expected widespread interest in its content and its easy to read style, this book is recommended for most public and all college and university libraries."
— *E-Streams, Feb '01*

"Recommended for public libraries."
— *Reference & User Services Quarterly, American Library Association, Spring 2000*

"Recommended reference source."
— *Booklist, American Library Association, Feb '00*

"A wealth of information, useful statistics, references are up-to-date and extremely complete. This wonderful collection of data will help students who are interested in a career in any type of forensic field. It is a great resource for attorneys who need information about types of expert witnesses needed in a particular case. It also offers useful information for fiction and nonfiction writers whose work involves a crime. A fascinating compilation. All levels." — *Choice, Association of College and Research Libraries, Jan 2000*

"There are several items that make this book attractive to consumers who are seeking certain forensic data.... This is a useful current source for those seeking general forensic medical answers."
— American Reference Books Annual, 2000

Gastrointestinal Diseases & Disorders Sourcebook

Basic Information about Gastroesophageal Reflux Disease (Heartburn), Ulcers, Diverticulosis, Irritable Bowel Syndrome, Crohn's Disease, Ulcerative Colitis, Diarrhea, Constipation, Lactose Intolerance, Hemorrhoids, Hepatitis, Cirrhosis, and Other Digestive Problems, Featuring Statistics, Descriptions of Symptoms, and Current Treatment Methods of Interest for Persons Living with Upper and Lower Gastrointestinal Maladies

Edited by Linda M. Ross. 413 pages. 1996. 0-7808-0078-8.

". . . very readable form. The successful editorial work that brought this material together into a useful and understandable reference makes accessible to all readers information that can help them more effectively understand and obtain help for digestive tract problems."
— Choice, Association of College & Research Libraries, Feb '97

SEE ALSO Diet & Nutrition Sourcebook, Digestive Diseases & Disorders, Eating Disorders Sourcebook

---

Genetic Disorders Sourcebook, 3rd Edition

Basic Consumer Health Information about Hereditary Diseases and Disorders, Including Facts about the Human Genome, Genetic Inheritance Patterns, Disorders Associated with Specific Genes, Such as Sickle Cell Disease, Hemophilia, and Cystic Fibrosis, Chromosome Disorders, Such as Down Syndrome, Fragile X Syndrome, and Turner Syndrome, and Complex Diseases and Disorders Resulting from the Interaction of Environmental and Genetic Factors, Such as Allergies, Cancer, and Obesity

Along with Facts about Genetic Testing, Suggestions for Parents of Children with Special Needs, Reports on Current Research Initiatives, a Glossary of Genetic Terminology, and Resources for Additional Help and Information

Edited by Karen Bellenir. 777 pages. 2004. 0-7808-0742-1.

ALSO AVAILABLE: Genetic Disorders Sourcebook, 1st Edition. Edited by Karen Bellenir. 642 pages. 1996. 0-7808-0034-6.

Genetic Disorders Sourcebook, 2nd Edition. Edited by Kathy Massimini. 768 pages. 2001. 0-7808-0241-1.

"Recommended for public libraries and medical and hospital libraries with consumer health collections."
— E-Streams, May '01

"Recommended reference source."
— Booklist, American Library Association, Apr '01

"Important pick for college-level health reference libraries."
— The Bookwatch, Mar '01

"Provides essential medical information to both the general public and those diagnosed with a serious or fatal genetic disease or disorder."
— Choice, Association of College and Research Libraries, Jan '97

Head Trauma Sourcebook

Basic Information for the Layperson about Open-Head and Closed-Head Injuries, Treatment Advances, Recovery, and Rehabilitation

Along with Reports on Current Research Initiatives

Edited by Karen Bellenir. 414 pages. 1997. 0-7808-0208-X.

Headache Sourcebook

Basic Consumer Health Information about Migraine, Tension, Cluster, Rebound and Other Types of Headaches, with Facts about the Cause and Prevention of Headaches, the Effects of Stress and the Environment, Headaches during Pregnancy and Menopause, and Childhood Headaches

Along with a Glossary and Other Resources for Additional Help and Information

Edited by Dawn D. Matthews. 362 pages. 2002. 0-7808-0337-X.

"Highly recommended for academic and medical reference collections."
— Library Bookwatch, Sep '02

Health Insurance Sourcebook

Basic Information about Managed Care Organizations, Traditional Fee-for-Service Insurance, Insurance Portability and Pre-Existing Conditions Clauses, Medicare, Medicaid, Social Security, and Military Health Care

Along with Information about Insurance Fraud

Edited by Wendy Wilcox. 530 pages. 1997. 0-7808-0222-5.

"Particularly useful because it brings much of this information together in one volume. This book will be a handy reference source in the health sciences library, hospital library, college and university library, and medium to large public library."
— Medical Reference Services Quarterly, Fall '98

Awarded "Books of the Year Award"
— American Journal of Nursing, 1997

"The layout of the book is particularly helpful as it provides easy access to reference material. A most useful addition to the vast amount of information about health insurance. The use of data from U.S. government agencies is most commendable. Useful in a library or learning center for healthcare professional students."
— Doody's Health Sciences Book Reviews, Nov '97

Health Reference Series Cumulative Index 1999

A Comprehensive Index to the Individual Volumes of the Health Reference Series, Including a Subject Index, Name Index, Organization Index, and Publication Index

Along with a Master List of Acronyms and Abbreviations

Edited by Edward J. Prucha, Anne Holmes, and Robert Rudnick. 990 pages. 2000. 0-7808-0382-5.

"This volume will be most helpful in libraries that have a relatively complete collection of the Health Reference Series." —*American Reference Books Annual, 2001*

"Essential for collections that hold any of the numerous *Health Reference Series* titles." —*Choice, Association of College and Research Libraries, Nov '00*

◼

Healthy Aging Sourcebook

Basic Consumer Health Information about Maintaining Health through the Aging Process, Including Advice on Nutrition, Exercise, and Sleep, Help in Making Decisions about Midlife Issues and Retirement, and Guidance Concerning Practical and Informed Choices in Health Consumerism

Along with Data Concerning the Theories of Aging, Different Experiences in Aging by Minority Groups, and Facts about Aging Now and Aging in the Future; and Featuring a Glossary, a Guide to Consumer Help, Additional Suggested Reading, and Practical Resource Directory

Edited by Jenifer Swanson. 536 pages. 1999. 0-7808-0390-6.

"Recommended reference source." —*Booklist, American Library Association, Feb '00*

SEE ALSO *Physical & Mental Issues in Aging Sourcebook*

◼

Healthy Children Sourcebook

Basic Consumer Health Information about the Physical and Mental Development of Children between the Ages of 3 and 12, Including Routine Health Care, Preventative Health Services, Safety and First Aid, Healthy Sleep, Dental Care, Nutrition, and Fitness, and Featuring Parenting Tips on Such Topics as Bedwetting, Choosing Day Care, Monitoring TV and Other Media, and Establishing a Foundation for Substance Abuse Prevention

Along with a Glossary of Commonly Used Pediatric Terms and Resources for Additional Help and Information.

Edited by Chad T. Kimball. 647 pages. 2003. 0-7808-0247-0.

"It is hard to imagine that any other single resource exists that would provide such a comprehensive guide of timely information on health promotion and disease prevention for children aged 3 to 12."

—*American Reference Books Annual, 2004*

"The strengths of this book are many. It is clearly written, presented and structured." —*Journal of the National Medical Association, 2004*

◼

Healthy Heart Sourcebook for Women

Basic Consumer Health Information about Cardiac Issues Specific to Women, Including Facts about Major Risk Factors and Prevention, Treatment and Control Strategies, and Important Dietary Issues

Along with a Special Section Regarding the Pros and Cons of Hormone Replacement Therapy and Its Impact on Heart Health, and Additional Help, Including Recipes, a Glossary, and a Directory of Resources

Edited by Dawn D. Matthews. 336 pages. 2000. 0-7808-0329-9.

"A good reference source and recommended for all public, academic, medical, and hospital libraries." —*Medical Reference Services Quarterly, Summer '01*

"Because of the lack of information specific to women on this topic, this book is recommended for public libraries and consumer libraries." —*American Reference Books Annual, 2001*

"Contains very important information about coronary artery disease that all women should know. The information is current and presented in an easy-to-read format. The book will make a good addition to any library." —*American Medical Writers Association Journal, Summer '00*

"Important, basic reference." —*Reviewer's Bookwatch, Jul '00*

SEE ALSO *Heart Diseases & Disorders Sourcebook, Women's Health Concerns Sourcebook*

◼

Heart Diseases & Disorders Sourcebook, 2nd Edition

SEE *Cardiovascular Diseases & Disorders Sourcebook, 3rd Edition*

◼

Hepatitis Sourcebook

Basic Consumer Health Information about Hepatitis A, Hepatitis B, Hepatitis C, and Other Forms of Hepatitis, Including Autoimmune Hepatitis, Alcoholic Hepatitis, Nonalcoholic Steatohepatitis, and Toxic Hepatitis, with Facts about Risk Factors, Screening Methods, Diagnostic Tests, and Treatment Options

Along with Information on Liver Health, Tips for People Living with Chronic Hepatitis, Reports on Current Research Initiatives, a Glossary of Terms Related to Hepatitis, and a Directory of Sources for Further Help and Information

Edited by Sandra J. Judd. 597 pages. 2005. 0-7808-0749-9.

Household Safety Sourcebook

Basic Consumer Health Information about Household Safety, Including Information about Poisons, Chemicals, Fire, and Water Hazards in the Home

Along with Advice about the Safe Use of Home Maintenance Equipment, Choosing Toys and Nursery Furniture, Holiday and Recreation Safety, a Glossary, and Resources for Further Help and Information

Edited by Dawn D. Matthews. 606 pages. 2002. 0-7808-0338-8.

"This work will be useful in public libraries with large consumer health and wellness departments."
— *American Reference Books Annual, 2003*

"As a sourcebook on household safety this book meets its mark. It is encyclopedic in scope and covers a wide range of safety issues that are commonly seen in the home." — *E-Streams, Jul '02*

Hypertension Sourcebook

Basic Consumer Health Information about the Causes, Diagnosis, and Treatment of High Blood Pressure, with Facts about Consequences, Complications, and Co-Occurring Disorders, Such as Coronary Heart Disease, Diabetes, Stroke, Kidney Disease, and Hypertensive Retinopathy, and Issues in Blood Pressure Control, Including Dietary Choices, Stress Management, and Medications

Along with Reports on Current Research Initiatives and Clinical Trials, a Glossary, and Resources for Additional Help and Information

Edited by Dawn D. Matthews and Karen Bellenir. 613 pages. 2004. 0-7808-0674-3.

Immune System Disorders Sourcebook, 2nd Edition

Basic Consumer Health Information about Disorders of the Immune System, Including Immune System Function and Response, Diagnosis of Immune Disorders, Information about Inherited Immune Disease, Acquired Immune Disease, and Autoimmune Diseases, Including Primary Immune Deficiency, Acquired Immunodeficiency Syndrome (AIDS), Lupus, Multiple Sclerosis, Type 1 Diabetes, Rheumatoid Arthritis, and Graves Disease

Along with Treatments, Tips for Coping with Immune Disorders, a Glossary, and a Directory of Additional Resources

Edited by Joyce Brennfleck Shannon. 671 pages. 2005. 0-7808-0748-0.

ALSO AVAILABLE: *Immune System Disorders Sourcebook.* Edited by Allan R. Cook. 608 pages. 1997. 0-7808-0209-8.

Infant & Toddler Health Sourcebook

Basic Consumer Health Information about the Physical and Mental Development of Newborns, Infants, and Toddlers, Including Neonatal Concerns, Nutrition Recommendations, Immunization Schedules, Common Pediatric Disorders, Assessments and Milestones, Safety Tips, and Advice for Parents and Other Caregivers

Along with a Glossary of Terms and Resource Listings for Additional Help

Edited by Jenifer Swanson. 585 pages. 2000. 0-7808-0246-2.

"As a reference for the general public, this would be useful in any library." — *E-Streams, May '01*

"Recommended reference source."
— *Booklist, American Library Association, Feb '01*

"This is a good source for general use."
— *American Reference Books Annual, 2001*

Infectious Diseases Sourcebook

Basic Consumer Health Information about Non-Contagious Bacterial, Viral, Prion, Fungal, and Parasitic Diseases Spread by Food and Water, Insects and Animals, or Environmental Contact, Including Botulism, E. Coli, Encephalitis, Legionnaires' Disease, Lyme Disease, Malaria, Plague, Rabies, Salmonella, Tetanus, and Others, and Facts about Newly Emerging Diseases, Such as Hantavirus, Mad Cow Disease, Monkeypox, and West Nile Virus

Along with Information about Preventing Disease Transmission, the Threat of Bioterrorism, and Current Research Initiatives, with a Glossary and Directory of Resources for More Information

Edited by Karen Bellenir. 634 pages. 2004. 0-7808-0675-1.

Injury & Trauma Sourcebook

Basic Consumer Health Information about the Impact of Injury, the Diagnosis and Treatment of Common and Traumatic Injuries, Emergency Care, and Specific Injuries Related to Home, Community, Workplace, Transportation, and Recreation

Along with Guidelines for Injury Prevention, a Glossary, and a Directory of Additional Resources

Edited by Joyce Brennfleck Shannon. 696 pages. 2002. 0-7808-0421-X.

"This publication is the most comprehensive work of its kind about injury and trauma."
— *American Reference Books Annual, 2003*

"This sourcebook provides concise, easily readable, basic health information about injuries. . . . This book is well organized and an easy to use reference resource suitable for hospital, health sciences and public libraries with consumer health collections."
— *E-Streams, Nov '02*

Kidney & Urinary Tract Diseases & Disorders Sourcebook, 1st Edition

SEE Urinary Tract & Kidney Diseases & Disorders Sourcebook, 2nd Edition

Learning Disabilities Sourcebook, 2nd Edition

Basic Consumer Health Information about Learning Disabilities, Including Dyslexia, Developmental Speech and Language Disabilities, Non-Verbal Learning Disorders, Developmental Arithmetic Disorder, Developmental Writing Disorder, and Other Conditions That Impede Learning Such as Attention Deficit/ Hyperactivity Disorder, Brain Injury, Hearing Impairment, Klinefelter Syndrome, Dyspraxia, and Tourette Syndrome

Along with Facts about Educational Issues and Assistive Technology, Coping Strategies, a Glossary of Related Terms, and Resources for Further Help and Information

Edited by Dawn D. Matthews. 621 pages. 2003. 0-7808-0626-3.

ALSO AVAILABLE: Learning Disabilities Sourcebook, 1st Edition. Edited by Linda M. Shin. 579 pages. 1998. 0-7808-0210-1.

"The second edition of *Learning Disabilities Sourcebook* far surpasses the earlier edition in that it is more focused on information that will be useful as a consumer health resource."
— *American Reference Books Annual, 2004*

"Teachers as well as consumers will find this an essential guide to understanding various syndromes and their latest treatments. [An] invaluable reference for public and school library collections alike."
— *Library Bookwatch, Apr '03*

Named "Outstanding Reference Book of 1999."
— *New York Public Library, Feb 2000*

"An excellent candidate for inclusion in a public library reference section. It's a great source of information. Teachers will also find the book useful. Definitely worth reading."
— *Journal of Adolescent & Adult Literacy, Feb 2000*

"Readable . . . provides a solid base of information regarding successful techniques used with individuals who have learning disabilities, as well as practical suggestions for educators and family members. Clear lan-

Leukemia Sourcebook

Basic Consumer Health Information about Adult and Childhood Leukemias, Including Acute Lymphocytic Leukemia (ALL), Chronic Lymphocytic Leukemia (CLL), Acute Myelogenous Leukemia (AML), Chronic Myelogenous Leukemia (CML), and Hairy Cell Leukemia, and Treatments Such as Chemotherapy, Radiation Therapy, Peripheral Blood Stem Cell and Marrow Transplantation, and Immunotherapy

Along with Tips for Life During and After Treatment, a Glossary, and Directories of Additional Resources

Edited by Joyce Brennfleck Shannon. 587 pages. 2003. 0-7808-0627-1.

"Unlike other medical books for the layperson, . . . the language does not talk down to the reader. . . . This volume is highly recommended for all libraries."
— *American Reference Books Annual, 2004*

Liver Disorders Sourcebook

Basic Consumer Health Information about the Liver and How It Works; Liver Diseases, Including Cancer, Cirrhosis, Hepatitis, and Toxic and Drug Related Diseases; Tips for Maintaining a Healthy Liver; Laboratory Tests, Radiology Tests, and Facts about Liver Transplantation

Along with a Section on Support Groups, a Glossary, and Resource Listings

Edited by Joyce Brennfleck Shannon. 591 pages. 2000. 0-7808-0383-3.

"A valuable resource."
— *American Reference Books Annual, 2001*

"This title is recommended for health sciences and public libraries with consumer health collections."
— *E-Streams, Oct '00*

"Recommended reference source."
— *Booklist, American Library Association, Jun '00*

Lung Disorders Sourcebook

Basic Consumer Health Information about Emphysema, Pneumonia, Tuberculosis, Asthma, Cystic Fibrosis, and Other Lung Disorders, Including Facts about Diagnostic Procedures, Treatment Strategies, Disease Prevention Efforts, and Such Risk Factors as Smoking, Air Pollution, and Exposure to Asbestos, Radon, and Other Agents

Along with a Glossary and Resources for Additional Help and Information

Edited by Dawn D. Matthews. 678 pages. 2002. 0-7808-0339-6.

"This title is a great addition for public and school libraries because it provides concise health information on the lungs."
— *American Reference Books Annual, 2003*

"Highly recommended for academic and medical reference collections." — *Library Bookwatch, Sep '02*

■

Medical Tests Sourcebook, 2nd Edition

Basic Consumer Health Information about Medical Tests, Including Age-Specific Health Tests, Important Health Screenings and Exams, Home-Use Tests, Blood and Specimen Tests, Electrical Tests, Scope Tests, Genetic Testing, and Imaging Tests, Such as X-Rays, Ultrasound, Computed Tomography, Magnetic Resonance Imaging, Angiography, and Nuclear Medicine

Along with a Glossary and Directory of Additional Resources

Edited by Joyce Brennfleck Shannon. 654 pages. 2004. 0-7808-0670-0.

ALSO AVAILABLE: *Medical Tests, 1st Edition.* Edited by Joyce Brennfleck Shannon. 691 pages. 1999. 0-7808-0243-8.

"Recommended for hospital and health sciences libraries with consumer health collections."
— *E-Streams, Mar '00*

"This is an overall excellent reference with a wealth of general knowledge that may aid those who are reluctant to get vital tests performed."
— *Today's Librarian, Jan 2000*

"A valuable reference guide."
— *American Reference Books Annual, 2000*

■

Men's Health Concerns Sourcebook, 2nd Edition

Basic Consumer Health Information about the Medical and Mental Concerns of Men, Including Theories about the Shorter Male Lifespan, the Leading Causes of Death and Disability, Physical Concerns of Special Significance to Men, Reproductive and Sexual Concerns, Sexually Transmitted Diseases, Men's Mental and Emotional Health, and Lifestyle Choices That Affect Wellness, Such as Nutrition, Fitness, and Substance Use

Along with a Glossary of Related Terms and a Directory of Organizational Resources in Men's Health

Edited by Robert Aquinas McNally. 644 pages. 2004. 0-7808-0671-9.

ALSO AVAILABLE: *Men's Health Concerns Sourcebook, 1st Edition.* Edited by Allan R. Cook. 738 pages. 1998. 0-7808-0212-8.

"This comprehensive resource and the series are highly recommended."
— *American Reference Books Annual, 2000*

"Recommended reference source."
— *Booklist, American Library Association, Dec '98*

■

Mental Health Disorders Sourcebook, 3rd Edition

Basic Consumer Health Information about Mental and Emotional Health and Mental Illness, Including Facts about Depression, Bipolar Disorder, and Other Mood Disorders, Phobias, Post-Traumatic Stress Disorder (PTSD), Obsessive-Compulsive Disorder, and Other Anxiety Disorders, Impulse Control Disorders, Eating Disorders, Personality Disorders, and Psychotic Disorders, Including Schizophrenia and Dissociative Disorders

Along with Statistical Information, a Special Section Concerning Mental Health Issues in Children and Adolescents, a Glossary, and Directories of Resources for Additional Help and Information

Edited by Karen Bellenir. 661 pages. 2005. 0-7808-0747-2.

ALSO AVAILABLE: *Mental Health Disorders Sourcebook, 1st Edition.* Edited by Karen Bellenir. 548 pages. 1995. 0-7808-0040-0.

ALSO AVAILABLE: *Mental Health Disorders Sourcebook, 2nd Edition.* Edited by Karen Bellenir. 605 pages. 2000. 0-7808-0240-3.

"Well organized and well written."
— *American Reference Books Annual, 2001*

"Recommended reference source."
— *Booklist, American Library Association, Jun '00*

■

Mental Retardation Sourcebook

Basic Consumer Health Information about Mental Retardation and Its Causes, Including Down Syndrome, Fetal Alcohol Syndrome, Fragile X Syndrome, Genetic Conditions, Injury, and Environmental Sources

Along with Preventive Strategies, Parenting Issues, Educational Implications, Health Care Needs, Employment and Economic Matters, Legal Issues, a Glossary, and a Resource Listing for Additional Help and Information

Edited by Joyce Brennfleck Shannon. 642 pages. 2000. 0-7808-0377-9.

"Public libraries will find the book useful for reference and as a beginning research point for students, parents, and caregivers."
— *American Reference Books Annual, 2001*

"The strength of this work is that it compiles many basic fact sheets and addresses for further information in one volume. It is intended and suitable for the general public. This sourcebook is relevant to any collection providing health information to the general public."
— *E-Streams, Nov '00*

"From preventing retardation to parenting and family challenges, this covers health, social and legal issues and will prove an invaluable overview."
— *Reviewer's Bookwatch, Jul '00*

Movement Disorders Sourcebook

Basic Consumer Health Information about Neurological Movement Disorders, Including Essential Tremor, Parkinson's Disease, Dystonia, Cerebral Palsy, Huntington's Disease, Myasthenia Gravis, Multiple Sclerosis, and Other Early-Onset and Adult-Onset Movement Disorders, Their Symptoms and Causes, Diagnostic Tests, and Treatments

Along with Mobility and Assistive Technology Information, a Glossary, and a Directory of Additional Resources

Edited by Joyce Brennfleck Shannon. 655 pages. 2003. 0-7808-0628-X.

". . . a good resource for consumers and recommended for public, community college and undergraduate libraries."

— American Reference Books Annual, 2004

Muscular Dystrophy Sourcebook

Basic Consumer Health Information about Congenital, Childhood-Onset, and Adult-Onset Forms of Muscular Dystrophy, Such as Duchenne, Becker, Emery-Dreifuss, Distal, Limb-Girdle, Facioscapulohumeral (FSHD), Myotonic, and Ophthalmoplegic Muscular Dystrophies, Including Facts about Diagnostic Tests, Medical and Physical Therapies, Management of Co-Occurring Conditions, and Parenting Guidelines

Along with Practical Tips for Home Care, a Glossary, and Directories of Additional Resources

Edited by Joyce Brennfleck Shannon. 577 pages. 2004. 0-7808-0676-X.

Obesity Sourcebook

Basic Consumer Health Information about Diseases and Other Problems Associated with Obesity, and Including Facts about Risk Factors, Prevention Issues, and Management Approaches

Along with Statistical and Demographic Data, Information about Special Populations, Research Updates, a Glossary, and Source Listings for Further Help and Information

Edited by Wilma Caldwell and Chad T. Kimball. 376 pages. 2001. 0-7808-0333-7.

"The book synthesizes the reliable medical literature on obesity into one easy-to-read and useful resource for the general public."

— American Reference Books Annual 2002

"This is a very useful resource book for the lay public."

— Doody's Review Service, Nov '01

"Well suited for the health reference collection of a public library or an academic health science library that serves the general population." *— E-Streams, Sep '01*

"Recommended reference source."

— Booklist, American Library Association, Apr '01

" Recommended pick both for specialty health library collections and any general consumer health reference collection." *— The Bookwatch, Apr '01*

Ophthalmic Disorders Sourcebook, 1st Edition

SEE Eye Care Sourcebook, 2nd Edition

Oral Health Sourcebook

SEE Dental Care & Oral Health Sourcebook, 2nd Ed.

Osteoporosis Sourcebook

Basic Consumer Health Information about Primary and Secondary Osteoporosis and Juvenile Osteoporosis and Related Conditions, Including Fibrous Dysplasia, Gaucher Disease, Hyperthyroidism, Hypophosphatasia, Myeloma, Osteopetrosis, Osteogenesis Imperfecta, and Paget's Disease

Along with Information about Risk Factors, Treatments, Traditional and Non-Traditional Pain Management, a Glossary of Related Terms, and a Directory of Resources

Edited by Allan R. Cook. 584 pages. 2001. 0-7808-0239-X.

"This would be a book to be kept in a staff or patient library. The targeted audience is the layperson, but the therapist who needs a quick bit of information on a particular topic will also find the book useful."

— Physical Therapy, Jan '02

"This resource is recommended as a great reference source for public, health, and academic libraries, and is another triumph for the editors of Omnigraphics."

— American Reference Books Annual 2002

"Recommended for all public libraries and general health collections, especially those supporting patient education or consumer health programs."

— E-Streams, Nov '01

"Will prove valuable to any library seeking to maintain a current, comprehensive reference collection of health resources. . . . From prevention to treatment and associated conditions, this provides an excellent survey."

— The Bookwatch, Aug '01

"Recommended reference source."

— Booklist, American Library Association, July '01

SEE ALSO Women's Health Concerns Sourcebook

Pain Sourcebook, 2nd Edition

Basic Consumer Health Information about Specific Forms of Acute and Chronic Pain, Including Muscle and Skeletal Pain, Nerve Pain, Cancer Pain, and Disorders Characterized by Pain, Such as Fibromyalgia, Shingles, Angina, Arthritis, and Headaches

Along with Information about Pain Medications and Management Techniques, Complementary and Alternative Pain Relief Options, Tips for People Living with Chronic Pain, a Glossary, and a Directory of Sources for Further Information

Edited by Karen Bellenir. 670 pages. 2002. 0-7808-0612-3.

ALSO AVAILABLE: Pain Sourcebook, 1st Edition.
Edited by Allan R. Cook. 667 pages. 1997. 0-7808-0213-6.

"A source of valuable information. . . . This book offers help to nonmedical people who need information about pain and pain management. It is also an excellent reference for those who participate in patient education."
— *Doody's Review Service, Sep '02*

"The text is readable, easily understood, and well indexed. This excellent volume belongs in all patient education libraries, consumer health sections of public libraries, and many personal collections."
— *American Reference Books Annual, 1999*

"A beneficial reference." — *Booklist Health Sciences Supplement, American Library Association, Oct '98*

"The information is basic in terms of scholarship and is appropriate for general readers. Written in journalistic style . . . intended for non-professionals. Quite thorough in its coverage of different pain conditions and summarizes the latest clinical information regarding pain treatment." — *Choice, Association of College and Research Libraries, Jun '98*

"Recommended reference source."
— *Booklist, American Library Association, Mar '98*

◼

Pediatric Cancer Sourcebook

Basic Consumer Health Information about Leukemias, Brain Tumors, Sarcomas, Lymphomas, and Other Cancers in Infants, Children, and Adolescents, Including Descriptions of Cancers, Treatments, and Coping Strategies

Along with Suggestions for Parents, Caregivers, and Concerned Relatives, a Glossary of Cancer Terms, and Resource Listings

Edited by Edward J. Prucha. 587 pages. 1999. 0-7808-0245-4.

"An excellent source of information. Recommended for public, hospital, and health science libraries with consumer health collections." — *E-Streams, Jun '00*

"Recommended reference source."
— *Booklist, American Library Association, Feb '00*

"A valuable addition to all libraries specializing in health services and many public libraries."
— *American Reference Books Annual, 2000*

◼

Physical & Mental Issues in Aging Sourcebook

Basic Consumer Health Information on Physical and Mental Disorders Associated with the Aging Process, Including Concerns about Cardiovascular Disease, Pulmonary Disease, Oral Health, Digestive Disorders, Musculoskeletal and Skin Disorders, Metabolic Changes, Sexual and Reproductive Issues, and Changes in Vision, Hearing, and Other Senses

Along with Data about Longevity and Causes of Death, Information on Acute and Chronic Pain, Descriptions of Mental Concerns, a Glossary of Terms, and Resource Listings for Additional Help

Edited by Jenifer Swanson. 660 pages. 1999. 0-7808-0233-0.

"This is a treasure of health information for the layperson." — *Choice Health Sciences Supplement, Association of College & Research Libraries, May 2000*

"Recommended for public libraries."
— *American Reference Books Annual, 2000*

"Recommended reference source."
— *Booklist, American Library Association, Oct '99*

SEE ALSO Healthy Aging Sourcebook

◼

Podiatry Sourcebook

Basic Consumer Health Information about Foot Conditions, Diseases, and Injuries, Including Bunions, Corns, Calluses, Athlete's Foot, Plantar Warts, Hammertoes and Clawtoes, Clubfoot, Heel Pain, Gout, and More

Along with Facts about Foot Care, Disease Prevention, Foot Safety, Choosing a Foot Care Specialist, a Glossary of Terms, and Resource Listings for Additional Information

Edited by M. Lisa Weatherford. 380 pages. 2001. 0-7808-0215-2.

"Recommended reference source."
— *Booklist, American Library Association, Feb '02*

"There is a lot of information presented here on a topic that is usually only covered sparingly in most larger comprehensive medical encyclopedias."
— *American Reference Books Annual 2002*

◼

Pregnancy & Birth Sourcebook, 2nd Edition

Basic Consumer Health Information about Conception and Pregnancy, Including Facts about Fertility, Infertility, Pregnancy Symptoms and Complications, Fetal Growth and Development, Labor, Delivery, and the Postpartum Period, as Well as Information about Maintaining Health and Wellness during Pregnancy and Caring for a Newborn

Along with Information about Public Health Assistance for Low-Income Pregnant Women, a Glossary, and Directories of Agencies and Organizations Providing Help and Support

Edited by Amy L. Sutton. 626 pages. 2004. 0-7808-0672-7.

ALSO AVAILABLE: Pregnancy & Birth Sourcebook, 1st Edition. Edited by Heather E. Aldred. 737 pages. 1997. 0-7808-0216-0.

"A well-organized handbook. Recommended."
— *Choice, Association of College and Research Libraries, Apr '98*

"Recommended reference source."
— *Booklist, American Library Association, Mar '98*

"Recommended for public libraries."
— *American Reference Books Annual, 1998*

SEE ALSO Congenital Disorders Sourcebook, Family Planning Sourcebook

Prostate Cancer Sourcebook

Basic Consumer Health Information about Prostate Cancer, Including Information about the Associated Risk Factors, Detection, Diagnosis, and Treatment of Prostate Cancer

Along with Information on Non-Malignant Prostate Conditions, and Featuring a Section Listing Support and Treatment Centers and a Glossary of Related Terms

Edited by Dawn D. Matthews. 358 pages. 2001. 0-7808-0324-8.

"Recommended reference source."
— Booklist, American Library Association, Jan '02

"A valuable resource for health care consumers seeking information on the subject. . . .All text is written in a clear, easy-to-understand language that avoids technical jargon. Any library that collects consumer health resources would strengthen their collection with the addition of the *Prostate Cancer Sourcebook.*"
— American Reference Books Annual 2002

■

Public Health Sourcebook

Basic Information about Government Health Agencies, Including National Health Statistics and Trends, Healthy People 2000 Program Goals and Objectives, the Centers for Disease Control and Prevention, the Food and Drug Administration, and the National Institutes of Health

Along with Full Contact Information for Each Agency

Edited by Wendy Wilcox. 698 pages. 1998. 0-7808-0220-9.

"Recommended reference source."
— Booklist, American Library Association, Sep '98

"This consumer guide provides welcome assistance in navigating the maze of federal health agencies and their data on public health concerns."
— SciTech Book News, Sep '98

■

Reconstructive & Cosmetic Surgery Sourcebook

Basic Consumer Health Information on Cosmetic and Reconstructive Plastic Surgery, Including Statistical Information about Different Surgical Procedures, Things to Consider Prior to Surgery, Plastic Surgery Techniques and Tools, Emotional and Psychological Considerations, and Procedure-Specific Information

Along with a Glossary of Terms and a Listing of Resources for Additional Help and Information

Edited by M. Lisa Weatherford. 374 pages. 2001. 0-7808-0214-4.

"An excellent reference that addresses cosmetic and medically necessary reconstructive surgeries. . . . The style of the prose is calm and reassuring, discussing the many positive outcomes now available due to advances in surgical techniques."
— American Reference Books Annual 2002

"Recommended for health science libraries that are open to the public, as well as hospital libraries that are open to the patients. This book is a good resource for the consumer interested in plastic surgery."
— E-Streams, Dec '01

"Recommended reference source."
— Booklist, American Library Association, July '01

■

Rehabilitation Sourcebook

Basic Consumer Health Information about Rehabilitation for People Recovering from Heart Surgery, Spinal Cord Injury, Stroke, Orthopedic Impairments, Amputation, Pulmonary Impairments, Traumatic Injury, and More, Including Physical Therapy, Occupational Therapy, Speech/ Language Therapy, Massage Therapy, Dance Therapy, Art Therapy, and Recreational Therapy

Along with Information on Assistive and Adaptive Devices, a Glossary, and Resources for Additional Help and Information

Edited by Dawn D. Matthews. 531 pages. 1999. 0-7808-0236-5.

"This is an excellent resource for public library reference and health collections."
— American Reference Books Annual, 2001

"Recommended reference source."
— Booklist, American Library Association, May '00

■

Respiratory Diseases & Disorders Sourcebook

Basic Information about Respiratory Diseases and Disorders, Including Asthma, Cystic Fibrosis, Pneumonia, the Common Cold, Influenza, and Others, Featuring Facts about the Respiratory System, Statistical and Demographic Data, Treatments, Self-Help Management Suggestions, and Current Research Initiatives

Edited by Allan R. Cook and Peter D. Dresser. 771 pages. 1995. 0-7808-0037-0.

"Designed for the layperson and for patients and their families coping with respiratory illness. . . . an extensive array of information on diagnosis, treatment, management, and prevention of respiratory illnesses for the general reader."
— Choice, Association of College and Research Libraries, Jun '96

"A highly recommended text for all collections. It is a comforting reminder of the power of knowledge that good books carry between their covers."
— Academic Library Book Review, Spring '96

"A comprehensive collection of authoritative information presented in a nontechnical, humanitarian style for patients, families, and caregivers." *— Association of Operating Room Nurses, Sep/Oct '95*

SEE ALSO Lung Disorders Sourcebook

Sexually Transmitted Diseases Sourcebook, 2nd Edition

Basic Consumer Health Information about Sexually Transmitted Diseases, Including Information on the Diagnosis and Treatment of Chlamydia, Gonorrhea, Hepatitis, Herpes, HIV, Mononucleosis, Syphilis, and Others

Along with Information on Prevention, Such as Condom Use, Vaccines, and STD Education; And Featuring a Section on Issues Related to Youth and Adolescents, a Glossary, and Resources for Additional Help and Information

Edited by Dawn D. Matthews. 538 pages. 2001. 0-7808-0249-7.

ALSO AVAILABLE: *Sexually Transmitted Diseases Sourcebook, 1st Edition.* Edited by Linda M. Ross. 550 pages. 1997. 0-7808-0217-9.

"Recommended for consumer health collections in public libraries, and secondary school and community college libraries."
— *American Reference Books Annual 2002*

"Every school and public library should have a copy of this comprehensive and user-friendly reference book."
— *Choice, Association of College & Research Libraries, Sep '01*

"This is a highly recommended book. This is an especially important book for all school and public libraries." — *AIDS Book Review Journal, Jul-Aug '01*

"Recommended reference source."
— *Booklist, American Library Association, Apr '01*

"Recommended pick both for specialty health library collections and any general consumer health reference collection." — *The Bookwatch, Apr '01*

Skin Disorders Sourcebook, 1st Edition

SEE *Dermatological Disorders Sourcebook, 2nd Edition*

Sleep Disorders Sourcebook, 2nd Edition

Basic Consumer Health Information about Sleep and Sleep Disorders, Including Insomnia, Sleep Apnea, Restless Legs Syndrome, Narcolepsy, Parasomnias, and Other Health Problems That Affect Sleep, Plus Facts about Diagnostic Procedures, Treatment Strategies, Sleep Medications, and Tips for Improving Sleep Quality

Along with a Glossary of Related Terms and Resources for Additional Help and Information

Edited by Amy L. Sutton. 567 pages. 2005. 0-7808-0745-6.

ALSO AVAILABLE: *Sleep Disorders Sourcebook, 1st Edition.* Edited by Jenifer Swanson. 439 pages. 1998. 0-7808-0234-9.

"This text will complement any home or medical library. It is user-friendly and ideal for the adult reader."
— *American Reference Books Annual, 2000*

"A useful resource that provides accurate, relevant, and accessible information on sleep to the general public. Health care providers who deal with sleep disorders patients may also find it helpful in being prepared to answer some of the questions patients ask."
— *Respiratory Care, Jul '99*

"Recommended reference source."
— *Booklist, American Library Association, Feb '99*

Smoking Concerns Sourcebook

Basic Consumer Health Information about Nicotine Addiction and Smoking Cessation, Featuring Facts about the Health Effects of Tobacco Use, Including Lung and Other Cancers, Heart Disease, Stroke, and Respiratory Disorders, Such as Emphysema and Chronic Bronchitis

Along with Information about Smoking Prevention Programs, Suggestions for Achieving and Maintaining a Smoke-Free Lifestyle, Statistics about Tobacco Use, Reports on Current Research Initiatives, a Glossary of Related Terms, and Directories of Resources for Additional Help and Information

Edited by Karen Bellenir. 621 pages. 2004. 0-7808-0323-X.

Sports Injuries Sourcebook, 2nd Edition

Basic Consumer Health Information about the Diagnosis, Treatment, and Rehabilitation of Common Sports-Related Injuries in Children and Adults

Along with Suggestions for Conditioning and Training, Information and Prevention Tips for Injuries Frequently Associated with Specific Sports and Special Populations, a Glossary, and a Directory of Additional Resources

Edited by Joyce Brennfleck Shannon. 614 pages. 2002. 0-7808-0604-2.

ALSO AVAILABLE: *Sports Injuries Sourcebook, 1st Edition.* Edited by Heather E. Aldred. 624 pages. 1999. 0-7808-0218-7.

"This is an excellent reference for consumers and it is recommended for public, community college, and undergraduate libraries."
— *American Reference Books Annual, 2003*

"Recommended reference source."
— *Booklist, American Library Association, Feb '03*

Stress-Related Disorders Sourcebook

Basic Consumer Health Information about Stress and Stress-Related Disorders, Including Stress Origins and Signals, Environmental Stress at Work and Home, Mental and Emotional Stress Associated with Depression, Post-Traumatic Stress Disorder, Panic Disorder, Suicide, and the Physical Effects of Stress on the Cardiovascular, Immune, and Nervous Systems

Along with Stress Management Techniques, a Glossary, and a Listing of Additional Resources

Edited by Joyce Brennfleck Shannon. 610 pages. 2002. 0-7808-0560-7.

"Well written for a general readership, the *Stress-Related Disorders Sourcebook* is a useful addition to the health reference literature."
— *American Reference Books Annual, 2003*

"I am impressed by the amount of information. It offers a thorough overview of the causes and consequences of stress for the layperson. . . . A well-done and thorough reference guide for professionals and nonprofessionals alike." — *Doody's Review Service, Dec '02*

Stroke Sourcebook

Basic Consumer Health Information about Stroke, Including Ischemic, Hemorrhagic, Transient Ischemic Attack (TIA), and Pediatric Stroke, Stroke Triggers and Risks, Diagnostic Tests, Treatments, and Rehabilitation Information

Along with Stroke Prevention Guidelines, Legal and Financial Information, a Glossary, and a Directory of Additional Resources

Edited by Joyce Brennfleck Shannon. 606 pages. 2003. 0-7808-0630-1.

"This volume is highly recommended and should be in every medical, hospital, and public library."
— *American Reference Books Annual, 2004*

Substance Abuse Sourcebook

Basic Health-Related Information about the Abuse of Legal and Illegal Substances Such as Alcohol, Tobacco, Prescription Drugs, Marijuana, Cocaine, and Heroin; and Including Facts about Substance Abuse Prevention Strategies, Intervention Methods, Treatment and Recovery Programs, and a Section Addressing the Special Problems Related to Substance Abuse during Pregnancy

Edited by Karen Bellenir. 573 pages. 1996. 0-7808-0038-9.

"A valuable addition to any health reference section. Highly recommended."
— *The Book Report, Mar/Apr '97*

". . . a comprehensive collection of substance abuse information that's both highly readable and compact. Families and caregivers of substance abusers will find the information enlightening and helpful, while teachers, social workers and journalists should benefit from the concise format. Recommended."
— *Drug Abuse Update, Winter '96/'97*

SEE ALSO *Alcoholism Sourcebook, Drug Abuse Sourcebook*

Surgery Sourcebook

Basic Consumer Health Information about Inpatient and Outpatient Surgeries, Including Cardiac, Vascular, Orthopedic, Ocular, Reconstructive, Cosmetic, Gynecologic, and Ear, Nose, and Throat Procedures and More

Along with Information about Operating Room Policies and Instruments, Laser Surgery Techniques, Hospital Errors, Statistical Data, a Glossary, and Listings of Sources for Further Help and Information

Edited by Annemarie S. Muth and Karen Bellenir. 596 pages. 2002. 0-7808-0380-9.

"Large public libraries and medical libraries would benefit from this material in their reference collections."
— *American Reference Books Annual, 2004*

"Invaluable reference for public and school library collections alike." — *Library Bookwatch, Apr '03*

Thyroid Disorders Sourcebook

Basic Consumer Health Information about Disorders of the Thyroid and Parathyroid Glands, Including Hypothyroidism, Hyperthyroidism, Graves Disease, Hashimoto Thyroiditis, Thyroid Cancer, and Parathyroid Disorders, Featuring Facts about Symptoms, Risk Factors, Tests, and Treatments

Along with Information about the Effects of Thyroid Imbalance on Other Body Systems, Environmental Factors That Affect the Thyroid Gland, a Glossary, and a Directory of Additional Resources

Edited by Joyce Brennfleck Shannon. 599 pages. 2005. 0-7808-0745-6.

Transplantation Sourcebook

Basic Consumer Health Information about Organ and Tissue Transplantation, Including Physical and Financial Preparations, Procedures and Issues Relating to Specific Solid Organ and Tissue Transplants, Rehabilitation, Pediatric Transplant Information, the Future of Transplantation, and Organ and Tissue Donation

Along with a Glossary and Listings of Additional Resources

Edited by Joyce Brennfleck Shannon. 628 pages. 2002. 0-7808-0322-1.

"Along with these advances [in transplantation technology] have come a number of daunting questions for potential transplant patients, their families, and their health care providers. This reference text is the best single tool to address many of these questions. . . . It will be a much-needed addition to the reference collections in health care, academic, and large public libraries."
— *American Reference Books Annual, 2003*

"Recommended for libraries with an interest in offering consumer health information." — *E-Streams, Jul '02*

"This is a unique and valuable resource for patients facing transplantation and their families."
— *Doody's Review Service, Jun '02*

Traveler's Health Sourcebook

Basic Consumer Health Information for Travelers, Including Physical and Medical Preparations, Transportation Health and Safety, Essential Information about Food and Water, Sun Exposure, Insect and Snake Bites, Camping and Wilderness Medicine, and Travel with Physical or Medical Disabilities

Along with International Travel Tips, Vaccination Recommendations, Geographical Health Issues, Disease Risks, a Glossary, and a Listing of Additional Resources

Edited by Joyce Brennfleck Shannon. 613 pages. 2000. 0-7808-0384-1.

"Recommended reference source."
— *Booklist, American Library Association, Feb '01*

"This book is recommended for any public library, any travel collection, and especially any collection for the physically disabled."
—*American Reference Books Annual, 2001*

■

Urinary Tract & Kidney Diseases & Disorders Sourcebook, 2nd Edition

Basic Consumer Health Information about the Urinary System, Including the Bladder, Urethra, Ureters, and Kidneys, with Facts about Urinary Tract Infections, Incontinence, Congenital Disorders, Kidney Stones, Cancers of the Urinary Tract and Kidneys, Kidney Failure, Dialysis, and Kidney Transplantation

Along with Statistical and Demographic Information, Reports on Current Research in Kidney and Urologic Health, a Summary of Commonly Used Diagnostic Tests, a Glossary of Related Terms, and a Directory of Resources for Additional Help and Information

Edited by Ivy L. Alexander. 625 pages. 2005. 0-7808-0750-2.

ALSO AVAILABLE: Kidney & Urinary Tract Diseases & Disorders Sourcebook, 1st Ed. Edited by Linda M. Ross. 602 pages. 1997. 0-7808-0079-6.

■

Vegetarian Sourcebook

Basic Consumer Health Information about Vegetarian Diets, Lifestyle, and Philosophy, Including Definitions of Vegetarianism and Veganism, Tips about Adopting Vegetarianism, Creating a Vegetarian Pantry, and Meeting Nutritional Needs of Vegetarians, with Facts Regarding Vegetarianism's Effect on Pregnant and Lactating Women, Children, Athletes, and Senior Citizens

Along with a Glossary of Commonly Used Vegetarian Terms and Resources for Additional Help and Information

Edited by Chad T. Kimball. 360 pages. 2002. 0-7808-0439-2.

"Organizes into one concise volume the answers to the most common questions concerning vegetarian diets and lifestyles. This title is recommended for public and secondary school libraries." — *E-Streams, Apr '03*

"Invaluable reference for public and school library collections alike." — *Library Bookwatch, Apr '03*

"The articles in this volume are easy to read and come from authoritative sources. The book does not necessarily support the vegetarian diet but instead provides the pros and cons of this important decision. The *Vegetarian Sourcebook* is recommended for public libraries and consumer health libraries."
— *American Reference Books Annual, 2003*

■

Women's Health Concerns Sourcebook, 2nd Edition

Basic Consumer Health Information about the Medical and Mental Concerns of Women, Including Maintaining Health and Wellness, Gynecological Concerns, Breast Health, Sexuality and Reproductive Issues, Menopause, Cancer in Women, the Leading Causes of Death and Disability among Women, Physical Concerns of Special Significance to Women, and Women's Mental and Emotional Health

Along with a Glossary of Related Terms and Directories of Resources for Additional Help and Information

Edited by Amy L. Sutton. 748 pages. 2004. 0-7808-0673-5.

ALSO AVAILABLE: Women's Health Concerns Sourcebook, 1st Edition. Edited by Heather E. Aldred. 567 pages. 1997. 0-7808-0219-5.

"Handy compilation. There is an impressive range of diseases, devices, disorders, procedures, and other physical and emotional issues covered . . . well organized, illustrated, and indexed." — *Choice, Association of College and Research Libraries, Jan '98*

SEE ALSO Breast Cancer Sourcebook, Cancer Sourcebook for Women, Healthy Heart Sourcebook for Women, Osteoporosis Sourcebook

■

Workplace Health & Safety Sourcebook

Basic Consumer Health Information about Workplace Health and Safety, Including the Effect of Workplace Hazards on the Lungs, Skin, Heart, Ears, Eyes, Brain, Reproductive Organs, Musculoskeletal System, and Other Organs and Body Parts

Along with Information about Occupational Cancer, Personal Protective Equipment, Toxic and Hazardous Chemicals, Child Labor, Stress, and Workplace Violence

Edited by Chad T. Kimball. 626 pages. 2000. 0-7808-0231-4.

"As a reference for the general public, this would be useful in any library." —*E-Streams, Jun '01*

"Provides helpful information for primary care physicians and other caregivers interested in occupational medicine. . . . General readers; professionals."
— *Choice, Association of College & Research Libraries, May '01*

"Recommended reference source."
— *Booklist, American Library Association, Feb '01*

"Highly recommended." — *The Bookwatch, Jan '01*

Worldwide Health Sourcebook

Basic Information about Global Health Issues, Including Malnutrition, Reproductive Health, Disease Dispersion and Prevention, Emerging Diseases, Risky Health Behaviors, and the Leading Causes of Death

Along with Global Health Concerns for Children, Women, and the Elderly, Mental Health Issues, Research and Technology Advancements, and Economic, Environmental, and Political Health Implications, a Glossary, and a Resource Listing for Additional Help and Information

Edited by Joyce Brennfleck Shannon. 614 pages. 2001. 0-7808-0330-2.

"Named an Outstanding Academic Title." *—Choice,*
Association of College & Research Libraries, Jan '02

"Yet another handy but also unique compilation in the extensive Health Reference Series, this is a useful work because many of the international publications reprinted or excerpted are not readily available. Highly recommended." *—Choice, Association of College*
& Research Libraries, Nov '01

"Recommended reference source."
—Booklist, American Library Association, Oct '01

Teen Health Series

Helping Young Adults Understand, Manage, and Avoid Serious Illness

List price $65 per volume. **School and library price $58 per volume.**

Alcohol Information for Teens

Health Tips about Alcohol and Alcoholism

Including Facts about Underage Drinking, Preventing Teen Alcohol Use, Alcohol's Effects on the Brain and the Body, Alcohol Abuse Treatment, Help for Children of Alcoholics, and More

Edited by Joyce Brennfleck Shannon. 370 pages. 2005. 0-7808-0741-3.

Asthma Information for Teens

Health Tips about Managing Asthma and Related Concerns

Including Facts about Asthma Causes, Triggers, Symptoms, Diagnosis, and Treatment

Edited by Karen Bellenir. 386 pages. 2005. 0-7808-0770-7.

Cancer Information for Teens

Health Tips about Cancer Awareness, Prevention, Diagnosis, and Treatment

Including Facts about Frequently Occurring Cancers, Cancer Risk Factors, and Coping Strategies for Teens Fighting Cancer or Dealing with Cancer in Friends or Family Members

Edited by Wilma R. Caldwell. 428 pages. 2004. 0-7808-0678-6.

"Recommended for school libraries, or consumer libraries that see a lot of use by teens."
— *E-Streams, May 2005*

"A valuable educational tool."
— *American Reference Books Annual, 2005*

"Young adults and their parents alike will find this new addition to the *Teen Health Series* an important reference to cancer in teens."
— *Children's Bookwatch, February 2005*

Diet Information for Teens

Health Tips about Diet and Nutrition

Including Facts about Nutrients, Dietary Guidelines, Breakfasts, School Lunches, Snacks, Party Food, Weight Control, Eating Disorders, and More

Edited by Karen Bellenir. 399 pages. 2001. 0-7808-0441-4.

"Full of helpful insights and facts throughout the book. ... An excellent resource to be placed in public libraries or even in personal collections."
— *American Reference Books Annual 2002*

"Recommended for middle and high school libraries and media centers as well as academic libraries that educate future teachers of teenagers. It is also a suitable addition to health science libraries that serve patrons who are interested in teen health promotion and education."
— *E-Streams, Oct '01*

"This comprehensive book would be beneficial to collections that need information about nutrition, dietary guidelines, meal planning, and weight control. ... This reference is so easy to use that its purchase is recommended."
— *The Book Report, Sep-Oct '01*

"This book is written in an easy to understand format describing issues that many teens face every day, and then provides thoughtful explanations so that teens can make informed decisions. This is an interesting book that provides important facts and information for today's teens."
— *Doody's Health Sciences Book Review Journal, Jul-Aug '01*

"A comprehensive compendium of diet and nutrition. The information is presented in a straightforward, plain-spoken manner. This title will be useful to those working on reports on a variety of topics, as well as to general readers concerned about their dietary health."
— *School Library Journal, Jun '01*

Drug Information for Teens

Health Tips about the Physical and Mental Effects of Substance Abuse

Including Facts about Alcohol, Anabolic Steroids, Club Drugs, Cocaine, Depressants, Hallucinogens, Herbal Products, Inhalants, Marijuana, Narcotics, Stimulants, Tobacco, and More

Edited by Karen Bellenir. 452 pages. 2002. 0-7808-0444-9.

"A clearly written resource for general readers and researchers alike."
— *School Library Journal*

"The chapters are quick to make a connection to their teenage reading audience. The prose is straightforward and the book lends itself to spot reading. It should be useful both for practical information and for research, and it is suitable for public and school libraries."
— *American Reference Books Annual, 2003*

"Recommended reference source."
— *Booklist, American Library Association, Feb '03*

"This is an excellent resource for teens and their parents. Education about drugs and substances is key to discouraging teen drug abuse and this book provides this much needed information in a way that is interesting and factual." —*Doody's Review Service, Dec '02*

Eating Disorders Information for Teens

Health Tips about Anorexia, Bulimia, Binge Eating, and Other Eating Disorders

Including Information on the Causes, Prevention, and Treatment of Eating Disorders, and Such Other Issues as Maintaining Healthy Eating and Exercise Habits

Edited by Sandra Augustyn Lawton. 337 pages. 2005. 0-7808-0783-9.

Fitness Information for Teens

Health Tips about Exercise, Physical Well-Being, and Health Maintenance

Including Facts about Aerobic and Anaerobic Conditioning, Stretching, Body Shape and Body Image, Sports Training, Nutrition, and Activities for Non-Athletes

Edited by Karen Bellenir. 425 pages. 2004. 0-7808-0679-4.

"This book will be a great addition to any public, junior high, senior high, or secondary school library."
—*American Reference Books Annual, 2005*

Learning Disabilities Information for Teens

Health Tips about Academic Skills Disorders and Other Disabilities That Affect Learning

Including Information about Common Signs of Learning Disabilities, School Issues, Learning to Live with a Learning Disability, and Other Related Issues

Edited by Sandra Augustyn Lawton. 337 pages. 2005. 0-7808-0796-0.

Mental Health Information for Teens

Health Tips about Mental Health and Mental Illness

Including Facts about Anxiety, Depression, Suicide, Eating Disorders, Obsessive-Compulsive Disorders, Panic Attacks, Phobias, Schizophrenia, and More

Edited by Karen Bellenir. 406 pages. 2001. 0-7808-0442-2.

"In both language and approach, this user-friendly entry in the *Teen Health Series* is on target for teens needing information on mental health concerns." —*Booklist, American Library Association, Jan '02*

"Readers will find the material accessible and informative, with the shaded notes, facts, and embedded glossary insets adding appropriately to the already interesting and succinct presentation."
—*School Library Journal, Jan '02*

"This title is highly recommended for any library that serves adolescents and parents/caregivers of adolescents." —*E-Streams, Jan '02*

"Recommended for high school libraries and young adult collections in public libraries. Both health professionals and teenagers will find this book useful."
—*American Reference Books Annual 2002*

"This is a nice book written to enlighten the society, primarily teenagers, about common teen mental health issues. It is highly recommended to teachers and parents as well as adolescents."
—*Doody's Review Service, Dec '01*

Sexual Health Information for Teens

Health Tips about Sexual Development, Human Reproduction, and Sexually Transmitted Diseases

Including Facts about Puberty, Reproductive Health, Chlamydia, Human Papillomavirus, Pelvic Inflammatory Disease, Herpes, AIDS, Contraception, Pregnancy, and More

Edited by Deborah A. Stanley. 391 pages. 2003. 0-7808-0445-7.

"This work should be included in all high school libraries and many larger public libraries. . . . highly recommended."
—*American Reference Books Annual 2004*

"Sexual Health approaches its subject with appropriate seriousness and offers easily accessible advice and information." —*School Library Journal, Feb. 2004*

Skin Health Information for Teens

Health Tips about Dermatological Concerns and Skin Cancer Risks

Including Facts about Acne, Warts, Hives, and Other Conditions and Lifestyle Choices, Such as Tanning, Tattooing, and Piercing, That Affect the Skin, Nails, Scalp, and Hair

Edited by Robert Aquinas McNally. 429 pages. 2003. 0-7808-0446-5.

"This volume, as with others in the series, will be a useful addition to school and public library collections."
—*American Reference Books Annual 2004*

"This volume serves as a one-stop source and should be a necessity for any health collection."
—*Library Media Connection*

Sports Injuries Information for Teens

Health Tips about Sports Injuries and Injury Protection

Including Facts about Specific Injuries, Emergency Treatment, Rehabilitation, Sports Safety, Competition Stress, Fitness, Sports Nutrition, Steroid Risks, and More

Edited by Joyce Brennfleck Shannon. 405 pages. 2003. 0-7808-0447-3.

"This work will be useful in the young adult collections of public libraries as well as high school libraries."
— *American Reference Books Annual 2004*

■

Suicide Information for Teens

Health Tips about Suicide Causes and Prevention

Including Facts about Depression, Risk Factors, Getting Help, Survivor Support, and More

Edited by Joyce Brennfleck Shannon. 368 pages. 2005. 0-7808-0737-5.

Health Reference Series